THE PUBLIC/PRIVATE MIX FOR HEALTH

The relevance and effects
of change

THE PUBLIC/PRIVATE MIX FOR HEALTH

The relevance and effects of change

ESSAYS BY
A. J. CULYER · GORDON FORSYTH
RUDOLF KLEIN · ALAN MAYNARD
GORDON McLACHLAN
ALBERT VAN DER WERFF & FRANS RUTTEN
ROBERT VAN DEN HEUVEL & ANDRÉE SACREZ
FRITZ BESKE · JEAN-FRANÇOIS LACRONIQUE
VICTOR G. RODWIN
WALTER J. McNERNEY · ROBERT G. EVANS
JOHN S. DEEBLE

EDITED BY GORDON McLACHLAN
AND ALAN MAYNARD

THE NUFFIELD PROVINCIAL
HOSPITALS TRUST

Published by
The Nuffield Provincial Hospitals Trust
3 Prince Albert Road, London NW1 7SP

ISBN 0 900574 38 0

© The Nuffield Provincial Hospitals Trust 1982

Designed by Bernard Crossland
Printed and bound in Great Britain
by Burgess & Son (Abingdon) Ltd, Station Road,
Abingdon, Oxfordshire

Prefatory note

By the Chairman of the
Nuffield Provincial Hospitals Trust

From the days of David Lloyd George those politicians responsible for finding the money to care for the nation's health have seldom been loath to look abroad for models which might be copied, by adaptation, for our own righteous purposes. So it was no surprise when a Secretary of State having chosen amongst the deliberations of the Trust that which then most interested him, that we should find ourselves investigating not only the workings of 'the public/private mix' in this country but also how they order such matters in other places. Just as the exigencies of the NHS have enforced a search for supplementary financial provision alongside taxation, so a comparable turn of events has swung the Trust into a new way of tackling the tasks laid upon it at its inception. When the NHS and the Trust were, comparatively, well-found, there was virtue in our making grants for 'study, experiment and demonstration'; but these if successful, tended to create an expensive need no longer to be catered for in the mounting recurrent expenditure of the NHS. So the Trust, with new tailoring, has come to examine and stress how best, or even how more economically the service might be run and has become, as a consequence, a purposeful research bureau, its deliberations assayed in selective seminar, its results made available by publication. Since, it is supposed, ugly publications gain few readers, the emphasis has been upon agreeable presentation (for which the Trust is again most grateful to Mr Bernard Crossland). The public is therefore offered this book, which derives from the enthusiastic drive of the Secretary of the Trust (whose name appears as one of the editors) and the

v

willingness of those he has come to know in sundry places, to apply their thinking to their own arrangements, so that we may all see what emerges from the tested comparison. There is of course no attempt to temper the conclusions of the varying contributors or for the Trustees to draw their own. They are grateful to those who have been persuaded to put their offerings into the common pool, and to their Secretary, once again, for his urgency and skill in constructing it for us all.

E.T.W.

August 1982

Contents

Contents

PART 2

THE WESTERN EUROPEAN EXPERIENCE

The Netherlands, Belgium, The Federal Republic of Germany
and France

x   *Contents*

Unscrambling the omelet: Public and private
health care financing in Australia   425
JOHN S. DEEBLE
Abstract, 427. Introduction, 428. Background, 428. Results, 438. Conclusions, 451. Notes and references, 462. Appendix 1, 465.

PART 4
FINALE

Prologue: Reviewing the evidence   469

The regulation of public and private health care
markets   471
ALAN MAYNARD
Abstract, 473. Introduction, 474. The ideology and the objectives of the
reformers, 478. The nature of the health care market, 483. The characteristics of the alternative scenarios, 488. Conclusion, 508. References, 509.

The public/private mix in health care: The
emerging lessons   513
GORDON McLACHLAN AND ALAN MAYNARD
Abstract, 515. Analysing the dilemma, 516. The similarity of policy goals
across health care systems, 518. Altering the mix, 525. The effects of
altering the mix, 530. The future: common challenges to the public and
private sectors, 540. Research priorities, 548. Overview, 553. Postscript,
555. Notes and references, 557.

Author, country, and subject index   559

Introduction

GORDON McLACHLAN

GORDON McLACHLAN

Gordon McLachlan has been Secretary of the Nuffield Provincial Trust since 1956. He is General Editor of Trust publications and Editor of many books on their List. He was Joint Editor of the International Survey *Health Service Prospects* published to commemorate the 150th anniversary of *The Lancet* in 1973. A long-term observer of the American scene he was a Consulting Editor of the American *Health Services Journal* 1966–74, and has been a consultant to the American Hospitals Association (citation for meritorious service 1976), a member of the Council of the Hospital Research and Educational Trust, and the Parker B. Francis Distinguished Lecturer of the American College of Hospital Administrators. He was elected to Membership of the Institute of Medicine of the National Academy of Sciences, Washington D.C. in 1974. He has been a Consultant to WHO (Europe) for their publication policy and edited two of their recent publications concerned with Planning and Health Information Systems, as well as being Rapporteur for the European Technical Assembly in 1978. A graduate of Edinburgh University and a Chartered Accountant by discipline, he is an honorary LLD of the University of Birmingham and an honorary Fellow of the Royal College of General Practitioners.

Introduction

The public/private mix

In most countries there is inevitably always a mix of public and private interests in health affairs generally and in health care specifically. The distinction is important because, while there has long been a recognition of environmental factors in the health of populations, which came to the fore in the emergence of the Public Health movement in Western countries in the nineteenth century, it is only in more recent years with the universal attention paid to policies designed to improve the distribution and access to health care facilities, that there has been a focussing on the role of government in the provision and regulation of health services. Of course the constituents of the public/private mix varies considerably from country to country, since they are rooted in social and economic history and progress. The relative strength of each sector is also subject to change but the conservative nature of health services ensures brakes on radical change.

As long as the boom in the provision of health care as an integral part of social services continued, not much attention was paid to the character of this mix, particularly because for many years following the second World War there was sufficient elasticity in the sources of funds available for development in both public and private sectors for it to be largely academic to raise the fundamental issue of how to accommodate the hard choices which invariably stem from deciding priorities with limited resources. In recent years however, a range of questions common certainly to the Western democracies has emerged out of the emotional mists which tend to envelop health care when questions of resources arise. 'Value for money', 'optimum use of resources',

3

'equity in care', and 'equity of access', etc. etc. are some of
the battle cries which are bandied about, when the anguish
arising from the inability easily to answer the ever-rising
demands for desirable development to meet ever-increasing
expectations bites deep into the social and political consci-
ousness of nations. Central governments in retreat to their
economic citadels, stoutly fend off appeals for direct relief.
Over-simple solutions rooted in economic theories with only
limited practical application to the complexities involved
in the provision of health services in the modern world,
are championed in the political arena as alternatives, and
the frustrations which arise from the revelation of their
insubstantiality are expressed in every kind of rhetoric: and
sometimes regrettably they express themselves in social and
political conflict and strife.

The problem of demand exceeding supply in the health
service field is indeed world-wide. Because of the unique
arrangements of the NHS however, in which for all practical
purposes the whole of the stock of hospitals in the UK in
July 1948 was nationalized to provide both hospital and
specialist services and cover was provided for the whole
population for primary care, with the financial provision
largely coming from tax revenues of one sort or another, the
public/private mix is relatively easy to identify and the
gradient of change since 1948 simple to gauge. Thus, the
major problems concerned with relative flexibilities and ca-
pabilities for change in the public/private mix can be seen
possibly more clearly in the UK than anywhere else in the
world, since the specificity of the several mixtures in many
countries is obscured by the mélanges of public, private not-
for-profit hospitals, private for-profit hospitals, etc., together
with a range of insurance arrangements for financing the cost
of health care which are bewildering in their complexities.
Even the residue of idealogical criticism of the NHS left over
from 1948, has not been of much account until recently,
when the much publicised increase over the years in the
number of people insuring themselves and their families for
private medical care because of their apparent dissatisfaction
(particularly with aspects of access to the hospital and specialist services), has caused the ember to smoulder to the

emission of both smoke and heat. It has also given rise to the speculation whether there are options open for greater official encouragement to the private sector and especially to those who can afford it, to make provision for care privately rather than accepting what is publicly available. This speculation does, however, tend to obscure how the priorities for general provision identified over the years of the NHS, should be achieved if the mix was to change radically.

The future of the NHS and its financing

Recently there have been expressions of considerable uneasiness about the future of the NHS. Principally this is a reflection of the economic climate in the country which generates the uncertainty about whether there is likely to be any significant increase in resources available for development of services believed necessary to apply and encourage advances in medicine in the near future. Indeed with a largely centralized financial system if improvement has to depend on an *increased share for the NHS of static or falling GDP,* the questions which arise from scarcity of resources, have even greater political edge than applies to those arguments which have been put in the past in support of the case for maintaining a *constant proportion of an increasing GDP,* since the prospect for either or both of these policies at present seem bleak. In the present economic and political atmosphere it might be some years before any significant increase in funds for morale-boosting development, from public sources is possible. That of course does not mean that the system itself as it stands, is not capable of being rationalized for more efficient operation, which is increasingly being seen as a challenge to management to enable resources to be released for fresh development. Indeed it is often claimed that the history of the NHS, for which since its inception, there has each year inevitably been a clamour for increased resources, suggests that for achieving value for money, and to reduce the likelihood of instant reaction to transient fashion (which in health care exists no less than in other parts of the economy) pressures for better use of restricted resources are no bad thing.

The Royal Commission set up to look at the question of financing the NHS and reporting in 1979, did little to allay fears that with the present arrangements there is a prospect of insufficient funding for development, for in effect it dismissed the feasibility of radical changes incorporating either a supplementary scheme or possible alternatives as substitutions, whose aim would be to tap additional sources in order to add extra finance for the development of services.

It is also especially relevant with the apparent outlook of the Conservative Government which took office in 1979 that although hitherto there has been all-party support for the notion of the NHS, there has always been some criticism of it on ideological grounds. The accent on the individual, making provision for himself and family is often linked with the belief in the greater effectiveness of the 'market' as applied to health care, on the assumption that such care is a commodity in the economic spectrum and that the laws of supply and demand will take care of establishing appropriate levels of provision in the social system. Such a notion is of course regarded in many quarters, by no means labelled as collectivist, as an outrageously over-simplification of an approach to a complex of important personal services, but however one views health care, it is incontestable that given the emotion engendered by health matters, there is a resources problem now, likely to be more acute in the near future when the financing of desirable developments in the health service has to be faced. It is in consequence of this, that there has been no little speculation whether it is possible by means other than increased taxation—which at the moment seems unlikely—for example, by insurance options, to increase the resources available for health care, without surrendering the principal ideals of welfare and many of the better features of the existing NHS which for all its imperfections has undoubtedly had its great successes in terms of social equity, distribution of skills, and quality of care. Indeed, for all its having been ignored by the Royal Commission of 1979 the question of public policy related to alternative means of financing health care services and the effect any change will have on the relative public/private mix, is unlikely to go away and will remain as a possible source of undesirable conflict unless all possible options with all their attendant side-effects, are more fully and soberly explored than has been the case hitherto.

Alternative insurance bases

It is of course not unduly difficult to set out the lines of available options for the financing of health services in a different way to that at present existing in the UK, since in the West the only real alternatives either in whole or in part, are through the use of insurance systems, public, private, or mixtures of both.

Broadly these follow two main lines. The *first* can probably best be characterized under the term 'social insurance' which embraces systems regulated by government and financed through a pay-roll tax. With both employer and employee contributing by this means the money is made to flow to accredited intermediaries of the Friendly society type (e.g. Sickness Funds, 'Mutualités' etc.). There can of course be variations of this and indeed in France there is a quango-type organization in the shape of the 'Caisse Nationale' (CNAMTS) which, while by far the main agent, has not an altogether exclusive monopoly but allows a small part of the stage to a number of 'Mutualités', some of them large and powerful, based on professional groups, such as teachers. The social insurance line in one form or another is illustrated by the systems in such Western European countries as the Netherlands, Belgium, the Federal Republic of Germany, and France.

The *second* involves a variety of insurance options for individuals or groups acting on behalf of individuals to supplement whatever is provided by the state through some insurance provision, either by means of 'indemnity' insurance as exemplified in the case in the UK in the Provident Association arrangements, which enables the insurer to buy services in the private sector, or as in France to reinsure for the 'shortfall' in the public scheme through a 'Mutualité'. There is also another important form, the 'service'-type insurance as exists in the Blue Cross and Blue Shield Plans in the USA, by which the carrier enters into contracts for particular levels of service with the providers such as hospitals and physicians. While there is a lively indemnity insurance sector in the US, the bulk of health insurance, including that through government programmes such as Medicaid (for the poor) and Medicare (for the aged) is provided by service contracts mainly through the Blue Cross and Blue Shield arrangements. Here the third-party, the 'carrier' has a special interest in the basic hospital-based service provided, and contracts for the cost of the service that has to be negotiated periodically. This interest entails a complex series of rules to which the individual and providers are subject including those for reimbursement of outlays. The carriers too are publicly regulated. It is hardly surprising that as a result of such complications, fairly heavy administrative expenditure is borne at the carrier and provider levels.

The politics of health care provision

Because of somewhat loose political talk and in consequence of much comment in the media, there has been uncertainty during the last year or so about the government's intentions with regard to changing the basis of financing the NHS. This has been reflected in somewhat wild and ill-judged comments in the media, founded largely on reported statements at Ministerial level. Thus Dr Vaughan, the Minister of State at the time, in the summer of 1981 talked optimistically of possible change, if only partly to an insurance-based system, and in particular was reported as saying that 'Ministers preferred to look across the Channel (i.e. presumably to the "social insurance" option) rather than across the Atlantic'. This could not have been regarded by those promoting the expansion of the Provident Association movements in the UK as too happy an observation, inasmuch as the Associations are almost exclusively in the indemnity insurance business. It seemed clear that there was some confusion about the means of effecting change, if not the end, which was presumably to stimulate an increase in the stake of the private sector and consequently some relief to the public purse. At the same time it was known through answers to Parliamentary Questions that a Departmental Working Party had been set up, with the addition of two outside advisers with some experience of the private sector.

Despite the somewhat hysterical flurries of rhetoric in reaction to the vague references to possible changes, about the possibility of the 'dismantling' of the NHS as well as the consequences of a 'major expansion' of private medicine to the public sector, an estimate of which seemed to be arrived at by an over-simple projection of the implication of the apparently large increase in recent years in the number of people insured through the Provident schemes, the evidence of the likelihood of major change was still slight to anyone interested in hard facts. Indeed, in February 1982 the Chief Executive of BUPA categorically stated that he and his colleagues never thought that the prophets who twelve months before talked confidently of one in five of the population being privately insured by 1985 were right. A slow growth if any growth at all seemed to be the consensus of the cautious and better informed about the future of private insurance. It might also be remarked that the 'private' sector covers 'providers', institutional as well as professionals in private practice, together with insurers, but there still does not seem as yet common policies embracing all parties.

The options

It was also evident to anyone who had studied the matter closely that it was unlikely that the 'social insurance' option was a likely 'starter' in the conceivable future for adoption in the UK. The reality from any other than a superficial reconnaissance is that a change to such a system would have enormous consequences, for apparently little effect. Thus, because a national insurance system was already in being, while it would be easy enough to adjust national insurance contributions and to separate out the cascade of money which would flow through national insurance funding between social security and health, there would be a host of political considerations which would be likely to cause any government, however powerful, to pause, unless they had a consensus of both sides of industry and business generally. The likely effect too on the management of hospitals and the structure of health administration would make the problems of the 1974 and 1982 Health Service reforms seem like minor dislocations. Nor is it easy to see any parallels with sectors of the economy which have been denationalized. There is certainly no simple route to privatization by, say, selling off assets. Nor is management of the existing system with a different form of financing likely to be very simple, or be effected without an increase in manpower. The effect of any change in this direction would also be regressive on individuals, and cause not a few problems in the business world because of its likely immediate effect on costs and prices at a time of economic uncertainty, to say nothing of labour relations. In the preliminaries to this study the impressions that a change to a social insurance system is unlikely was strengthened with the knowledge that for all the talk in the media about Ministerial working parties reporting to the Secretary of State about all the possible options as a preliminary to a White Paper, it seems that during 1981 the Confederation of British Industries had not been consulted by the government either as to detail or even principle. It is thus hardly surprising in the light of the current industrial climate to discover that it seemed the CBI were not considering any major insurance option along the social insurance lines at all, although they have views about 'excessive' manpower in the NHS.

A little better perspective to what might be in Ministers' minds was gained early in 1982 when, through the means of an interview with *The Times* Political correspondent, the Secretary of State effectively dismissed the social insurance option, and talked warmly of encouraging the development of the existing insurance system through the non-profit Provident Association movement. This confirmed the thesis that it would be likely to be this policy in one way or another that would be favoured as a potential option by the government certainly for the life of this Parliament and possibly beyond.

Nevertheless, in this book we felt we ought to get examples of the present position of social insurance systems and in our conclusions are not only going to speculate about the options open, say, by encouraging the expansion (*inter alia*, through fiscal support) of the Provident type of insurance schemes, which have shown a marked expansion over the last few years without much fiscal encouragement, but also to look at how other countries are faring with other alternatives which provide public funding in whole or in part. An important part of this will be to try to understand what such possible changes might entail materially to individuals, to providers, to carriers, and to the bureaucracy required to oversee health arrangements, *especially* the effect of the controls and regulations which now feature greatly in all health economies whatever the method of funding. Since there is a great deal of evidence available from the experience of other countries, it was felt worthwhile to explore the way in which policies operate for the development of health services in a range of countries with broadly the same health objectives and subject to similar democratic (and professional) pressures. Above all, it would be foolish in this sophisticated age to consider alternative schemes of financing for health care, without examining them against the perspective of public expectations and an appreciation of the key elements in health policies generally which apply to most Western countries. It is also essential to speculate from the experience of other countries where insurance arrangements operate, about the likely effects of changes in the very complex systems which comprise modern health services in which in all countries, central government and public authorities at various levels play paramount roles in the mix of public and privately operated services. They also have to be considered against some of the notions of the welfare state, which in the event have ruled in one way or another in the countries in Western Europe since the Second World War, and continue to affect the attitudes as well as the lives of most of the population.

Foreign experience

Thus, as has been remarked, despite the seeming acknowledgement by Ministers of the overriding political difficulties that would be involved in changes to a 'social insurance' form of system, the book incorporates a special look at the implications of this option by relevant reference to the up-to-date experience of other countries with such schemes. This is largely because the subject of how to improve the basis of financing of health services in the UK in periods of financial restraint, will continue to be a matter for debate, and it is important to explore the implications of all the options to distinguish the practical possibilities from the myths which surround the hopes and fears of possible radical change. Above all hovers the fact that many of the problems which arise in most countries have common characteristics whatever the funding base or historical perspective. Again, contrary to what is frequently assumed in ignorance of local requirements, insurance-based systems are subject to regulations and controls, similar (sometimes greater) in effect to those that apply here. Again in the UK, except for the relatively small private sector and for NHS charges, we have practically no experience for over thirty years of the effect of a cash nexus between individual and provider and we ought to be aware of the implications. It is the case that some of the lessons specific to the principle of cash payments by patients, to be learnt from foreign experience under social insurance systems, are applicable to insurance systems based on indemnity or service contracts. It is also evident that a major feature at the present time of most foreign systems which have a social insurance base or otherwise, is the similarity of the aim of many of the measures which are being taken in deliberate attempts by governments to constrain *total* health expenditure whether public or private. In some of the financial reforms being currently mooted and explored abroad, the defined aim is certainly to restrict those public expenditures and commitments which are virtually open-ended. It is specially notable that this inevitably includes the implication that doctors' incomes will be constrained, an objective which should not be lost on those who extol the virtue of a move to fee schedules on an insurance base. The simple fact is that in such systems there has always had to be bargaining between the paymasters, either with the government as principal or as a powerful party in the background, and the medical profession.

Expenditure control—a universal problem

Indeed, seeking to avoid a study which could be construed either as a 'Pilgrims' Progress' or 'Gulliver's Travels', we sought comments on the general theme from a band of acknowledged experts and it is extraordinary how the several pictures reveal slightly depressed health sectors from every direction abroad which are not dissimilar to that in the UK. However much health systems and policies may seem to differ from country to country, all current policies have one common major aim, cost containment which is an omnibus description of policies—to contain not just *unit costs* but also *total* expenditure in both public and private sectors—in the public because of the spectre of an uncontrolled Public Sector Borrowing Requirement or its equivalent in other economies, in the private because of the inflationary effect of health care costs on the economy as a whole. There is a striking similarity in each system of the effect of the economic controls sought and applied in all the parties concerned in health care contracts. In the European countries studied: the Netherlands, Belgium, the Federal Republic of Germany and France, the packages of financial reforms are all designed to control expenditure, principally public but affecting private too.

Across the Atlantic in Canada, some centralized control is exercised through the system of global budgets, which is a principle not far removed from that practised here. In the US, true to its tradition of veering away from Federal direct action, the policies being suggested are to restrain costs and utilization by means of 'cost-sharing' (which can in effect be construed as an euphemism for 'co-payments' or 'charges') or through 'consumer choice' and 'competition'. 'Deregulation' (at least on some accounts) is part of this philosophical package but it is not always what the rhetoric seems to imply. The other devices explored in the US are of more recent vintage, but are based on the theory that consumer choice can be a dampener to cost and that for-profit 'providers', i.e. hospitals, can provide services at cheaper prices than those in the NHS, or indeed as is claimed than not-for-profit companies.

Competition with and 'taxing' the private sector

In the UK, for all the unease about the NHS, the 'collective' ideal has hardly been dented, far less breached by the notion of competition although the combination of limited resources and resource reallocation on some seemingly more equitable basis may change that subtly. The NHS has always, of course, been a sensitive area in which politicians tread warily because changes affecting it (and moves towards even the encouragement of the private sector are believed to come into that category), have to be rationalized to avoid political problems. This is possibly the reason for the government now seemingly recognizing that in health care there are elements of cost which are financed at the moment exclusively by the massive public sector by one Department of State or another, and which do not appear in the private sector. Among these are the costs of training and education of nurses and doctors. It is believed that there have already been representations to the carriers that the public sector should receive some recompense from the private sector for these costs, possibly by way of levies on insurers. However reasonable this might seem to be—and it is possible to see the analogy with the levies for industrial training, to implement such a policy would require a complex mechanism. But the industrial training levy is unpopular and there is a real fear in the case of the private health sector that if this principle is conceded by any part of it, it will be a mechanism that can be turned to frequently and affect all constituent parts. Inevitably too, it could open the door to the notion of levying balancing charges to be laid on private hospitals for other purposes, in order to make the 'competition' between public and private hospitals more equitable.

The plan of the book

This book comprises a series of commissioned essays following on a preliminary study directed towards the major criticisms of the economics of the NHS which have been made over the years, and of the relevant experiences in other countries using different methods and systems of finance to those applying here. Good descriptions of the health care systems of those countries are available to fill out those features referred to in the essays. The text as a whole is designed to provide a mosaic of discussion within the framework of this Introduction and the Finale of most of the elements which are frequently assumed would be part of any system which could conceivably be regarded as an option open to a British Government set on reforming the finances of the NHS. In particular what was specially notable in the preliminary reconnaissance was the extent of control and regulation which had become almost universally applicable to health service systems here and abroad. Special attention was accordingly paid to this feature in the commissions for the essays, which present the experiences of other countries in the public/private mix for health.

The UK scene

The essays in *Part 1* deal exclusively with the UK scene and together are designed to give a current perspective and an appraisal of the literature of criticism by policy analysts published over the last few years. The *first* essay by *Culyer* discusses the myths and realities of the 'market' position on health including the question of control with an analysis of the objectives or policy goals for alternative systems based on that theory, as alternatives to the NHS and the means of achieving these. The theoretical and empirical validity of the 'market' position for health which is prominent as a reason for seeking alternatives, is discussed along with the administrative and other changes probably necessary if the market is to work efficiently. There is also some speculation on the important question of whether the resultant health care 'market' will meet the desirable policy objectives of a health care system which thirty *plus* years of the NHS have pinpointed fairly clearly. The *second* essay by *Forsyth* explores the convoluted semantics of health which tend to confuse the present picture of health care systems and the likely impact of a stronger private sector on the still dominant public sector. There is also some discussion of what may be involved in terms of control by government of private provision as necessary public policy. This essay too raises the question of the social objectives of health care policy against the notions of the welfare state which still rule. It also poses the question of policies designed to reconcile the efficient use of resources and the achievement of equity for the whole population; and to what extent it is possible to achieve these objectives without recourse to the kind of regulation and bureaucracy which makes for inflexibility. We live in a consumer age and the *third* essay by *Klein* seeks to explore implications of the rise of consumerism and the kind of consumer protection which seems likely to be implicit in a privately financed sector of the health economy. This also being a planning age with some experience in the UK of the limitations of planning with regard to health, it discusses how effectively a planning system for the optimum use of *total* health care resources can be applied. Finally in the *fourth* essay *Maynard* analyses the implications of the recent history of the private insurance schemes in the UK and the problems to which they are currently and potentially subject, with special reference to the largest of these, BUPA, where expansion has been greatest, but which to the surprise of many, for the first time reported an operating loss in 1981. There is also a discussion of the characteristics and limitations of the insurance options which seem open to the government.

The health world outside the UK and its relevance

It is a common human weakness that, beset with our own troubles we tend to ignore the evidence of external trends, which apply elsewhere in societies similar to our own. Yet there is no doubt that anxieties about costs and the resultant policies for constraints in expenditure for health services are features which are of universal concern at the moment. That this is part of the whole question of health service financing in which the appropriate mix of public and private contributions towards health services is a matter for concern in every country in the West is indisputable.

The major elements of this concern are identified in *Part 2* through essays from expert observers in other countries in Western Europe with social insurance systems. The mosaic of these essays, constructed out of a variety of experiences, presents the implications of the options open in the perspective of the current political, economic, social, and cultural circumstances of the UK.

It cannot be stressed too much that in all countries the great complexity of health services makes for an innate conservatism in form which practically ensures the inevitability of only gradual change in societies unused to revolutionary change. A struggle for freedom within a developing efficient health economy can be identified as a major objective but it is alas true, that the more one observes, the more evident it is that each system has its own band of regulations and controls, which the indigenous actors—providers, professionals, populations—have come to tolerate within their own social and professional systems, but which in other societies would be regarded as irritating and mean.

Thus there is an attempt in these essays to set out accounts by experts of a variety of disciplines, of the objectives and nature of controls and regulations in certain Western European insurance-based health care markets and their relationship to health objectives. In this connection, regulation is defined as activity by public or private institutions which affect or seek to affect the price, quantity, quality, and distribution of health care finance and provision. This of course covers both public and private regulatory activity and where it bears significantly on individuals, institutions and professions. In this way it is hoped that the differentiation between the nature, public, private or joint, of the control and regulatory processes will be revealed.

The essays in *Part 3* have been commissioned to illuminate what is happening in the health care economies in the English speaking countries with which the UK has close ties. Thus, for the USA the essay by *McNerney* deals with the theories of competition, consumer choice, and cost-sharing, policies which exercise their own form of controls and regulations. Again, whether in the wake of the collapse of the Voluntary Effort and the advent of Reaganomics, there is a likelihood of other mandated controls operating, is also explored. Similarly we have gone beyond Europe to look at the experience of two Commonwealth countries. *Evans* places the Canadian experience of controls by a system of global budgets in the context of North American attitudes. *Deeble* gives an account of the current scene in Australia which has recently denationalized its insurance-based health care financing arrangements and on the face of it at least has returned to the use of 'Funds', which while notionally private are tightly regulated.

The Finale

Part 4 seeks to raise the major issues which emerge from the previous essays for which however there is no substitute for studying closely for analogies. *Maynard* discusses the various issues of control and regulation which apply universally in relation to the objectives of health care which tend to be common ground for governments. The final essay by *the Editors,* in addition to setting out the various practical options open, explores some of the myths of the objectives and effects which surround the general subject of change. It also indicates the priorities for research and action which seem to arise if any government is realistic about seeking *the optimum* combination of public and private systems which together can best attain with efficiency the broad objectives common to most health systems in the modern world. The principal of these are justice, equity, and accessibility to all sections of the population, while at the same time permitting economic and professional flexibility as well as reasonable freedom in order to give satisfaction to the population at large.

REFERENCES

DAMERELL, DEREK V. Letter to *The Times,* 9 February 1982.
DEITCH R. (1981). 'Government intensifies search for options in health care financing', *Lancet,* ii, 481.
Facts(1981). (National Centre for Health Statistics: Washington, D.C.).
FLETCHER, DAVID, *Daily Telegraph,* 5 February 1982.
FORSYTH, G. (ed.) (1975). *Prelude to Harmony on a Community Theme.* (Oxford University Press for the Nuffield Provincial Hospitals Trust).
HAVILAND, JULIAN *The Times,* 28 January 1982.
HENKE, DAVID *Guardian,* 1 December 1981.
HICKS, RON (1981). *Rum, Regulation, and Riches.* (Australian Hospitals Association: Sydney, N.S.W.).
TRAHAN, MICHAEL (1981). *Health Insurance in France, Australia, and Canada.* (Department of National Health and Welfare: Ottawa).

PART

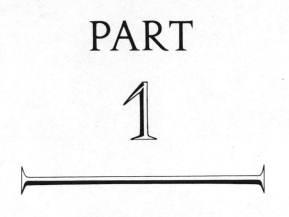

1

The UK
scene

The UK scene: current perspectives

The market for health care in all countries is complex and dominated by powerful interest groups. These interest groups and the complexity of financing and providing care transcend any differences and indeed changes in institutional structures. Neither does organizational change and any alterations in the public-private mix alter the fundamental nature of the health care market.

This section consists of analyses, from four different viewpoints describing various aspects of the existing public/private mix in Britain, and discussing possible effects of alternative mixes. The underlying theses explored by the authors are that if the mix is altered, one set of policy problems is likely to be exchanged for another. The characteristics of these problems may not always be attractive and indeed may make the attainment of the goals of public policy concerning health generally more difficult. The existing health care system is not without its flaws and in common with most institutions has to be kept under review. It would be naive however to believe that 'privatization' of the NHS or any part of it, would take Britain to some Utopia of health care. Any different mix of public and private activity would be likely to generate new problems, and new responses by the actors in the health care market to these problems. Some provider and consumer groups would gain and others would lose. At the same time there is no escape from regulation and control. It is likely that one type of regulatory environment would be exchanged for another: with any major increase in the private sector, the role of regulation (by which is meant the manipulation of the price as well as the quality and quantity of health care) would almost inevitably increase with regard to private institutions. Such institutions would have to develop the means—not necessarily simple—of responding to the challenges of this complex market in ways similar to those after which the NHS has groped for over thirty years.

21

The NHS and the market

Images and realities

A. J. CULYER

A. J. CULYER

Professor Tony Culyer is a professor of Economics at the University of York, England and Deputy Director of the Institute of Social and Economic Research at York. He is organizer of the UK Health Economists' Study Group, Scientific Adviser to the Chief Scientist of the DHSS, Honorary Adviser to the Office of Health Economics, Co-editor of the *Journal of Health Economics,* and has acted as consultant to the WHO, EEC, OECD and to governments and industry. Since he has been at York he has also been a Senior Research Associate at the Ontario Economic Council; a Visiting Professorial Lecturer at Queen's University, Kingston, Ontario, Canada; William Evans Visiting Professor at the University of Otago, New Zealand; and a Visiting Fellow, Australian National University.

He has published some 80 articles and pamphlets, many of them on health matters, and twelve books of which the most recent is *The Political Economy of Social Policy* (Oxford: Martin Robertson, 1980). Forthcoming books include a report on the proceedings of the European Workshop on Health Indicators (of which he was chairman) and the proceedings of the first European conference on the evaluation of medical technology (jointly chaired by him and Dr Bruno Horisberger of St Gallen, Switzerland).

Outside economics he is mainly occupied as organist and choirmaster in a rural parish church.

The NHS and the market
Images and realities

ABSTRACT

There is a robust tradition in economics that contrasts the
imperfect reality of Britain's NHS with a benchmark form of
social organization where all transactions are conducted in a
perfectly operating market. This paper argues that the tradition is unhelpful: partly because it is usually assumed too
readily that the *imperfect* markets of reality more completely
achieve effectiveness and efficiency than the NHS; partly
because the benchmark is far too general to be of much
practical help in redesigning the organization and finance of
health care in the UK; partly because the benchmark is, in
any case flawed on its own terms, and partly because it
distracts attention from the constructive contribution economics (in conjunction with other disciplines) may make to
important matters of policy and hence, at best, makes economics irrelevant and, at worst, brings it into disrepute. An
alternative, more pragmatic, economic approach to health
services research is proposed.

IMAGE AND REALITY

Image ... reality ...

It is hard to distinguish the two, since on the one hand our
images condition what we see (and what we look for) and
hence in part determine our realities, while on the other
hand the realities we have experienced can limit the alternative images that we might invent about 'how things might
be' in a reality yet to come. We are all slaves of both. Those
henceforth designated as 'marketeers' tend to possess an
image of a market with the sort of nobility described by
Adam Smith. Their perception of the realities of actual

25

markets in health care tends to focus on the desirable attributes of these realities at the expense of the less desirable,
whereas their perception of the realities of the NHS itself
focusses on some of its more objectionable features at the
expense of its accomplishments. The opposite is true of the
so-called 'antimarketeers'.

These fundamental differences in perception and observation cannot make for fruitful dialogue. If one adds to them
the slenderness of the available data for making many of the
relevant comparisons of realities to an ignorance of how
many of the key actors in any health care system operate,
what their aspirations are and how constrained they are in
achieving them, as well as the differences that are occasionally actually articulated about the appropriate objectives
served by systems of health care, then the stage is set not
merely for an unfruitful dialogue but for a dialogue of the
deaf: the opposing arguments come to pass one another like
ships in the night.

In this paper an attempt is made to explore some of these
differing images and realities, not with the hope of setting
out any 'correct' image or reality but rather with the intention of identifying as clearly as possible the nature of the
differences between images and the concordance—or lack of
it—between any image and any reality. The focus will
mainly be on the images of the marketeers—that is their
images of the market in health care and the NHS. Something
will also be said about some alternative images, though
whether these correspond to the images of the antimarketeers
is perhaps a moot question. The antimarketeers are less
homogeneous than the marketeers, since, whereas nearly all
marketeers have at root a liberal economic image of the
market, the antimarketeers include liberals, marxists, and a
host of other image-makers who are to be discovered both
within the liberal-marxist spectrum and within other spectra
differently defined. While our focus is on images of the
marketeers, and highly critical things may be said about
them, it is not part of the intention to proclaim an alternative let alone an inherently superior image of the NHS. Nor
do we seek to offer any 'truer' reality of the NHS. To expose
the weaknesses of the marketeers' images and realities is not

the same as to espouse the cause of any particular group of antimarketeers.[1]

The paper seeks to explain the key features of the marketeers' image of the market for health in contrast with the reality of the market. It goes on to discuss the marketeers' image of the NHS and to explore an alternative image—not of the NHS but of appropriate ways of putting economic analysis to work in the light of conclusions reached in the previous sections. The main conclusion is that *health care markets are always and everywhere so imperfect that the marketeers' image of the market for health is a completely irrelevant description of an unattainable Utopia.* The concluding section describes an economic approach to health care policy that is equally applicable to systems mainly organized in imperfect markets or by imperfect governmental procedures and that does not depend upon a Utopian vision of the ideal.

The reader looking for symmetry will note the absence of sections dealing with the reality of the NHS and the antimarketeers' images of the market and the NHS. The former of these aspects is partially treated in Culyer (1981). The latter was treated in Culyer (1971 and 1972). These two articles reached the kind of conclusion arrived at in the present paper, but were critical of the antimarketeers' image, as this is of that of the marketeers. All three strands of argument are omitted from the present paper since they are not required in order to reach the conclusions described later.

THE MARKETEERS' IMAGE OF THE MARKET

Voluntary contracting

The marketeers' image of the market is at root the view that the inherent rivalry of private interests can be reconciled by

1. The writer has in his time been as critical of antimarketeers as he now proposes to be about the marketeers. In some circles this earned him the reputation—quite inappropriately—of being a marketeer. He has not, therefore, now 'become' an antimarketeer! He merely remains an economist preoccupied with testing hypotheses and trying to make reasonable statements about familiar realities that may lead to modest—but real—improvements rather than describing the unobtainable and devising Nirvana solutions to present problems.

free (i.e. voluntary) contracting between interested parties. These interests need not, incidentally, be only *selfish* interests —it is a calumny to charge the marketeers with assuming the Mandevillian worst about human nature. If such contracting can take place, and be upheld by a system of enforcement (whether by custom or law), and can take place in all matters of mutual conflict, then the marketeers' argument is that resources will be allocated in such a fashion that no redistribution can take place that does not impose a net harm on someone. In this, it is assumed that conflict arises essentially out of the inadequacy of available resources to satisfy everyone's last want. In other words, benefits will be maximized over costs; moreover, they will be maximized by a procedure that preserves the libertarian view of freedom.

Efficient outcomes

The institutional counterpart to this image is that of a system of private property entitlements with the special —and crucial—characteristic that the entitlements, which specify who has the right to use resources in particular ways, may be exchanged between individuals if suitable compensation is forthcoming. The initial distribution of rights may be either equal or of increasing degrees of inequality; but whatever the nature of this distribution, the marketeers' basic vision is that free production and exchange will produce an *efficient* outcome—that is when all resources have been transferred to their most valued uses. Up to this point there are 'gains from trade'. It becomes a 'zero sum game' when the cake can be redistributed but its size cannot be larger. Questions about the justice of the initial distribution of rights and the justice of the final distribution are generally taken as independent issues. The marketeers' image of the market is separable from their image (which is not a unique one) of the justice of various distributions.

Income, or wealth, distributions are but a special case of the distribution of rights which would include *all* rights and entitlements, not just those that are commonly exchanged in markets and that therefore have price tags readily attached to them.

From this general image flows directly a number of specific images of how a health care system ought to run. But first it is desirable to consider an illustrative set of characteristic attitudes taken by marketeers about health services.

No free services

The notion that *health services should not be free of charge* follows directly from the proposition that the resources used by health services are scarce and from a well-established behavioural theorem that the lower any price the more of the priced good or service will be demanded. A zero money price (there may, of course, be time and other impediments to access) implies that more will be demanded of the service than is warranted. Resources will be drawn into the health care system the value of which will be increasing elsewhere since they are no longer available to satisfy other wants, but whose value in health care is falling. If the excess demands at zero price are met—or even partly met—it follows that the value of more resources in health care is less than their value elsewhere. This alternative use value is measured by what must be offered in compensation to those demanding their use elsewhere in the economy, as revealed in the markets for the various resources in question. In the economic sense, marginal cost exceeds marginal value. This is just as bad for efficiency as when marginal value exceeds marginal cost. The only way to get the two into equilibrium is to allow market trading to take place. As long as someone values a service at the minimum cost that someone else incurs to provide it, then it will be provided. If it is not provided, then no one can have valued it sufficiently.

The marketeers do not necessarily have to suppose that information about marginal values and costs is perfect—only that more information is more conducive to the efficient outcome than less and that markets generally produce more information about these things than nonmarkets in the form of prices of inputs and outputs. Since information is, moreover, valuable it will often pay people to specialize in information production and exchange (again in markets). According to this view, information that is not provided is not necessarily valueless, but its value will be less than its cost.

In the market, then, at the going price, those demanding goods or services will get as much as they demand, and this will be as much as suppliers want to supply. The health sector will be of the size at which these forces come into balance. Either a larger or a smaller one implies inefficiency. There will be no queues or complaints about underfinancing. Rationing will be entirely by price—not at the whim of someone with authority to determine 'needs'—a word on which marketeers tend to pour scorn. The outcome is efficient. Benefit over cost is at a maximum. The market procedure also minimizes the role of those who like arranging other people's lives, ('life-arranger' is another term of scorn used by marketeers) and is therefore conducive to freedom.

To the charge that the market may deny access to those with insufficient incomes, the marketeers' retort will be that an unjust income distribution is no more or less than that. Therefore the marketeer advocates corrective action by way of appropriate transfers of income. It is important, however, not to destroy the market.

No regulation

A favourite cry is *'Do not regulate'*. Regulation, according to the marketeers, is a simple way of accomplishing either one of two objectives, each of which is undesirable. The first is to give power to the 'life-arrangers' to determine what shall happen. This must be at the cost of those who voluntarily buy and sell in the market, otherwise there would be no demand to 'arrange' (or 'rearrange') other people's lives. The marketeers reject the idea that those with superior information or specially noble motives should be placed in a position to arrange the lives of those who have neither. They argue that the solution to inadequate information is not to hand decision-making over to somebody else but to provide more information. The idea that some people are better able to judge the welfare of others than the others are themselves is particularly objectionable to the marketeers who see the 'arrangers' as a species of censor (which, in a way, they are) and hence illiberal.

The other objective of regulation is to give monopoly power to particular groups. Marketeers are fond of observing how the ostensibly regulated, capture control of the regulatory mechanisms and use them to their advantage. Professional licensing is a classic case. In general, the claim is that competition in open markets produces both efficient resource allocation and freedom. Regulation nearly always imposes barriers to entry and jacks up the income of those who are thereby protected. Just as open markets harness self-interest to the common good, so self-interest often seeks to destroy the openness of markets. Constant vigilance is therefore required.

According to this line of argument anyone should be free to set up as a medical practitioner or supplier of medicines. Even the heavily regulated markets of today offer protection to those supplying quack remedies. The proper answer is to allow competitors to expose fraudulent claims and incompetence, permit markets in relevant information to develop, and to allow recourse to the courts in cases of negligence, incompetence, failure to deliver, etc.

No compulsory insurance

Yet another invocation is 'do not make insurance compulsory'. Most people dislike having to take risks. The financial risk of sickness is one such. In a market, in exchange for suitable compensation for bearing the risk, specialist agencies can arise to accept the financial consequences of an individual's falling sick. Under competition, the premium one pays will depend upon the sums insured and the probability of the events insured against occurring, together with the costs of the insurance agencies themselves. Those for whom the uncertain financial prospect of falling sick next year is worse than the financial prospect of paying a certain premium will therefore insure. Those for whom that is not true will not insure. To force the latter to insure is therefore to make them worse off since for them the cost is higher than the benefit.

Since attitudes to different kinds of risk differ and the financial consequences of any particular risk differ, and since individual probabilities of falling sick also differ, a wide variety of insurance policies will emerge catering to individual, family and group demands.

A place for profits

A high priority is given to a system that *permits profit-seeking.* Marketeers see wealth-seeking behaviour as the main motive that promotes efficient production and distribution of goods and services, including health services, information, and insurance. They also, however, allow that some non-profit agencies may naturally arise in markets (for example, charities). If these can compete with profit agencies, and survive, all well and good. If not, then they should die. There is no case for public subsidy in the form of subsidies or exemptions from taxation. Thus, if people wish to give their labour to a charity (as many do) they should be free so to do. Nor should profit agencies be protected from what they may see as 'unfair' competition. In general, however, marketeers expect non-profit activity to be relatively unimportant because it tends to be high-cost activity. The owners of non-profit agencies are typically unlike the owners (equity holders) of profit agencies in that they cannot signal approval or disapproval of the agency's work by buying or selling equity and thereby enhance or protect their wealth. In fact their personal wealth is rarely affected in any way by their role as trustees, managers, etc., which reduces the personal costs to them of inefficiency. Moreover inefficiency may bring other doubtful benefits (e.g. a congenial but ineffective set of colleagues and employees). Hence costs rise.

'Yes' to income redistribution but 'no' to market-rigging

Marketeers feel that bad income distributions should be put right by altering the distributions not by rigging the market. Since markets rigged in the various ways described produce inefficiency and harm freedom, bad income distributions remedied by market rigging achieve one good at the cost of acquiring a bad. Marketeers are not necessarily complacent about the income or wealth distribution (though many are) but they do argue the merits of changing it directly, thereby preserving the beneficial effects of market competition.

With health insurance, however, the marketeers will argue that distributional problems will be minimized. After all, an individual (or family) will not have to pay the medical bill, but only the insurance premium. A large though uncertain expenditure is transformed into a smaller certain expenditure. Moreover with risk pooling by insurance agencies, relatively high risks are subsidized by relatively low risks. Thus, those who would otherwise face high premiums may actually face lower ones. If, moreover, such high risks tend to be the poorer members of the community (as most evidence suggest they are) the distributional problem becomes even smaller.

No business protection

Finally, it is stoutly believed that *special pleading on the part of businesses seeking protection* should be resisted. Supplying agencies of all kinds often seek special protection arrangements by way of regulation that excludes competitors, provides subsidy, etc. These rarely have the effects intended and nearly always damage efficiency. Monopolies should be broken up (unless there are adequately compensating scale economies —and even this is a defence not all marketeers would admit) as should all monopolistic licensing arrangements. The marketeers are not particularly 'pro' big business—only efficient business.

These, then, are characteristic marketeers' images of how and why the market can and should be allowed to operate. The images could be elaborated further but it will be more useful to turn to the realities of the market, for the image is the image of an ideal and however attractive the description of the ideal might be, the reality is demonstrably remote from it. Indeed, it is possible that the marketeers' image of the market in health care is permanently unrealizable in existing markets. The imperfections of reality are not mere aberrations or temporary annoyances that can be put right by appropriate social engineering. Rigged markets, on the contrary, are a permanent and enduring feature of health care. The problem is not how to 'unrig' them but how best to live with them; ultimately to develop an image of what can be done to improve an inherently flawed market system for health or, in the case of the NHS, to develop an image of what can be done to improve an inherently flawed NHS.

THE REALITIES OF THE MARKET

The realities of facts

Some of the claims made in the preceding section are discussed in this section, though not in the same order for reasons which will become apparent. 'Realities' are not necessarily the same as 'concrete facts', for the latter are, in the end, not invariably of help in sorting out the current issues. A high point of absurdity was reached in the early days of battle between the marketeers and the antimarketeers (Titmuss, 1963; Lees, 1964) when Titmuss pointed to higher occupancy rates in British hospitals relative to American as evidence of waste in the US while Lees argued that the reality was that the higher occupancy occurred in the US, so that the waste was really in the NHS. About the same time Weisbrod (1964) demonstrated that US occupancy was almost certainly too high for efficiency. Hence, whether Lees or Titmuss was right about the 'concrete facts', they were *both wrong* in their interpretation of what the facts implied! Many 'realities' are in fact *'stylized facts'*, occasionally giving regrettably distorted views.

The realities of insurance

Insurance is equivalent to a price subsidy on health care. Suppose you are fully insured against the financial burden of whatever health care you may receive in the event of your falling sick. This means that when you fall sick, the price you confront is effectively zero. A fully insured person is thus in precisely the same position as one in a 'free' health care system. Since the demand for all forms of health care rises (though not proportionately) as price falls, a health system with insurance suffers from the same difficulty as a zero price system does. The main difference is that in an NHS-type system, whether the extra care demanded will be supplied depends upon the rationing method used, whereas in the market system the suppliers will be reimbursed by an insurance company. There is thus a built-in propensity for over-supply in an insurance-based system.

Another force also works towards oversupply: if one is insured, the financial burden of sickness is relieved, hence there is no urgent incentive to avoid a sick state. The probability of falling sick will therefore rise in so far as an individual's health state can be—if only in part—influenced by his own actions. This applies too in 'free' health systems. Both these effects are usually referred to by the quaint name 'moral hazard'; and they apply equally in a market with insurance, and in the NHS. A paradox begins to emerge as *the reality of the market* converges on the marketeers' *image of the NHS.*

Markets do evolve methods of mitigating moral hazard. All involve financial penalties for insured parties and hence reduce the benefits (for risk-averse people) of being insured, *viz: fixed indemnity* (a maximum level of benefit), that does nothing to affect behaviour leading to any expense less than this; *deductibles* (akin to the 'excess' in British motor vehicle insurance), which have little effect so long as expected expense exceeds the deductible; *co-insurance,* whereby the insurance company pays only a certain proportion of the medical bill above the deductible, and that clearly erodes the benefit of insurance. In general, then, the more complete one's insurance the more one is in the position leading to the inefficiency complained of by the marketeers. The more effectively moral hazard is curtailed the less the benefits of insurance: moral hazard is zero when coinsurance is 100 per cent but this is where one has no insurance at all!

Another difficulty with health insurance in the market is called 'adverse selection'. Insurance companies assess the probability that an individual will fall sick and make a claim upon broad classes of experience across groups of the population (so-called 'community rating'). Any individual who feels that the probability of his needing care is higher than that on which his insurer is assessing him will have an extra incentive to insure. Take a population of 100 people, 50 of whom on past history may be expected to pay £100 in medical fees, and 50 of whom may be expected to pay £300. The insurer offers premiums on the basis of the *average* risk so (ignoring the insurer's own operating costs) the premium will be set at £200 since £200 × 100 will just cover the expected pay-out of £100 × 50 + £300 × 50. This will seem an excessive premium to those expecting only £100 expenses, who will therefore not buy insurance unless they are quite extraordinarily averse to bearing the risk themselves. The insurer is left with the high risk cases insured at the risk calculated actuarially as low. In a pure market we therefore expect to see insurance agencies being forced away from community rating and having to tailor individual premiums more to individual risks.

In the USA, Blue Cross/Blue Shield originally adopted community rating such that all families of a given size paid the same premium. When commercial insurers entered the market they used 'experience rating' thereby offering probable low users more favourable premium terms than Blue Cross/Blue Shield, who in response and in order to maintain market shares had to modify their community rating basis for premium calculation.

This illustrates well the problem that competition creates in markets: it is less a problem of efficiency (for efficiency requires that premiums be proportional to risk) than of equity, for if premium averaging becomes impossible by pooling risks, the premiums for high risk groups, the chronic sick, etc., are likely to become sufficiently high for major distributive questions to be raised. Specific health subsidies for these groups will be demanded and with them the whole panoply of regulation, state finance, monitoring, and audit.

The realities of monopoly and regulation

Conducting health service policy on the assumption that monopoly and regulation will be swept away by appropriate policies is a doubtful procedure. It is enormously difficult either to prevent the growth of monopoly or to push it back once it has grown. But if it should not prove possible to eliminate monopoly and regulation for the sake of the regulated, then the rest of the marketeers' programme has to be called in question.

An obvious example occurs in the case of the medical profession, though as Dennis Lees has pointed out (Lees, 1966) the granting of professional licences has continued apace in Britain in many spheres including many ancillary to the doctors themselves (dentists, chiropodists, physiotherapists, dietitians, and lots more). The same appears to be true of all developed countries. It seems that a strongly organized professional monopoly that controls entry to the profession, terms of service, permitted forms of advertising, disciplinary procedure, etc., is a *universal* characteristic of all developed countries (wherever they lie on the liberal-collective spectrum). But if that is so, to advocate the market in *the rest* of health care activity no longer becomes an obvious logical corollary of the search for either efficiency or freedom. At the least, further regulation may become warranted (e.g. to limit and monitor abuse). Moreover there is at the least a *prima facie* case for introducing a countervailing bargaining power, in the form of the state, in the determination of wages and salaries.

Another good illustration comes from the history of the relationship between Blue Cross and the hospitals in the USA. Blue Cross was originally created by hospitals and the American Hospitals Association in the 1930s. The Blue Cross plans were quickly successful in gaining charitable status and exemption from state taxes in many states as well as from federal tax. This gave them an immediate competitive advantage over commercial insurers and it is not surprising that Blue Cross had 60 per cent of the hospital insurance market after the Second World War. This large proportion also enabled Blue Cross to negotiate favourable 'quantity discounts' with the hospitals.

A code of practice was at the same time established by the American Hospitals Association that patients should be free to receive care in the hospital of their choice, that any plan licensed to use the Blue Cross insignia had to have written agreements with at least three quarters of the non-federal

hospitals in its area, and that Blue Cross cost reimbursements
to hospitals could vary according to what the costs happened
to be. This effectively removed competitive incentives for
hospitals to provide efficient (i.e. least cost) care. Blue Cross,
with its implicit subsidies via its charitable status and the
bulk discounts, was able for a long time to fend off commercial competitors even though actual costs must have been
higher than a fully competitive system could have achieved.
The regulated had again effectively captured the regulatory
mechanism (in this case they invented it!) and used it to
destroy competition.

The theoretical advantages of a private property system
depend upon the existence of an appropriate economic environment. Without that, the differences in efficiency to be
expected between, say, privately owned and publicly owned
institutions begin to look rather small in terms of *efficiency* of
their operation. What may not be at all similar, of course, is
the resultant distribution of wealth. A monopolized insurance industry, a monopolized pharmaceutical industry, a
regulated hospital industry, and regulated medical professions are all likely to generate much higher wealth for their
members in a market system that has failed than in a truly
competitive market system or in a publicly owned system.
That, of course, is why it pays them to monopolize and
regulate. But this reality is a far cry from the image of the
marketeers' ideal markets.

The realities of freedom

The robust individualism of the marketeers betrays a naive
faith in the capacity of individuals to resolve their own
problems and neglects two crucial aspects of the demand for
health care, both of which are illustrated alike in market and
non-market health systems. These are two aspects of what
seems to be a fact: that there is a demand for 'life-arranging'.
The first aspect of this rather special kind of demand is that
individuals demand the services of professionals to advise
them and act for them as agents—interpreting both their
needs and arranging for them to be met where possible. The
second aspect is that individuals are manifestly not uninter-

ested in the health of their fellow citizens. Let us examine each aspect in turn.

The 'agency relationship' between a professional and his client has been much discussed in the literature and there has been no settled empirical conclusion to the question whether (in either market or the NHS) the nature of this relationship enables physicians so to manipulate consumer demand to their own financial benefit (see, for example, Evans, 1974; Newhouse, 1981). This power is evidently more exercisable where there is (as there invariably is) a strong professional monopoly that both controls entry to the profession and limits competition between professionals and information about the quality of one's competitors. For this reason alone, every society has seen the necessity to regulate the professional to protect the public from abuse. It seems clear that the incentive to induce (or discourage) demand depends upon the mode of payment of physicians. For example, fee for service payments provide a direct incentive to provide more services. A salaried form of employment provides no such incentive. A combination of part-time salary in the NHS *plus* private practice provides a direct incentive to generate NHS waiting lists in order to bolster demand for care in private beds. These distortions exist in *all* systems. Research (of which there is not enough in this territory) has not yet provided satisfactory answers to questions about the magnitude or desirability of the consequences of the behaviour changes induced by these employment conditions. What is clear is that the marketeers' image of a prototypical consumer shopping around for the best quality care at the least price, and getting it, is not a phenomenon that is anywhere actually going to be observed.

The second aspect of the 'life-arranging' argument casts further fundamental doubt on the adequacy of the marketeers' image. It will be recalled that the root of the marketeers' claim that the market will promote the efficient outcome depends upon the notion that marginal value and marginal cost will be brought into equilibrium in the market. Now suppose, however, that the value of a person's health, or of his health care received, is not only that which he himself places upon it. Suppose that others too place a value upon an individual's health—or consumption. (If this were not the case, who other than the very poor would ever advocate subsidizing the health care of the very poor? The remarkable fact is that almost the only people who do not actively advocate such subsidies are the poor themselves!). It immediately follows that the market will *undersupply* health (and/or health care) by failing to allow for the additional value placed upon it by people other than the direct consumer. Therefore, even within its own efficiency claims the market image fails, for a part of the value of health or health care must lie in the collective value placed upon the individual's health or health care consumption, and this value is *over and above* the value ascribed to the consumption by the direct consumer himself. The various forms this collective interest may take in the consumption of an individual have been explored recently (Culyer and Simpson, 1980) and applied in a wider context (Culyer, 1980).

Distributional questions

The theoretical advantages of private insurance from the distributional point of view are, as we have seen, likely to be eroded by actual insurance practice. With monopoly in the hospital industry and the insurance industry too, these advantages will be further eroded by premium 'loading', that is, the addition to premiums of costs of administration and the costs of the inefficiencies that monopoly makes possible.

A marketeer's response to such difficulties would characteristically be to arrange public subsidy for insurance premiums via tax deductions, vouchers, etc. For the chronic sick and uninsurable, special programmes may have to be devised. The state really has little option but to become involved not only in health care financing but possibly also in its provision. To the extent that it does *not* engage in the latter, it will have to finance services billed at inflated cost thanks to the effects discussed above: one has state interference *and* inefficient markets.

Conclusions

For a real market to approximate to the marketeers' image requires not only continual vigilance but a competition in technique between those whom it pays to subvert the market, and those with the responsibility of preventing such subversion. It is by no means apparent that the ingenuity and effective power of the latter is going to win out against that of the former. The result one normally expects will be, of course, a compromise. It is a compromise that means that the claims of the marketeers for the market must inevitably be qualified—and indeed probably heavily qualified. Not only will the reality not correspond with the image, it may, as I have already hinted, even begin to resemble the marketeers' image of the NHS!

THE MARKETEERS' IMAGE OF THE NHS

Since the marketeers' image of the NHS flows rather directly from their image of the market, it is convenient to follow through the same type of phenomena that were explored earlier. An early indictment was Jewkes and Jewkes (1962) but there have been others since that may be paraphrased.

Services free of charge

As was seen earlier the objection to zero charges lies in the arbitrary relation that marginal value will have to marginal cost. It may be just as bad to have marginal value less than marginal cost, as the other way around, for if the former implies a health sector that is too large the latter implies one that is too small. Abolishing price means we lack the necessary evidence to weigh value against cost. The upshot must be (a) a health sector of arbitrary size (depending on what —if any—nonprice rationing methods are used); (b) a chronic excess demand, in that users will always demand more than is supplied, leading to waiting lists and probably a continuing chorus of complaints about underfinancing; and (c) rationing of whatever is supplied according to the criteria of the suppliers rather than from those on the demand side (erosion of 'consumer sovereignty'). This latter point relates to a species of property right, namely that granted to the allocators of health resources to determine who shall receive what and when. This is not an exchangeable right, even though it is a private property right of those granted this authority.

Marketeers have mixed attitudes about whether the zero-price health system will be too small or too large, although they all agree that it will be of the right size only by accident. Some (for example, Buchanan, 1965) argue that ignorance by taxpayers of the tax price they pay leads them to understate the cost to them of the NHS, while the manifest benefits of a free service as and when they need it are clearly positive. The predicted outcome is a budget that is too large even if the system is technically efficient (which it is unlikely to be, see below). Others (for example, Lees, 1962; Lindsay, 1980) argue that the size of the system will be too small. All agree, however, that it will be arbitrary.

Waiting in queues will be an inevitable feature of the absence of prices. As Goodman (1980) says

> patients wait and wait and wait. They wait for an appointment with their doctors. They wait in doctors' offices. After being referred to a specialist, they wait again for an appointment. On the day of their appointment, they wait even more. And, if they get the OK for any serious medical treatment, the waiting *really* begins. Patients who are scheduled for operations, for example, can end up waiting for years. (p.31)

Thus,
> even under a system of 'free' health care, health care is not really free—even to the users. Those patients who actually receive care have to be willing to wait longer and bear more inconvenience than other patients. (p.41)

Other inefficiencies

A basic condition for efficiency is, as was seen above, that whatever is produced should be produced at least cost. Producers, in search of personal profit, have an incentive to keep production costs as low as possible. Those who are most successful at minimizing costs are also those who will compete most successfully for consumers by keeping prices low. Competition is absent in the NHS. It is for the most part a non-profit monopoly owned and operated by the government. Given this, the characteristic marketeer's conclusion is reached by Goodman 'the British do not get their money's worth for their tax dollars. They have less care and a lower quality of care than could be achieved for the same amount of spending'. (p.52).

Part of this inefficiency will lie in what Lindsay (1980) has called the 'invisible' characteristics of health.

> Medical attention is demanded for many reasons and people demand many characteristics predicted to be invisible if delivered by a government-organized health sector. They demand pleasant surroundings and prompt attention by their physician. They demand privacy in their hospital accommodation and answers to their questions about health. Even when well, they seek reassurance about troubling symptoms and ailing relations. Because it is not observed, this sort of medical care output will be given less attention in government medical care budgets. If financed, budgeters would have no way to verify that the resources were used for the purposes intended, so they are not even budgeted. Bureaucratic managers in their turn will devote fewer resources to providing this type of care because it cannot be counted and does not therefore reflect favourably on their recorded performance as managers. (p.56).

Another aspect of inefficiency will reflect in hospital procedures and hospital costs. One will expect hospital costs to fall as the management do not bother to hire staff to supply 'invisible' services (thus we would expect to see fewer, say, nurses per bed in the NHS than in a market). Since capital expenditure is politically determined and its outputs may become apparent only after a government has lost office, this form of expenditure will be pared back. Of course, there will be relatively little capital spending anyway on TVs, furnishings, personal telephones, etc. since these constitute 'invisible' services that no one in the NHS will have any reason to supply. Lengths of hospital inpatient stay will be higher than in a market because 'patient care' is a monitorable output of the system and the longer one keeps someone in hospital, the lower the cost per day. This leads to a rise in the cost per case above what would be observed in an efficient market (as well as meaning that fewer patients are treated than could be).

Emigration of doctors and nurses

As the monopoly power of the NHS as an employer becomes effective so professional salaries are likely to be squeezed —and may even be so squeezed that the net present value of a doctor's after-tax income is smaller than the equivalent value for manual workers. This will induce a net outward emigration of physicians and a shortage of individuals seeking training in the medical schools. Since foreign born and trained doctors may be willing to supply medical services at lower prices than locally trained doctors, these will be hired to replace emigrating locally born doctors and make up the shortfall in the output of the medical schools. Such doctors, however, will also offer lower quality of care, particularly in respect of the 'invisible' characteristics, for locally trained personnel will be regarded as 'better' doctors by patients. Moreover such doctors will have no linguistic communication problems. Similar phenomena, and for the same reasons, will characterize nursing and the other medical professions. Thus, while the NHS may be able to operate at a lower *per caput* expenditure rate, it does so only at the cost of shortages of manpower, of underpaying its manpower, and of offering an inferior quality of service.

Equality will not be achieved

One aim of the NHS is to achieve equality of health care consumption (Lees, 1962) for those with the same need. However 'need' is such a vague concept that it may scarcely be put in operational terms. The geographical distribution of resources is therefore unlikely to be related to 'need' nor will it approach equal availability *per caput*. Abolition of price is certainly not a sufficient reason for expecting equality of consumption between social classes and those of different incomes. Indeed, since waiting time impacts more harshly on wage earners than upon salary earners or those on unearned income, and middle and upper social classes are more articulate in making their demands effective, the NHS will tend to distribute resources *away* from the poorer members of the community and towards the better off.

The marketeers' image of the NHS need not be illustrated any more. Its essence is that the NHS must fail by comparison with the market outcome. It must also fail even by the NHS's own criteria. The indictment is complete and comprehensive. What is more, there is lots of evidence that the NHS does *not* perform as an ideal market would—even if it is not quite so bad as the critics cited here would have us believe. But is the criterion by which the NHS is being judged appropriate?

ALTERNATIVE IMAGES OF HEALTH SYSTEMS

False perspectives

It would be a devastating criticism of a health system to observe that its reality failed to match an image of it that its devisers, supporters, and customers themselves had. It is a much less damaging criticism to judge a system to be a failure by reference to an image that they do not have or to an image that has no corresponding reality in the world we know. We must therefore confront the issue of whether the marketeers' image is an appropriate one, either in the context of the NHS or, indeed, any other.

The way the marketeers' image has most frequently been promulgated implies clearly that it is *not* appropriate. The principal reason for this lies in the lack of correspondence between the image of the market and any known markets of reality. If it is correct to conjecture that any market in its reality must be highly imperfect (by comparison with the image), then the comparison of an image of the NHS with an *unattainable* market reality is not a relevant exercise. We can probably allow that the marketeers' image of the NHS exaggerates its shortcomings, but even if it does not exaggerate them it is quite clear that the differences between *either* the marketeers' image of the NHS *or* the NHS in reality, and the market in reality, are by no means as wide (or as predictable) as the difference between the marketeers' two images. Indeed, it is characteristic of all the marketeers' literature cited in this paper that the *reality of the market* is *never* compared either with the reality of the NHS or with the marketeers' image of the market. The task of comparing complex realities has been left to sceptics from whom the purpose of *a priori* images is to provide testable hypotheses about reality, not to prejudge it.

Instead of the rather empty posturing that has hitherto characterized much of this debate and that has shed desperately little light on either the causes of some of the systematic differences that *can* be observed or on questions concerning how the system might be changed for the better, it seems more constructive to seek our understanding by proceeding in a rather different way. This involves asking far more *specific* questions about observed differences or desired changes.

Consider, for example, the issue discussed above about the *size* of the health sector. There is not a great deal of point in asking whether any particular system allocates too much or too little to health care in general. On the other hand there *is* point in asking, for example, *why it is that different countries spend such different amounts* on their health care systems: or *what effect there would be on a population's health if expenditure patterns shifted away from health care* itself to, say, *preventive measures of specified types,* or *why the rate of surgical intervention in one country is so much higher than that in others.* Such questions are empirically researchable.

Indeed, the first of these questions has been fairly convincingly answered already by empirical research. It seems clear the amount of health care expenditure in any country has little to do with the degree of state involvement in finance and production, but it has a great deal to do with the level of national income (Abel-Smith, 1967; Kleiman, 1974; Newhouse, 1975; OECD, 1977; Abel-Smith and Maynard, 1978;

Newhouse, 1978; Maxwell, 1981). The observed variations in *per caput* health spending (public and private) vary by a factor of about five even in the developed world and can almost entirely be accounted for by variations in the various countries' national incomes. The studies are all agreed that a $1 increase in GDP will generate an 8 cent increase in health spending and that—at least in the 1970s—the developed world was, as a whole, moving towards a steady 8 per cent of GDP in health expenditure. This implies, of course, and has been corroborated from other studies, that the demand for health care (whether reflected in markets or by political processes) is income elastic, a rise in income always generates a rise in health care expenditure. Such specific hypotheses, substantiated by repeated factual testing, are a far cry from the complex ramifications of the marketeers' generalized propositions and offer genuine insights, unambiguous rebuttals (for example, of the view that health spending is a necessity determined by health 'needs'), and hence clearer understanding of the underlying determinants of the phenomena we observe. The second kind of question suggested above has less clear answers at the moment—but the strategy for finding answers is clear; one has to develop clearly specified propositions about what will affect what, with what time lags, identify acceptable measures of each of these, and then test the hypotheses against the appropriately assembled facts.

The third kind of question also suggested is again capable of more specific specification and empirical enquiry. For example, Vayda (1973) found that the 1968 rates of surgical intervention for men and women were 1·8 and 1·6 times higher in Canada than in England and Wales. If the two countries have basically the same needs (for example, if one has a similar disease prevalence to the other), then we would expect to see higher mortality rates in England and Wales in the potentially fatal disorders. But this is not so. For some conditions the mortality is in fact the other way about (possibly due to the surgical intervention itself). What is different between the two populations is the method of hospital physician payment: fee-for-service as against salary. Too much should not be read into this phenomenon or the apparent explanation, and much further research remains to be done. The question is, however, a manageable one and the mode of proceeding with it clear. It is empirical, requiring careful data collection rather than quotations from newspaper headlines or casual observation.

Economic causes of health problems

The same procedure seems appropriate for all 'problems' believed to have economic causes. Thus, we have seen that there are good *a priori* reasons for supposing both for-profit and non-profit health agencies (including health insurance agencies) to suffer from inefficiencies in both markets as they are in reality and in the NHS. The appropriate approach again is not to advocate a return to an image of a market that has never existed, nor ever will, but to ask explicit questions about how the system (whether market or NHS) can be expected to change in response to some variables which may be assumed to affect it. If, for example, one is concerned with a mainly market system one might ask, as has Enthoven (1978, 1980, 1981), what theory and evidence lead us to expect of measures that encourage the development of prepayment health maintenance organizations. One might ask for the effects on, say cost *per* case, hospitalization rates, health status, and patient satisfaction. If one is concerned instead with the NHS, an analogous set of questions can be asked of the effects of making hospital doctors budget holders (for example, Wickings, 1975). In each case, one *starts from where one is* and considers conceptually manageable changes that might be made to the existing system, *hypotheses* about their consequences and *tests of such hypotheses* by experiment and/or other observation.

Cost-sharing

Exactly the same procedure is appropriate even in the highly controversial area of introducing more user prices in the NHS. What financial burden would actually fall on intensive NHS users if a consultative charge were introduced? What substitution of private for NHS care might it induce? What reduction in NHS consultations might it bring about? What delays in identifying and treating disease would result? These are all empirical questions, answers to which can inform decisions about the desirability of such charges, their appropriate size, etc. Even in the UK there are sufficient money prices and non-money shadow prices for helpful answers to be obtained. In the grand ideological clash of rival images, however, such specific and empirical questions are rarely asked. Accordingly the real information that might aid any practical choice very rarely becomes available.

Specifics not generalities

What would be desirable is, of course, a rival image to those of the marketeers and the antimarketeers. It is a modest image about specifically productive economic research rather than generalized propaganda. Neither the marketeers nor the antimarketeers have satisfactory descriptions of the objectives of a health system. The former lack one because in the never-never land of their image of the market no such specification is needed: the outcomes will be whatever individuals want and are prepared to pay for. The latter lack one because they have chosen to talk about a romantic world in which men and women of goodwill set about meeting the reasonable needs of their clients, and have never addressed the question of the meaning of 'needs', what is 'reasonable', who the 'clients' should be, or how such 'needs' might best be met.

It is not the aim of this present paper to explore in detail how such objectives may be specified, although the irrelevance of the marketeers' image of a market makes it essential that this task be attempted at some stage. Nor is its aim to tackle the issue of how best objectives may, in defined instances, be attained. The objective has been instead to demonstrate the profound inadequacy of the marketeers' image of both the market and the NHS as a criterion for judging either its performance or how best that performance may be improved. In the next section some brief outline is offered of how a more fruitful economic research agenda might focus on various specifics.

CONCLUSIONS

The early debate between the marketeers and antimarketeers was initially centred around the question of whether health care was so very different from other goods that government provision and finance were necessary (for example, Mushkin, 1958; Titmuss, 1963). These special characteristics were hotly denied by others (especially Lees, 1960 and 1964) who attempted to show how markets could cope efficiently with each feature in turn. This stage of the debate was 'effectively terminated' (accordingly to Cullis and West, 1979) by an exhaustive discussion of how the parties to the debate had mistaken empirical issues for theoretical ones and had consequently sought theoretical answers to empirical questions (Culyer, 1971). With the advantage of hindsight and hence an ability to survey the debate relatively coolly, the emphasis could perhaps be put a little differently now. True, the issues *are* empirical at root but, notwithstanding this, considering what we *do* know and on any reasonable guess about what we do not, the chief conclusion to be drawn from this 'character of health' debate is not that government allocation is either appropriate or inappropriate, but that allocation by market forces must always and everywhere be severely flawed—not because the perfect market would necessarily produce poor results, but because only a parody of a market could ever, in 'reality', exist. Since the claims of the marketeers have always been based upon an image of the market rather than upon its reality, we are inexorably driven to the conclusion that their analysis is entirely irrelevant.

It follows from this that there is no need for us to explore the validity of their image of the NHS, for whether it is an accurate account of the reality or not (and it is often a grotesque parody (Culyer, 1981)), the account they give cannot tell us how much the NHS is worse—or even whether it is worse at all—than any markets in the realm of reality. For this reason the reader has been spared a blow-by-blow account of the deficiencies of the marketeers' image of the NHS. The reader is also relieved of the necessity of having to read any account of the antimarketeers' image of the NHS (though it could be asserted it has usually been as divorced from the reality of the NHS as the marketeers' image of the market is from the reality of the market).

The economic focus has therefore to be—and fortunately it has increasingly so become—more upon specific hypotheses that are subject to empirical measurement and test. We do not, or should not, ask what things would be like in a world that we know to be unattainable. We ask more specific questions about whether we could tell if we were accomplishing them better (or cheaper); also what changes—starting from where we are—we believe (together with the evidence for believing them) would bring us closer to accomplishing them.

Although there are innumerable potentially fruitful avenues for research there are two major ones that transcend organizational and financial arrangements and that should underlie the pattern of research in the next couple of decades. As a shorthand, these may be characterized as on the one hand *procedural evaluation* and, on the other, *behavioural modelling*. The first of these is concerned at one important level with the economic aspects of efficacy and effectiveness studies in clinical and epidemiological trials. It is well known that the 'technology matrix' (Russell, 1982) in medicine is in large part a 'black box': we simply lack systematic evidence, as distinct from case studies (which is merely a respectable term for 'anecdote'), about the impact that many measures in common practice (let alone those afforded by new technological advance) have upon the health and comfort of patients whether actual or potential. With the growth of scientific epidemiology the scene is set for fruitful collaboration between epidemiologists, clinicians, and economists for a major series of studies tackling the issue not only of effectiveness but also of cost-effectiveness. Clinical procedures are but one part of the 'black box'. The same is true of other aspects of medical practice: evaluation of the effectiveness of organizations (like health centres, solo practices, hospital departments, etc.) to determine the pay-off to alternative constellations of technical skills and divisions of responsibility for various aspects of care; evaluation of alternative locations of care (e.g. for the elderly); evaluation of information systems; evaluation of major health service investments. All are examples of types of study of which there are not nearly enough, where various mixes of research skills are needed and where single disciplinary hegemonies are unlikely alone to provide satisfactory illumination of the relevant 'black boxes'.

Alongside the evaluation of 'procedures' we need much more behavioural modelling both of the response of the client public to changes (e.g. in health education information, prices for care, demographic change, distance from facilities) and of the providers of care (e.g. the behavioural effects of introducing budgets for hospital teams of clinicians, of changes in the fees for various types of service—in medical, dental, and ophthalmic general practice), of changes in promotion prospects (e.g. by altering the ratio of consultant to junior hospital posts). In all these respects policy is largely conducted on a 'seat of the pants' basis, with desperately little systematic information for the basis of making predictions about 'what will happen if...' and disappointingly little experiment.

These types of enquiry are a far cry from the generalities of the marketeers' approach. Moreover, they begin by acknowledging our substantial ignorance about some crucial basic phenomena in the health services no matter how they are, in general, organized—whether, for example, they are in large part organized in or outside markets. These enquiries also immediately throw up the need for further fundamental research, both theoretical and applied, in matters such as the definition and measurement of 'health' itself—not as an exercise in vacuous slogan manufacturing but as an essential input into the evaluation of the services we have and of any changes that may be proposed. Again, merely to state the issue is to imply that its solution (or solutions) needs multidisciplinary endeavour—an endeavour in which economics has a necessary but by no means sufficient role to play.

This all amounts to a research programme in social science rather than Utopian political and economic philosophy. This is the nature of the 'images' we should be seeking. The images are, to be sure, theories. But they are theories that are manageable with our meagre intellectual resources; that are carefully specified enough to be applicable in concrete situations: that do not attempt to invent 'grand designs' whose (conceded) beauty is all too frequently matched by their total ambiguity as a guide to action, and whose validity is flawed by the necessity that their very grandeur has been purchased at the cost of an umpteenth removal from reality.

This alternative image is really an image writ small in contrast to the headline images of the marketeers and anti-marketeers. Like them we should care about the output of health services, but let us ask how we define and measure it—research questions that were never dreamed of in the heyday of the great debate. Like them we should care about the *value* of that output but let us ask how we define and measure that—in short certain research questions that have hardly ever been asked, let alone answered. Like them let us ask how outcomes are produced, how they may be produced most efficiently, a speculation which may take us outside the health sector as commonly conceived. Like them let us ask how individuals, whether patients or professionals, will react to changes in the circumstances that affect their behaviour; but let us do so in specific contexts of what exist in the real world rather than the abstract image of the world. Like them let us be concerned with equity—but let us ask what equity consists in, and how it may be measured, monitored, and achieved.

The market controversy is instructive: it not only failed to resolve any issue of any importance—no matter how remote; it also distracted attention and scarce research talent away from a meaningful research agenda. It has also— with a predictable lag—influenced a generation of undergraduates now become politicians (of all political hues) to raise to the centre of the political stage a set of issues that their university mentors have long since left on the shelf to gather dust. Let us then put them on a still higher shelf!

BIBLIOGRAPHY

ABEL-SMITH, B. (1967). *An International Study of Health Expenditure.* (WHO: Geneva).
— —, B. and MAYNARD, A. K. (1978). *The Organisation, Financing and Cost of Health Care in the European Community.* (EEC: Brussels).

BUCHANAN, J. M. (1965). *The Inconsistencies of the NHS.* (Institute of Economic Affairs).

CULLIS, J. G. and WEST, P. A. (1979). *The Economics of Health: An introduction.* (Martin Robertson).

CULYER, A. J. (1971). 'The nature of the commodity "health care" and its efficient allocation', *Oxf. Econ. Pprs.,* **23,** 189.

—— (1972). 'On the relative efficiency of the NHS', *Kyklos,* **25,** 266.

—— (1980). *The Political Economy of Social Policy.* (Martin Robertson).

—— (1981). 'Acht Trugschlüsse über das Britische Gesundheitswesen', *Medita,* **6,** 22.

—— and SIMPSON, H. (1980). 'Externality models and health; Rückblick over the last twenty years', *Econ. Rec.,* **56,** 222.

ENTHOVEN, A. C., (1978). 'Consumer choice health plans, Parts I and II', *N.E.J.M.,* **298,** 709.

—— (1980). *Health Plan: The Only Practical Solution to the Soaring Cost of Medical Care.* (Addison-Wesley: Reading, Mass.).

—— (1981). 'The behavior of health care agents: Provider behavior' in J. VAN DER GAAG and M. PERLMAN (eds.) *Health, Economics and Health Economics.* (North-Holland: Amsterdam).

EVANS, R. G. (1974). 'Supplier-induced demand: Some empirical evidence and implications' in M. PERLMAN (ed.) *Economics of Health and Medical Care.* (Macmillan).

GOODMAN, J. C. (1980). *National Health Care in Great Britain: Lessons for the USA.* (Fisher Institute: Dallas).

JEWKES, J. and S. (1962). *The Genesis of the British NHS.* (Basil Blackwell).

KLEIMAN, E. (1974). 'Determinants of National Outlay on Health' in M. PERLMAN, (ed.) op cit.

LEES, D. S. (1960). 'The Economics of Health Services', *Lloyds Bank Review,* **56,** 26.

—— (1962). 'The Logic of the British National Health Service', *J. Law & Econ.,* **5,** 111.

—— (1964). *Monopoly or Choice in Health Services?* (Institute of Economic Affairs).

—— (1966). *Economic Consequences of the Professions.* (Institute of Economic Affairs).

LINDSAY, C. M. (1980) *National Health Issues: The British Experience.* (Roche Laboratories).

MAXWELL, R. J. (1981). *Health and Wealth.* (Lexington: Mass.).

MUSHKIN, S. (1958). 'Towards a Definition of Health Economics', *Pub. Hlth. Rep.,* **73,** 785.

NEWHOUSE, J. P. (1975). 'Development and Allocation of Medical Care Resources', *Proc. 29th World Medical Assembly.* (Tokyo).

—— (1978). *The Economics of Medical Care: A Policy Perspective.* (Addison-Wesley: Reading, Mass.).

—— (1981). 'The Demand for Medical Care Services: A Retrospect and a Prospect' in J. VAN DER GAAG and M. PERLMAN (eds.), op cit.

OECD (1977). *Public Expenditure on Health.* (Paris).

TITMUSS, R. (1963), 'Ethics and Economics of Health Care' in *Medical Care*, reprinted as Chapter 21 in *Commitment to Welfare*. (Allen and Unwin, 1968).

VADYA, E. (1973). 'A Comparison of Surgical Rates in Canada and England and Wales', *N.E.J.M.*, **20**, 1224.

WEISBROD, B. A. (1964). 'Collective-consumption Sources of Individual-consumption Goods', *Q. J. Econ.*, **128**, 471.

WICKINGS, I., *et al.* (1975). *The Effect of Presenting Management Information to Clinically Accountable Teams*. (Health Information Unit, Brent Health District).

The semantics of
health care policy and the
inevitability of regulation

GORDON FORSYTH

GORDON FORSYTH

Gordon Forsyth is Professor of Health Service Studies and Director of the Health Services Management Unit in the Department of Social Administration at the University of Manchester. He was educated at Manchester Grammar School and at Manchester University (where he took first-class honours in economic and social studies). He has been engaged in operational studies of health services since 1956 when he carried out a case-load survey in the Barrow and Furness group of hospitals. This was one of a series of studies, sponsored by the Nuffield Provincial Hospitals Trust, which radically affected thinking about hospital planning in this country and led to the Ministry of Health's first ten-year building plan of 1962. In 1964 he established and directed the research branch of the Saskatchewan Medical Care Insurance Commission, the governing body of the first compulsory tax-supported Government medical care insurance scheme to be introduced in North America. In 1962, as a World Health Organization Travelling Fellow, he visited research centres in Canada and the USA, and in 1969 he was a WHO short-service consultant in public health administration training. By arrangement with the Ministry of Overseas Development through the Central Treaty Organization, he has acted as adviser on health insurance to the Government of Turkey. He is an Honorary Fellow of the Institute for Health Service Studies at the University of Leuven. He is author of *The Demand for Medical Care; Doctors and State Medicine: Gateway or Dividing Line?* and editor of *Prelude to Harmony on a Community Theme* by J. Van Langendonck, a study of health insurance policy in the EEC. He has contributed to several publications by the Nuffield Provincial Hospitals Trust.

The semantics of
health care policy and the
inevitability of regulation

ABSTRACT

Although the present Government has expressed interest in insurance-based health care systems and is broadly sympathetic to the private sector, no major specific measure has yet been taken radically to change the financial basis of the NHS. Reviewing the relationship between the NHS and private practice since 1948, and trends in insurance-based European systems, Gordon Forsyth suggests that regulation of providers of health services by public authorities is inevitable. It is argued further that the future expansion of voluntary hospital insurance may be less rapid than recent trends suggest and that the significant change since 1975 has been the emergence of the private hospital. Despite the Health Services Act of 1980, and the cessation of phasing private pay-beds out of NHS hospitals, there may have been no real change in central policy since the change in government in 1979, and the development of private facilities outside the NHS may still be favoured to the disadvantage of the NHS, the hospital consultants, and the voluntary insurance sector. The essay concludes by suggesting that it is in the interest of the voluntary insurance sector to contribute to the costs of nurse training by paying at local level sums that are calculated possibly on the numbers of nurses employed in private hospitals.

INTRODUCTION: THE ECONOMIC BACKGROUND AND PERSPECTIVE

The growth of public expenditure and policies for its containment

Between 1951 and 1975 (see Table 1) expenditure by public authorities in the UK expressed as a percentage of Gross National Product at factor cost rose from 44·9 to 57·9.

59

Table 1. *The growth of social expenditure in the UK.*

Per cent of GNP at factor cost:	1910	1921	1931	1937	1951	1961	1971	1975	New Basis 1975	New Basis 1980
All Social Services	4·2	10·1	12·7	10·9	16·1	17·6	23·8	28·8	28·1	28·9
Social Security		4·7	6·7	5·2	5·3	6·7	8·9	9·5	9·3	11·5
Welfare						0·3	0·7	1·1	1·0	1·1
Health		1·1	1·8	1·8	4·5	4·1	5·1	6·0	5·8	6·2
Education		2·2	2·8	2·6	3·2	4·2	6·5	7·6	7·2	6·5
Housing		2·1	1·3	1·4	3·1	2·3	2·6	4·6	4·7	3·7
Infrastructure	0·7	0·6	1·0	1·0	3·6	4·8	6·3	6·8	5·8	4·0
Industry and Employment	1·8	4·5	3·2	2·8	6·9	4·9	6·5	8·3	5·9	4·2
Justice and Law	0·6	0·8	0·8	0·7	0·6	0·8	1·3	1·5	1·5	1·7
Military	3·5	5·6	2·8	5·0	10·8	7·6	6·6	6·2	6·1	7·0
Debt Interest and Other	1·9	7·7	8·2	5·2	6·9	6·3	5·9	6·3	5·5	6·8
Total State Expenditure	12·7	29·4	28·8	25·7	44·9	42·1	50·3	57·9	54·2*	53·6*
Total State Revenue	11·0	24·4	25·0	23·8	42·7	38·5	48·6	46·6	45·1	47·7
Borrowing Requirement	1·7	5·0	3·8	1·9	2·2	3·6	1·7	11·3	9·1	5·9

Sources. I. Gough, *The Policital Economy of the Welfare State*, Macmillan, 1979, Table 5.1; National Income and Expenditure, 1981.

Notes. For more precise definitions of each term, see (I. Gough, 'State Expenditure in Advanced Capitalism', *New Left Review*, **92**, 1975, p.60). 'New Basis' for calculating public expenditure involves the following major changes:

(a) Only government lending to nationalized industries included, instead of their total capital expenditure under the old basis.

(b) Only that part of debt interest financing non-trading 'social capital' such as roads, schools and hospitals included, instead of total debt interest under old basis.

(c) Non-trading capital consumption (i.e. wear and tear of social capital such as hospitals) excluded from individual categories of social services; under old basis this included as 'imputed rent'. Now added at end to total state expenditure.

*Including non-trading capital consumption not shown in above figures.

Within this sum, expenditure on social services (social security, welfare, health, education, and housing) rose from 16·1 per cent to 28·8 per cent. In other words by 1975 public authorities accounted for nearly 60 per cent of GNP and half of that was accounted for by the 'Welfare State'.

During this period *taxation* did not keep pace with expenditure: total state revenue rose from 42·7 per cent in 1951 to 46·6 per cent in 1975 but the Public Sector borrowing requirement rose from 2·2 per cent to 11·3 per cent.

Since 1975 successive governments have sought to reduce public spending. It is said that had the public expenditure programme been allowed to proceed unchanged after 1975 then the cost, taken in conjunction with the statutory requirement to increase pensions (and consequently social security contributions) would have implied for the average wage-earner an effective marginal tax rate of 55 pence in the pound. Given the apparent general unwillingness to recognize the social wage as part of personal income (and in truth much of the social wage is somebody else's personal income, for example teachers, doctors, nurses, etc.) the Labour Government began the process of reducing public spending from 1976 and the succeeding Conservative administration pursued the same broad policy albeit with variations in emphasis.

By 1980 the PSBR had been reduced by 3·2 per cent. This was achieved by increasing total State revenue by 2·6 per cent rather than by a massive reduction in State spending (down by only 0·6 per cent). Expenditure on 'social welfare services' increased marginally between 1975 and 1980 by 0·9 per cent. Within this overall increase, however, social security rose by 2·3 per cent and the brunt of the cuts was thrust on housing and education.

Compared with education and housing the National Health Service has so far been considerably shielded from the worst of the economic chill. Between 1951 and 1975 expenditure on the NHS rose from 4·1 per cent of GNP to 6·0 per cent. During this period employment in the NHS doubled from half a million to over one million staff of all types and grades. The expansion was based on growth rates in real terms of between 3·0 per cent and 3·5 per cent per annum.

After 1975 the rate of growth was restricted to 1·5 per cent per annum until 1982, when the Public Expenditure White Paper set the growth rate for the NHS at 0·5 per cent.

Some effects of containment policies

At this rate of growth the level of service offered seems likely to decline. It is generally accepted that for technical reasons (largely the difficulty of increasing productivity in an essentially personal service) the NHS needs an extra 0·5 per cent annually to maintain services at a constant level and a further 0·8 per cent to compensate for the ageing of the population. For the first time since the inception of the NHS in 1948, therefore, there appears to be a real prospect of a decline in the volume and quality of service. At the same time the Secretary of State, Mr Norman Fowler, has committed himself to the policy of giving priority to services for the elderly and chronic sick, the mentally ill and the mentally handicapped. In February 1982 he announced that Chairmen of Regional Health Authorities would be accountable to him in ensuring that within their Regions there would be adherence to the central policy of discrimination in favour of community services and the care sector.

If the Secretary of State is successful in exerting greater central control over the use of NHS resources then the policy, combined with a rate of growth consistent with the maintenance of a constant level of service, must in theory imply a sharp deterioration in the general acute sector. Among other effects, waiting periods for elective repair surgery may lengthen and people will have an added incentive to take up voluntary health insurance. The events are probably not directly related—central governments rarely have a comprehensive strategy on these things—but in the budget of 1981 employees earning less than £8500 per annum who were enrolled in group voluntary health insurance schemes ceased to be liable to pay income tax on the value of their employer's contribution to such schemes. The Chancellor of the Exchequer has therefore forfeited some revenue to encourage elective repair surgery in the private sector which his colleague, the Secretary of State, might have used to improve services for the uninsurable long-term sick in the public sector.

Encouragement of the private sector?

The present Government is sympathetic to the private sector in health care. A former Minister, Dr Vaughan, forecast that by 1985 private insurance would cover 20 per cent of the population compared with the present figure of 6 per cent (1). It has also been estimated (2) that ultimately the private sector would contribute as much as £1000 million. This would imply an eight-fold expansion above the estimated private expenditure of £130m in 1980 (equivalent to about 1 per cent of NHS expenditure). Apart from the minor tax concession in 1981 the Government has taken no direct action to stimulate a major expansion of voluntary health insurance. It has taken the Provident Associations over thirty years to increase the beneficiaries covered by voluntary health insurance to 6 per cent of the population. In 1964 the Royal Commission on Health Services in Canada (3) noted that after thirty-five years of voluntary effort less than a third of the Canadian people were adequately covered, and went on to recommend the creation of a universal, comprehensive, tax-supported system under public agency control in each province.

No doubt the progress of voluntary health insurance has been slower in the UK because there has been a National Health Service adequate to the needs of most people—especially those seeking general acute services. Shall we be able to say that in thirty years' time?

The reduced rate of growth for the NHS in 1982 catches the new District Health Authorities mid-way through a ten-year planning cycle over which NHS Treasurers had been told they could assume annual growth rates of 1·5 per cent. Many authorities face the prospect of new district general hospitals coming on stream with insufficient revenue to run them fully. Again the indications are that potential patients will be put under increased pressure to seek private treatment and opt for voluntary health insurance.

Health care financing as a whole

The present Government's policy towards health care financing is not at all clear in any detail. Certainly there is a favourable attitude to the private sector but whether private insurance is seen as an additive or a serious alternative to the NHS is uncertain. The Government has also expressed interest in occupationally-based insurance systems of the kind prevailing in France, Luxembourg, Belgium, the Netherlands, and West Germany. It should not perhaps be overlooked that the Chancellor of the Exchequer, Sir Geoffrey Howe, was a member of a committee set up under the auspices of the British Medical Association to study health service financing and which in 1970 advocated a radical change (4). The scheme proposed envisaged a public sector funded by general taxation for the chronic sick, mentally ill and handicapped, and a two-tier insurance system for the general acute sector; compulsory insurance with per capita premiums related to national average earnings would confer entitlement to services described as 'adequate' while voluntary insurance at higher premiums would confer 'superior' services. Both compulsory and voluntary insurance premiums would be chargeable against income tax and voluntary insurance would confer exemption from payment of the compulsory premium.

Attention on this and other alternatives to financing the NHS out of general taxation has been sharpened not as yet by specific government action but by uncertainty about future policy and the lower plateau of NHS funding. In any case, whether the private sector is seen as a complement to the NHS or a competitor, an additive or an alternative, the private sector exists and its relationship to the NHS needs to be considered carefully. It was apparent long before the present Government took office that expenditure on the NHS could not continue to grow at the rates permitted between 1965 and 1975, in excess of the rate of growth of the economy generally. Reliance on general taxation in NHS financing was bound to be questioned, particularly by a government elected on promises of tax reduction and a much-reduced role for the State in everyday life. Nobody can seriously object to change. The important thing is that the implications of change are well understood and that the goals pursued are not illusory.

No dismantling of the Welfare State

So far, and despite allegations to the contrary, the present Government has done nothing to 'dismantle' the Welfare State. Retirement pensions are increased annually according to increases in the cost of living, rather than in line with increases in the cost of living or average earnings, whichever was the higher but they are still inflation-proofed. The Government has however withdrawn supplementary benefit from some young people, allowed child benefit to fall below its 1979 value, cut by 5 per cent the rise in unemployment benefit and denied the full rate of long-term supplementary benefit to the long-term unemployed—all matters of considerable concern to the Social Security Advisory Committee (5). Meanwhile, between 1978–9 and 1981–2, the combined social security and tax burden on those earning the average wage rose by 20 per cent: for those earning five times the average wage it fell by 5 per cent (6).

'FREEDOM, CHOICE, SOCIALIZED MEDICINE'

Attitudes to the Welfare State and the NHS

A survey of attitudes to and the use of social services conducted in the 1950s for Political and Economic Planning (7) found other aspects of the Welfare State overshadowed by the National Health service. Indeed in the eyes of most of the people interviewed the NHS had become synonymous with the Welfare State itself. Even so it is difficult to understand why the NHS should have attracted the consistent attention it has from those who either support or oppose 'the deliberate use of political power by the State to modify the play of market forces over an agreed range of activities' to use Asa Briggs' definition (8).

A health service free at the time of use was only one of the assumptions made by Beveridge, if social security in a free society were to be possible in post-war Britain; full employment, adequate housing at reasonable rents, and a system of family allowances were deemed no less important in eradicating poverty than a free NHS. Child poverty, housing, and unemployment have been the subject of discussion and legislation in this country, but one cannot recall anyone seriously advocating unemployment, demanding a housing shortage, urging unreasonable rents or proposing the abolition of child benefit (except as part of a general shift to negative income tax). Debates about these aspects of the Welfare State have usually been highly technical and concerned with greater efficiency of administration as well as giving greater help to those most in need. By contrast discussion about the NHS and its predominant Exchequer financing has largely been concerned with abolition of the service as we know it and its replacement by one based on voluntary insurance. The discussion is littered with abstract terms such as 'freedom', 'choice', 'consumer sovereignty', and 'the market', which seem to have little of substance for the practical man to grasp. Moreover some of the statements made are little short of bizarre. For example, John and Sylvia Jewkes, urging the reform of the NHS in 1980 (9) write:

> With a fresh and determined Government the greater part of the vast tangle of controlling legislation which, since 1945, has pushed us towards a servile state, might quickly be swept away ... these controls are progressively restricting personal freedom and eroding economic incentives ... Sudden and radical changes in the NHS is another matter. This, even under the most favourable circumstances, will be the hardest nut to crack ... reform will call for patience, step-by-step progress and the use of the thin end of the wedge.

A prime obstacle to reform, apparently, is 'the almost pathological obsession on the part of the British public, in the face of all fact and logic, with the indestructible virtues of a comprehensive and free NHS'. The authors go on to suggest that as a first step, voluntary health insurance premiums should be made deductible from taxable income. They conclude:

> And, since we all value most that which we pay for, it would help to sweep away, after 32 years, the most bizarre socialist dream that has ever bedevilled our people...that the State can provide all and every medical service and medicament...without discouraging economy, creating shortages, and debasing quality.

In the face of such sweeping condemnation one has to remind oneself that private practice and voluntary health insurance are not actually illegal in this country. Moreover the State does not provide 'all and every medical service and medicament'. There are many minor services (for example, pre-adoption medical examination) for which doctors are entitled to charge. Interestingly, in the field of personal medical services, the only agency under a statutory duty to do anything specific, is the Family Practitioner Committee, which must provide a patient with a general practitioner.

In less emotionally charged language D. S. Lees in 'Health Through Choice' (10) has suggested that there is essentially no difference between health services and other consumer services. Illness is as predictable as fire hazard and should be financed in the same way through insurance. Noting that Britain, in comparison with other advanced countries, devotes a smaller proportion of GNP to health services and the tendency as incomes rise for proportionately more to be allocated to health care he suggests that, had they been free to do so, the British people would have spent a higher proportion of GNP on health services than the Government had allocated to the NHS. Quoting Lionel Robbins that 'the market offers a daily referendum among consumers with provision for minority preferences', Lees suggests that if the object is to maximise consumer satisfaction, then the NHS should be replaced by a system based on voluntary insurance.

Some common catchwords and a few facts

Common to all the liberal economists' writings on the NHS is an emphasis on 'freedom', 'choice' and 'the market'. In practice, what do these things mean? The reality is that patients are free to register with general practitioners or not as they see fit. General practitioners similarly are free to enter into contracts with FPCs for restricted or unrestricted general practice. The FPC must provide the patients with a GP, but individual GPs can refuse to accept individuals on their lists and patients are free to change their doctor. Direct access to consultant services is not permitted; but this is a function of a strong code of medical ethics and the referral system which precedes the NHS by at least half a century and which applies to private practice as strictly as to NHS practice (11).

Despite the freedom of choice available to both patient and doctor, private general practice is virtually extinct in Britain. Only 5 per cent of family doctors have 100 or more private patients each, a third have none at all, and the rest rarely more than 20 (12). Three factors make any expansion most unlikely. *First* the private patient must face the full cost of drugs. *Secondly* the patient who pays directly or through insurance may demand more than the patient who pays through taxation. This can threaten the doctor's professional authority, requiring him for example to make unnecessary home visits and order his work schedule to suit the patient rather than himself. *Thirdly* as Mencher (13) has pointed out, without control over hospital beds the GP finds it difficult to offer the private patient anything markedly different from the service he offers the NHS patient.

The abortive attempt by Independent Medical Services to broaden the scope of private general practice is highly significant. IMS was planned by the Private Practice Committee of the BMA in 1965 to organize voluntary insurance for private general practice. Only 1 per cent of GPs joined and the scheme was wound up in 1969. If the 'market' consists of potential purchasers and potential vendors, then both have made it plain that they prefer the NHS system of organizing the financing of general practice. Much of the academic debate surrounding the appropriateness of the market as a mechanism for organizing health services finances has not been especially relevant because advocates of a radical departure from finance by general taxation have dwelt too much on international comparisons of the percentage of GNP allocated to health services. Inadequate attention has been paid to differential relative prices, input mixes, and other complicating factors which make simplistic comparisons dangerous, while outputs—however they might be defined —have been virtually ignored. Moreover the percentage of GNP spent on health services says nothing about how the services generated by that expenditure are concentrated or dispersed in different income or social class groups. The social distribution of health services in differing financial systems cannot be ignored particularly bearing in mind that the heaviest users of health services are likely to be the most vulnerable economically.

The realities of insurance and relevant comparisons

Insurance by definition is exclusive. To attract voluntary enrolment by the good risks, premiums must be kept low. Premiums can be kept low either by depressing the price demanded by suppliers (doctors' fees and hospital charges) or more probably by excluding bad risks such as the elderly or again by excluding services such as those for mental illness. Even non-profit insurance has to pursue the potentially conflicting goals of providing generous benefits, maintaining low premiums, and having minimal administrative costs. The dilemma was experienced by the friendly societies, which catered for the élite of the working class before Lloyd George's Health Insurance Act of 1911, just as it is experienced by the Provident Associations today. The dilemma is likely to be no less difficult in future. In *Better Medicine by Better Insurance* (14) Hugh Elwell, a former senior staff member of BUPA, now an adviser to PPP and one of the two advisers to the Government's working party on health insurance, offers the prospect of a much expanded health insurance market with profit-making companies entering the field.

> Virile competition will stimulate existing funds into rethinking the range of their product. As competition increases, insurance will be geared to the demands of different sectors of the market. To the traditional system of indemnity insurance will be added co-insurance

—where the insured person pays a given proportion of the cost of the service received, and a deductible system—where the insured pays a given initial sum before the insurance cover takes over.

The techniques are designed to protect the insurer's funds rather than protect the consumer against the costs of treatment needed during illness. The distribution of the various options by age and income group is a matter for conjecture, but it would be surprising if the most favourable financial options were concentrated in those most likely to need health services, the poor and the elderly.

As a funding mechanism the NHS accepts all risks and, although nobody is compelled to use the service, compels everyone to pay for the service through general taxation. The administrative cost of raising the money is very low compared with the administrative costs of the cash flow through insurance systems—a proportion of the cost of running the Inland Revenue—but the NHS cannot limit its liability except through devices such as waiting lists and other overt forms of rationing.

In a sense there are *deductibles* in the NHS. Certain classes of National Insurance beneficiary lose part of their benefit when in hospital beyond certain periods. Charges for prescriptions, dental treatment, spectacles, and so on are also 'deductibles' in the sense that they reduce the cost to the Exchequer. The administrative cost of levying these charges is minimal to the Exchequer—in practice the onus is put on dentists and chemists to collect the money which FPCs deduct from the payments made to the dentists and chemists. There is little doubt that if general practitioners and hospital doctors were paid on an item-of-service basis, then there would have been charges for hospital outpatient and GP surgery visits long before now, on the cold evidence the NHS is less 'free' and far more pragmatic than the liberal economists are apt to appreciate.

Professor Culyer has examined in his essay the realities of the 'health market' generally but the term 'health insurance market' when used in contradistinction to the NHS is misleading in at least two important respects. *Firstly*, health insurance in this country means hospital insurance for acute care. Options including GP services have been offered but low take-up led to their withdrawal. Of those covered by voluntary health insurance 96 per cent are registered with NHS GPs (15). The insurers recommend that a fee be paid to the GP as referral agent but they do not cover it. Voluntary health insurance is not therefore comprehensive. *Secondly*, the patient carrying voluntary health insurance is still entitled to admission and treatment in a NHS hospital as a NHS patient. In such cases it is not unknown for the insurer to make an *ex gratia* payment. Indeed it is difficult to discover the extent of this practice, but among other options more recently offered by the Provident Associations is one which offers cash payments on admission to a NHS hospital. It cannot therefore be claimed that expenditure by the insurers on hospital services wholly represents expenditure on behalf of private patients.

COMPULSORY AND VOLUNTARY INSURANCE

A (1970) suggestion for the UK

In 1970 a committee associated with the Private Practice Committee of the British Medical Association and chaired by Dr Ivor Jones advocated a radical adaptation of the present system of financing health services in this country (16). As noted earlier the committee included in its membership the present Chancellor of the Exchequer. The committee took the aim of achieving a substantial increase in the level of expenditure on health services and accepted that taxation had reached saturation point. They also accepted that the future of growth of the British economy would not be sufficient to permit the desired increase in resources for the NHS. Their conclusion was that money would have to be diverted from consumers' expenditure. The problem of the social distribution of services was faced by accepting existing inequalities and indeed codifying them. The committee recommended that a public sector, financed by general taxation, should be responsible for hospital capital costs, drugs, the most expensive procedures, and services for the chronic sick, the mentally ill, and the mentally handicapped. All other services would be financed by a two-tier insurance system. A compulsory system would provide adequate services with per capita premiums related to the average wage. 'Adequacy' was not defined. It would be possible to opt out of the compulsory system by taking out more expensive 'voluntary' insurance offering better services (these too were never defined). All insurance premiums would be deductible from taxable income.

The committee assumed that people would start opting for voluntary insurance at about national average earnings; but of course the per capita basis of the scheme would question the validity of this assumption. Obviously the decision would be affected by the size of family and number of dependents as much as, if not more than, the earning level of those employed.

Whatever might be said about the social divisiveness of this proposal the financial implications were somewhat unspectacular. Using the committee's own figures the scheme—once the costs of tax exemption were taken into account—would have added a mere £159m to health services expenditure in 1968/69. (In that year the NHS cost almost £1·500m).

Were a system of the kind advocated by the Jones Committee enacted, the liberal economists' demand for 'freedom' would hardly be satisfied. Nor would the decision on how much to spend on health services be determined by 'consumers in the market'. In fact health service finance would enjoy the status presently accorded to social security—ear-marked taxation—as in the insurance-based health service systems operating in France, Belgium, Luxembourg, and Federal Republic of Germany (17).

The European model and the current scene

At first sight some features of the European systems must appear attractive to those seeking a major reduction in Exchequer funding and a reduced role for central government in the planning and control of health services: pluralist systems, with compulsory membership of hundreds of sickness insurance funds which collect income-related premiums from employer and employee as well as from individuals such as the self-employed, and negotiate contracts with public and private hospitals and with doctors. Appearances can be deceptive. The reality is that while most of the discussion about the NHS focusses on 'under-spending' the major problem in the European systems is the acute concern with 'over-spending'. In Britain, central control over resource allocation backed by the enforcement of strict cash limits allows political decisions to be made so that public expenditure on the NHS can be related to the state of the economy and related also to other perceived needs such as the encouragement of industrial investment or the creation of work-experience schemes for unemployed youth. In Europe, governments of countries with insurance-based health service systems are not yet in a position to control costs. They have, however, found themselves subsidizing health insurance and paying directly for health service costs to an increasing extent and have used an extending range of administrative devices to establish a greater degree of public control over systems which are rapidly losing some of their 'voluntary' attributes, while retaining the outward characteristics of an insurance system.

Coverage in foreign systems

Although the European systems differ in detail there are certain common features. As in Britain, virtually 100 per cent of the population are protected against the costs of sickness. There are two exceptions. In West Germany, students and the top 10 per cent of self-employed income earners are excluded from membership of the State scheme and must rely on private insurance or pay direct. In the Netherlands 50 per cent of the population are compulsorily and 20 per cent voluntarily enrolled in one scheme, but all Dutch residents must subscribe to a separate 'catastrophic risks' scheme which pays for residence in nursing homes and hospital costs beyond the first year's stay. In the Netherlands too, employees earning more than a wage-ceiling are excluded from the other State-subsidized scheme.

Typically the medical services, permitted drugs, prostheses, and so on are specified; but in practice there are few exclusions and the range of services provided under the insurance systems is much the same as that available under the NHS. Ensuring that the services are paid for under insurance is, however, more complicated. Entitlement to benefit must be established. In *France,* for example, the employed patient must have worked 200 hours in the three months preceding the date of treatment. In *Belgium* there are three conditions: six months membership of the scheme with 120 days of actual work, proof of payment of minimum contributions, and proof that the illness is covered by the insurance. Usually the insurer's permission must be sought before treatment is given or the patient is admitted to hospital. In cases of emergency admission the insurer must be notified within so many days or the patient will have to pay the costs himself.

Claims for reimbursement or partial reimbursement of payments, arguments with insurers over eligibility and entitlement, disputes with doctors about the cost of every item of service, all these are reflected in the high administrative costs which are characteristic of the European systems. The important issue is not the percentage of the population entitled to benefit but the way in which those entitled obtain their rights.

Some common characteristics of foreign systems

In principle the method of financing is common, although there are many variations in detail. *Essentially* the Europeans pay a percentage of gross wages or salary *before* tax. For *employed people* the premium is shared in varying proportions between employer and employee. In West Germany the premium is shared equally between the two parties, but in France the burden falls much more heavily on the employer and increases in the premium are reflected much more sharply on industrial labour costs. For *retired people* the premium is often on a flat-rate basis, with government subsidy, and is usually related to the value of state retirement pensions. Premiums for the *unemployed* are paid by public authorities. Rising unemployment in Europe has increased

dramatically the involvement of public funds in health insurance—one of several factors which have sharpened interest in
closer public control of health insurance costs. Generally the
premium covers the contributor and his immediate dependents, although there are exceptions in some countries where
the self-employed have to pay a premium for each dependent. For employed people the premium covers cash benefits
during absence from work through sickness, as well as hospital and medical services.

Apart from small charges for drugs and appliances health
services are generally free at the time of use, *apart from France
and Belgium*. In these countries the insurance will cover the
full cost of major surgery in hospital, but co-insurance applies to all other services and the patient will be reimbursed
at 80 per cent of the cost. In practice he may have to pay
more than 20 per cent because the reimbursement rate is
calculated on the officially approved fee schedule and the
doctor may charge at higher rates. The deterrent effect of co-
insurance is dubious since in France, for example, over half
the population insure against the 20 per cent direct charge.

The premiums are paid to sickness funds of which there
are many hundreds in most countries. In practice the funds
operate through smaller numbers of national organizations.
Within a legal framework the funds negotiate charges and
fees with hospitals and doctors. Increases in charges and fee
schedules have to be sanctioned by the relevant Minister. In
effect the funds have the power to levy taxation, since a
system which most people must join by law, financed
by levying a percentage of gross wages and salaries before
tax, is essentially being funded by general but ear-marked
taxation.

Given this funding mechanism the amount of money
available for health insurance has risen as incomes have risen
with inflation. Unfortunately the costs of health insurance
have risen faster than incomes because the costs of health
services, particularly hospital costs, have accelerated much
faster than national income. The actual percentage of wages
and salaries levied for health insurance has had to be increased from time to time, adding to industry's costs, and
leading trade unions to press for wage increases. Increasingly

governments have found themselves paying a greater proportion of costs. A striking feature of the European insurance-
based systems within the last decade is the similarity of
devices used in an attempt to control costs. Employers have
been required to give paid sick leave outside the insurance
system. The *per diem* charges in hospital used to include
depreciation and capital development but in every country
now these have been taken out of insurance and are paid for
directly by public authorities. And with increasing government financial involvement, has grown increased control.
Every Western European country now has a regional plan for
hospitals and all hospitals, public and private, must conform
to it. If a hospital wishes to develop or extend a service then
permission must be sought; and if new equipment is involved
then an authorizing certificate must be obtained from the
regional office of the relevant Ministry.

Control by incentives

It is apparent that in the insurance-based systems the incentives lie in the wrong direction. Paying hospitals on a *per
diem/* per patient basis encourages admission and keeping the
hospital beds occupied. Paying doctors by item of service
(not all but most European doctors are) encourages surgical
and other procedures and stimulates the general volume of
services and costs. Certainly there is no encouragement to
economize. Health service systems tend to adapt very slowly,
but it will be surprising if there is not a further extension of
regulation by public authorities in the European systems.
Indeed, having developed regional plans to control hospitals
there is interest already in developing control over the services outside hospital which affect the demand for and use of
hospitals. The Europeans appear to be moving along the
route taken by Britain between 1948 and 1974: moving from
hospital planning to comprehensive planning. The fact that
the system adopted in 1974 failed to achieve the desired
result does not make the pursuit of that goal irrational.

A cliché with a universal application

If *'socialized medicine'* means the collective protection of families and individuals against the costs of illness, requiring people to pay while they are well and working, for services they will want when they are ill and not able to work, with the State or State-regulated agencies acting as the fund holder, *then the European systems are just as 'socialist' as the NHS.* If the term 'socialized medicine' is intended to imply strict government control over total spending on health services then there is no such system anywhere in the world. There is some private practice even in the USSR and patients dissatisfied with their treatment at one polyclinic can go to another and pay extra. If it means government control over *public* spending on health services then this so far applies to the UK and not to the other European systems. No government anxious to tackle inflation can afford to ignore the biggest employer of labour in the country, particularly bearing in mind that the health care industry consumes wealth and does not create it. It is as important to control expenditure on health services as expenditure on local government services.

On the other hand if 'socialized medicine' is intended to suggest a system in which doctors are not free to exercise independent judgement in treating their patients then it patently misrepresents the facts. Only in West Germany is there indirect pressure on doctors to limit the volume of service they give to patients collectively, but the system is operated by the doctors themselves. There the sick funds pay on a capitation basis to the Association of Sick Funds Physicians. The Association pays doctors on an item-of-service basis and those who greatly exceed their peers in the cost or volume of service provided are at risk to be fined.

Under the NHS GP's can have remuneration witheld for over-prescribing but this is rare and can hardly be held to constitute an infringement of clinical freedom. There is nothing comparable in the hospital service. Interest in medical audit has arisen from within the medical profession in Britain (18) but it reflects a concern over *quality* rather than cost. There has been no development in Britain of the utilization review system, tissue committees, and professional activity studies developed in the USA, where the insurance funders have been much harder taskmasters on doctors than the DHSS or health authorities have been, or the provident movement might well be.

Pragmatism and health insurance policy

It was pragmatism, not ideology, which led to the abandonment of pluralism in Britain in 1948. And the insurance principle in health care was rejected in 1946 because its inefficiency had brought it into disrepute. By 1945 half the population (twenty four million people) were compulsorily insured under the National (Health) Insurance Act of 1911. Unlike the compulsory insurance systems operating in Europe today the British system was neither universal nor comprehensive. The retired, the middle-class, and the wives and dependent children of the insured were excluded from benefit. The benefits were in practice restricted for most of the insured to cash payments during sickness, absence from work, GP treatment and drugs. The system was funded by flat-rate contributions from employer, employee, and government to funds operated by commercial insurance concerns, trade unions, and friendly societies registered as Approved Societies under the Act. Quinquennially, if monies were left over after the payment of sickness absence benefits, then these could be used to pay for additional benefits such as payments towards the cost of stay in hospital, convalescent home, and so on. The approved societies, however, tended to be specialized occupationally and geographically and, given differential morbidity experience among their membership, had differential expenditures. The extra benefits therefore were available least to those who required them most. Not that the extra benefits were significantly available at all. In 1939 for example, when the system covered 17 million workers, only 1·6 million could have had their hospital costs paid under compulsory insurance. At that time the British system had the highest administrative costs and offered the poorest benefits of any compulsory insurance system in Europe.

The position of hospitals

Voluntary hospitals derived little from the system and given their charitable tradition ran into deficit and (except for those associated with medical schools) failed to match their facilities to the growing development of medical technology. In 1938, outside London, only 12 voluntary hospitals had pathology laboratories, and these were the hospitals associated with the 12 provincial medical schools. For the most part the municipal hospitals were specialized in infectious disease, mental illness, maternity, and chronic sickness, with few providing for the general acute section. But for the threat of the Second World War, and the creation of the Emergency Medical Service, the duplication, overlap and waste involved in a system of 3000 autonomous independent hospitals might have continued. As it happened, the NHS Act 1946 provided for most of the measures advocated by the Dawson Committee in 1920 (19), regional authorities to plan and co-ordinate hospitals, district general hospitals, and health centres. The reality of the NHS was determined by the medical profession, not by Beveridge.

THE NHS AND THE PRIVATE SECTOR

A peaceful coexistence

The pragmatism which led to public ownership of hospitals in Britain was reflected in the attitude to private practice. The relationship has not been studied very much and is therefore not well understood. From 1948 to 1975 the official attitude to private practice within NHS hospitals was that it was neither to be discouraged nor encouraged. The provision of private pay-beds within NHS hospitals was in part a concession to the consultant specialists who wanted part-time contracts with the NHS. But it was also justified on the grounds that if the best specialists did not join, then the public hospital service might develop as a second-rate rather than a first-rate service.

Ironically the voluntary hospital insurance system underwent the same process of rationalization and concentration as the hospitals. The market for private surgery needed to be efficiently organized and those who had assisted in delineating the hospital regions were instrumental in reorganizing voluntary insurance. The British United Provident Association for example was created in 1947 by the amalgamation of a large number of small Provident Associations. The Western Provident Association and Private Patients Plan were formed in 1950. The trades unions and friendly societies had the opportunity to participate but did not. Some of them, as contributory associations, offered their members cash payments towards the cost of private consultation and the incidental expenses of admission to hospital, such as pyjamas, toothbrush, etc.

Until 1966 the fee a surgeon might charge a private patient was restricted (50 guineas or 75 guineas in cases of exceptional difficulty) and covered pre- and post-operative work as well as the actual surgical procedure. The Provident Associations were therefore somewhat protected. This ceiling was removed by the then Minister, Mr Kenneth Robinson. By agreement with the medical profession the same Minister reduced the private bed *capacity* with the NHS from 5 per cent of the total beds to 1 per cent (occupancy was low and there was some agreed relocation to where demand was higher). During the same Minister's administration the seeds of the dispute which erupted in 1975 were sown.

The harvest of a doubtful policy

In 1965 the Minister sought to give priority, when new appointments were being made to consultant posts, to those prepared to work on a whole-time basis. In the event there was a compromise. Successful applicants would not be required to specify the nature of their contract until they had been offered the post. In return the Joint Consultants' Committee agreed that consultants working maximum part-time (9/11) could be required to work an additional unpaid session. This arrangement eventually bore most heavily on the provincial consultant working maximum part-time. Growing resentment was fuelled by the implementation of a new contract for GPs after 1966 and the impact of incomes policy. Between 1965 and 1975 the real net-of-tax earnings of consultants fell by 14 per cent while those for the average manual worker went up by 13 per cent (20).

The proposal therefore in 1975 to remove private pay-beds from NHS hospitals could not have come at a worse time. There was little to be said for the proposal in principle and even less in practice. Removing 1 per cent of the beds from private practice would hardly reduce waiting-periods significantly for those on NHS waiting lists. With no private bed capacity outside the NHS in many parts of the country many of the consultants working maximum part-time were faced with the prospect of having to accept full-time NHS contracts with the loss of the tax advantages available when employed part-time.

In the event, as a result of the Health Service Acts of 1976 and 1977, and the amending Act of 1980, the position of private practice within the NHS is not all that different. In general, when a change in the number of private pay-beds in an NHS hospital is being sought, authorization by the Secretary of State will be refused if the change will either to a significant extent interfere with services to NHS patients or to a significant extent operate to the disadvantage of NHS patients.

The question of the consultants' contract has also been resolved, with *maximum part-time becoming 10/11* and even full-timers being able to undertake private work. The *whole-time consultant* can privately earn up to 10 per cent of his NHS earnings over a three-year period (one effect has been to increase the number of domiciliary consultations within the NHS).

But the events of 1974, and the pay-beds dispute, have created a new situation in that the voluntary insurance organizations were stimulated into expanding private bed capacity outside the NHS. Moreover the entry into the field of profit-making health insurance concerns and profit-seeking hospitals has major implications for the private sector itself as well as for the NHS.

Some emerging issues

The major issues for consideration are interrelated. The size of population covered by voluntary health insurance will depend in part on the extent to which the government *discriminates against the general acute sector in the NHS* as well as the extent to which voluntary insurance is subsidized through the tax system (including the granting of charitable status to non-profit Provident Associations). It will also depend *on the costs of voluntary health insurance* and the way these are affected by the *movement of costs in the private hospitals.* The scale private hospital capacity reaches before 'significantly interfering with the operation of the NHS' will be determined largely by the scale of voluntary insurance and the costs of private treatment and the way the regulatory powers of the Secretary of State are exercised. The location of the private capacity, that is, whether it is mainly located inside the NHS or outside the NHS may well be affected by the capacity of NHS hospitals to compete successfully for private patients.

It was noted earlier that it took from 1947 to 1980 for voluntary health insurance to attract about 1·5 million subscribers and cover about 5 million people, 96 per cent of whom are registered with NHS GPs. They may opt out of the NHS hospital service *but the NHS cannot opt out of treating them* should they so choose. *Moreover they can use the NHS hospitals* as NHS patients, and *derive cash payments* from the insurance carrier. Much has been made recently of the sharp increase in those covered by voluntary insurance (rather less is made of the *lapse* rates which also fluctuate). In particular much emphasis has been put on the fact that over half the new subscribers are in group or occupational schemes. A great deal of publicity was given to a scheme negotiated with employers by a section of the ETU under which the employer was to pay voluntary insurance premiums as a fringe benefit. In fact the workers had the choice either of having a generous cash payment or admission to hospital as a private patient. If the main interest were to avoid admission to NHS hospitals, why was the cash option included in the scheme? Schemes of this kind clearly cannot be interpreted as evidence that manual workers are increasingly interested in opting out of the NHS.

The *tax concession in the budget of 1981* to those earning less than £8500 per annum may well have stimulated a further expansion of occupational schemes but how these schemes are used will be affected by any out-of-pocket payment the insured has to make. Although the Provident Associations cover the full amount of NHS and private hospital charges (the limit is in reality set by the costs of private accommodation in NHS teaching hospitals) they cannot guarantee to pay the full amount of the surgeons' fees. In practice they suggest appropriate schedules of fees but there is no mechanism to prevent the surgeon from charging outside the scale and the patient has to pay the difference. Experience therefore may make private insurance less attractive because of the 'cost-sharing' concept.

Tax subsidies

Tax subsidies to voluntary health insurance put the government in an invidious position. The private sector is largely catering for elective repair surgery in non-urgent cases. Any government which, as a matter of public policy, discriminates in favour of the 'care' sector and at the same time foregoes tax revenue to encourage private non-urgent repair surgery is inviting ridicule from the public and inducing cynicism among those within the NHS who have to implement the government's guidelines on policy. A policy favouring the chronic sick, mentally ill, and handicapped, at a time of general restraint on growth, must mean longer waiting for non-urgent surgery. Those who escape the inconvenience of waiting should do so at their own expense and not at the expense of those who lack the means. With tax subsidy, those who use the private sector are not reducing the waiting period for those who depend on the NHS; they are benefiting at the expense of the chronic sick, and the mentally ill, and handicapped.

The desirability of a stable private sector

Even without tax subsidy the government probably has a vested interest in a stable rather than an expanding private sector, especially if that expansion is financed by industry. Fiscal aid to industry and employment takes many forms and in 1980 such grants by public authorities amounted to 4·2 per cent of GNP. Industry through the CBI and other bodies, is not hesitant in pressing for financial assistance and if industrial costs rise because some firms offer their employees private health insurance it is difficult for a government to be selective and refuse aid to firms who have added to their costs. As Rudolph Klein points out elsewhere in this collection of essays, the effect of putting short-term sickness costs on to industry was probably nullified by other concessions to industry. As it is, the ability of employers to charge the costs of health insurance as a labour cost against Corporation Tax is of the same dubious inconsistency as the income tax concession of 1981.

The cost of voluntary health insurance therefore depends to a considerable extent on central government action. The costs are not likely to be reduced by *competition*. There is a firm expectation now that public authorities will protect the consumer in the private sector if not always the public sector and experience in the fields of motor insurance, package holidays, and estate agencies has led to public control either directly or indirectly through voluntary guarantees that bankruptcies will not seriously jeopardize the consumer. Competition in the field of voluntary health insurance cannot be left unrestricted and predictably there will be Department of Trade requirements for minimum levels of funds. Price competition is therefore likely to be restricted.

Competition, consumer choice, and risk

As it is, the recent *price competition* between the existing Provident Associations (21) has been tempered by economic reality. For example, BUPA and PPP were competing for the allegiance of university teachers and in 1981 PPP offered group plans at 50 per cent of the normal premium. It was understood that the premium would be reviewed in the light of the group's utilization. The scheme began in October 1981 but by December 1981 members of the group were informed that the premium would rise by 50 per cent from April 1982, that there had been insufficient time to assess utilization on a group basis and that the increase was based on utilization by individual subscribers. It would be interesting to know the lapse for this group scheme.

The advertised benefits of voluntary health insurance are *choice of consultant, privacy, and no waiting* (or, more strictly, admission at a time of convenience). One presumes that the first of these advantages has to be qualified according to the advice of the referring GP. The third implies excess capacity, which has a cost. At present the private hospitals are occupied below capacity level but will this situation persist as demand rises? Potentially also the private hospitals are *at risk to cost increases* in excess of increases within the NHS. Clearly it is in the consultants' interest to see the development of one-day surgery but those who have paid voluntary insurance may in fact insist on a few days' rest in relative comfort.

More important is the question of full-time medical cover. The present arrangements seem to vary and thus do the *risks*. In some private hospitals the consultant will come to attend to his private patients in an emergency. In others an emergency service is being created and doctors will be available to attend when required. They may well take on this task on a temporary basis, possibly while in transition from one NHS hospital to another. The cover is certainly less than that provided by the NHS, with the arrangements for on duty and on call work by junior hospital doctors. The inadequacy of medical cover in the private hospitals was one of the limiting factors on the proposal of the former Secretary of State (Mr Patrick Jenkin) that health authorities might reduce NHS waiting lists by making contractual arrangements with private hospitals for the admission of NHS patients. From the private hospitals' point of view, who would be sued if something went wrong? Clearly the health authority would not allocate its own junior medical staff to the private hospitals.

Unless they are prepared to see their costs (and the costs of health insurance) rise, the private hospitals will continue to be at *risk*. And at risk they are. Decisions at common law in the USA and Britain tend to follow the same principles (22).

In 1965 the Supreme Court of Illinois upheld the award of punitive damages against a voluntary hospital, despite the absence of a contract with the plaintiff (23). The case of Darling v the Charleston Community Memorial Hospital concerned an eighteen-year old college student who broke his leg playing football. During the night he complained to nursing staff at the hospital but no immediate action was taken and by the time his doctor was called in, the leg had become gangrenous and subsequently had to be amputated below the knee. The boy's father sued for damages and doctors involved in the case settled out of court. Liability was imposed on the hospital on the grounds of independent negligence. It was held:

> that the hospital had a duty of care in connection with supervising and reviewing the attending physician's treatment of the patient; that the standard of care could properly be evaluated in the light of . . . the standard of custom of other hospitals in the community and that the hospital was guilty of negligence in connection with the failure of its nurses properly to observe and report the condition of the plantiff.

In the case of Garfield Memorial Hospital v Marshall in 1953 (24) a voluntary hospital was adjudged guilty of contributory negligence in failing to provide medical attention. A woman in the seventh month of pregnancy was not believed by a resident doctor when she said she was in labour. When she gave birth—without the attendance of an obstetrician—the two resident doctors were dealing with another patient having triplets. The hospital was judged negligent in failing to call the patient's private physician, or an associated obstetrician, who was available.

Contributory negligence on the part of a voluntary hospital was also adjudged in Mundt v Alta Bates Hospital in 1963 (25). Here injury resulted when fluid being infused into a patient's vein was allowed to infiltrate the surrounding tissue and the leg swelled to twice its normal size. Nurses and the attending physician communicated by telephone and subsequently both doctor and the hospital were adjudged negligent for failing to observe and examine the patient's condition.

These cases illustrate the danger of relying on anything less than twenty-four hour medical cover of an acceptable standard, given that the patient's private consultant in the nature of things will not always be available in an emergency.

The private hospital in Britain will be at greater risk as the scale of provision grows.

The advantage of Section 5 beds

The better medical cover within the NHS makes NHS private pay-beds more attractive to consultants than private hospitals. In Central Manchester, for example, which has a NHS Private Patients Home and two private hospitals (one profit-seeking) the consultants have indicated that if the PPH is improved to match the best NHS standards (the luxurious standards of the private hospitals being beyond reach) then they will encourage their private patients to be admitted there. Following discussions with all staff interests, the District Health Authority has resolved, over the next two years, *to invest £120,000 in upgrading the private pay facility*. At current prices the annual return to the authority is £40,000 in income from private patients which the authority can of course, use as part of its general funds and possibly apply to the community and other services so much in the forefront of government policy. The example demonstrates that if they wish to, health authorities can compete with the private hospitals to the advantage of the NHS in general.

Potential problems of private sector

Consultant preferences are not the only factor to be considered but equally they cannot be ignored. The private hospitals in a real sense use the NHS to determine which doctors can admit patients to them. The rule seems to be that any doctor who is or has been an NHS consultant can have access. At the present low occupancy there is no pressure on consultants to discharge their patients other than the awareness of mounting insurance costs. But if the desired occupancy rate is achieved what are the prospects for the development of practices common in the USA with pressure to reduce length of stay? Developments of this kind may well reinforce the consultants' preference for NHS private pay-beds.

All private hospitals are profit-seeking. Even those run by BUPA must achieve an operating surplus. There is, however, a difference between those run by non-profit bodies and those run by commercial organizations. The accommodation charges advertised to the private patient are the same as for private accommodation in the NHS. There can, however, be other charges. One non-profit hospital charges at the rate of £45 for an operating theatre session of an hour and a half. In the same town another (profit) hospital charges at the rate of £240 per hour and a half.

The impact of differential costs has sharpened, too, the rivalry between the non-profit and commercial insurance organizations. Group plans whose members have used the commercial hospitals have had their premiums increased—in at least one case the employer has advised staff not to use certain hospitals or risk withdrawal of coverage by the group scheme. Clearly competition does not always widen consumer choice.

Competitiveness between the providers of private hospitals can have unfortunate consequences in the location of hospitals, despite provision for public control established in 1977. In Manchester, for example, a 'gentleman's agreement' between BUPA and American Medical International (Europe) that only one of them would attempt to develop a private hospital in the area was not honoured and there are now two private hospitals in addition to NHS private pay-bed capacity. Consultants using all three types of hospital are understandably interested in encouraging the development of emergency cover at the two private hospitals. The former Health Services Board approved the private developments.

Control and regulation by the Secretary of State

Since 1980 powers exercised by the former Health Services
Board have passed to the Secretary of State who has the
ability to control changes in NHS private bed capacity, but
only partial control over the private hospital capacity. The
1980 Act does in fact restrict the Secretary of State's powers
to revoke the authorization of private NHS beds. Authorization can only be revoked if he is satisfied that there are
available alternative facilities, *whether in the private sector or the
NHS,* sufficient to meet the reasonable demand for private
practice in the area served by the hospital in question. This is
a very important change and could well mean that the dice
are loaded against expansion of NHS private beds and in
favour of the expansion of private hospitals. For one thing,
existing private hospitals are included in the list of local
bodies which should be consulted by District Health Authorities when proposals for changes in NHS private provision
are being considered. But in the case of increases in private
hospital capacity the legislation does not apply to hospitals
with less than 120 beds. Moreover those with 120 or more
beds need not seek authorization for expansion if the increase
does not exceed twenty per cent over a three-year period.

There is a crucial qualification to all this, however. The
Secretary of State has discretionary power to designate districts and areas so that any private hospital development or
expansion requires authorization.

One can only hope that the power to regulate the scale of
the private sector, such as it is, will be used in the spirit of
pragmatism which characterized the public-private relationship from 1948 to 1975. It would be sad indeed if a Conservative administration emulated their Labour predecessors
and discriminated against private practice inside the NHS
and in favour of it outside the NHS. Both NHS and the
private sector are here to stay and the situation has an
inherent conflict. Social values cannot be ignored. We all
accept that access to health services should be determined by
need and not the ability to pay, but we all equally value the
freedom to spend our after-tax income on that which we
choose. A balance has to be struck. It is important that the

resources for private practice are efficiently organized. The surplus achieved even by the non-profit bodies who organize the private market is impressive and could even perhaps be looked at as a possible source of extra revenue for the NHS. Not that BUPA and the other Provident Associations should be taken into public ownership, but they might be required to contribute to the NHS which has in no small measure helped to sustain the fabric of a liberal democratic society which permits individual choices to be made.

It is surely in the interest of those who value private hospital care to ensure that antipathy to it is dissipated. To some extent the antipathy is based on the belief that private hospitals are subsidized by the NHS. The private hospitals rely on medical and nursing skills developed largely within the NHS but contribute nothing to the costs of medical and nursing education. Since ultimately the costs of training doctors and nurses fall largely on the Exchequer, it is relevant to note that organizations, such as BUPA, which enjoy the tax advantages of charitable status, are particularly well favoured. When considering the mechanism for imposing a levy on the private sector, however, it is essential to recognize that where staff are diverted from the NHS the impact is experienced locally and not nationally. Private hospitals tend to be located near teaching hospitals and to be concentrated in particular areas—Westminster, for example, has twenty private hospitals. Any levy on the private sector should therefore be allocated locally to the District Health Authority and might be related, for example, to the numbers of nurses employed in the private hospitals. Where subsidy in the other direction can be quantified and costed, then the value should be deducted from the annual levy. Unfortunately these reverse subsidies are often intangible. For example, the provision of a private hospital might conceivably make an area more attractive to prospective consultants and improve the number and calibre of applicants for vacant posts.

It might be argued that private hospitals help the NHS hospitals by reducing waiting lists for NHS beds and insurance organizations ought not therefore be required to compensate the NHS in any way. The central point is, however, that the NHS is a system which seeks to allocate services to patients according to individual assessments made by clinicians. In theory waiting times reflect those assessments and at best the NHS seeks to provide treatment at the time of relative need and not at a time of convenience. The waiting period in the acute sector will lengthen as the system overall determines that the chronic sick have a higher priority. Those who tacitly reject the decision to give greater priority to the long-term sick and insist on treatment in the acute sector at a time of greater convenience clearly must be free to make that choice, but they should surely be required to pay the full cost and accept that a levy on the insurance organizations might mean higher premiums.

An important asset

As Paul Torrens (26) pointed out, 'Health insurance is an immensely powerful vehicle—socially, economically, and organizationally. It can be an important asset in the future development of health services in Britain if properly directed and integrated into the total health care life of the country'. There is nothing new about voluntary health insurance. From early in the nineteenth century at least, ordinary working people in this and other European countries protected themselves collectively against the hazards of income loss during illness and in the process secured primary medical services. As we have seen, the NHS emerged as a mechanism for collectively organizing the funding of a comprehensive health service at minimal administrative cost. The provision for private treatment in hospital played a constructive role in the development of the public hospital service after 1948 and until 1975 the balance between public and private provision was not an issue of major concern.

Developments since the mid-1970s pose a new situation. The NHS hospitals can no longer anticipate financial resources to increase at the rates experienced before 1975, and the priorities policy will hardly leave the acute hospitals in a stable state. Voluntary health insurance has expanded its coverage but not yet at all spectacularly and forecasts of future expansion need to be modified. On the one hand there is the possibility that pressure on acute hospital provision will give added incentive to those who are able, either individually or through their employment, to insure against the costs of elective repair surgery, to do so. Pulling against this, however, is the probability that insurance costs will increase and employers particularly will seek compensation from public funds if their labour costs rise as they take on more of the burden of social provision. The central government can itself therefore to some extent determine the future of health insurance.

Central government policy itself was responsible for what may have been the most important new factor in the new public-private relationship—the emergence of private capacity outside the NHS hospitals. There are important issues of consumer protection here and given the surer medical cover in NHS hospitals, convenience for consultant staff, the ability of NHS private capacity to yield a profit at the local level for public services in general, a policy of discrimination in favour of NHS private-pay facilities would seem to be indicated when the Secretary of State—who has considerable regulatory powers—comes to consider changes in the level of private facilities in particular local circumstances.

The present government has made a minor tax concession to voluntary hospital insurance. As yet it has done nothing to suggest that its policy towards private practice differs substantially from that of its predecessor which, by discouraging private practice within the NHS, stimulated developments outside and thereby damaged (marginally) the NHS itself.

Interest in radical financial change has not been productive and does not constitute a policy. The reality is that both NHS and the private sector are here to stay and it is within the power of the Secretary of State to ensure that the NHS and private insurance are complementary. It is the private hospital which makes the two competitive.

REFERENCES

1. *Health and the Public Sector* (1981). (Adam Smith Institute).
2. *The Sunday Times*, 14 February 1982.
3. *Royal Commission on Health Services in Canada* (1964). (The Queen's Printer: Canada).
4. BRITISH MEDICAL ASSOCIATION (1970). *Health Services Financing*.
5. SOCIAL SECURITY ADVISORY COMMITTEE (1982). *First Report*. (HMSO).
6. *The Guardian*, 22 February 1982.
7. POLITICAL AND ECONOMIC PLANNING (1961). *Family Needs and the Social Services*. (George Allen and Unwin).
8. BRIGGS, A. (1977). 'The welfare state in historical perspective' in SHOTTLAND, C. (ed.) *The Welfare State*. (Harper & Row).
9. JEWKES, J. and S. (1980). 'A strategy for reform' in SELDON, A. (ed.) *The Litmus Papers*. (Centre for Policy Studies).
10. LEES, D. S. (1961). *Health Through Choice*. (Institute of Economic Affairs).
11. LEWIS, E. B. (1981). 'Private practice', *Brit. med J.*, **1**, 841.
12. CARTWRIGHT, A. (1967). *Patients and their Doctors*. (Routledge & Kegan Paul).
13. MENCHER, S. (1967). *Private Practice in Britain*. (G. Bell & Sons).
14. ELLWELL, H. (1980). 'Better Medicine by Better Insurance' in SELDON, A. (ed.), op. cit.
15. FORSYTH, G. (1967), 'Is the Health Service doing its Job?' *New Society*, **10**, 545.
16. BRITISH MEDICAL ASSOCIATION (1970). *Health Services Financing*.
17. LANGENDONCK, J. VAN (1973). *Prelude to Harmony on a Community Theme*. (Oxford University Press for the Nuffield Provincial Hospitals Trust).
18. DOLLERY, C. T. (1971). 'The quality of health care' in McLACHLAN, G. (ed.) *Challenges for Change*. (Oxford University Press for the Nuffield Provincial Hospitals Trust).
19. MINISTRY OF HEALTH (1920). *Interim Report of the Consultative Committee on Medical and Allied Services*. (HMSO).
20. NEWBOULD, C. D. (1977). 'Comparisons of medical and industrial salaries in UK, 1965–76', *Brit. med. J.*, **1**, 526.
21. *The Guardian*, 27 October 1981.
22. SOUTHWICK, A. F. JR. (1967). *The Doctor, The Hospital and The Patient in England*. (University of Michigan: Ann Arbor).
23. AMERICAN LAW REPORTS (1965). 'Darling v The Charleston Community Memorial Hospital', *14 American Law Reports*, **3rd**, 860.
24. ——(1953). 'Garfield Memorial Hospital v Marshall' (92 App. DC 234), *37 American Law Reports*, **2nd**, 1270.
25. ——(1963). 'Mundt v Alta Bates Hospital (223 Cal. App.)', *American Law Reports*, **2nd**, 413.
26. TORRENS, P. R. (1981). 'Some potential hazards of unplanned expansion of private health insurance in Britain', *Lancet*, **i**, 29.

Private practice and public policy
Regulating the frontiers

RUDOLF KLEIN

RUDOLF KLEIN

Rudolf Klein is Professor of Social Policy, and Director of the Centre for the Analysis of Social Policy at the School of Humanities and Social Sciences, University of Bath.

He was educated at Bristol Grammar School and Merton College, Oxford. For twenty years he was a journalist, latterly with the *Observer* where he was at various times Chief Leader Writer, Editor of the Leader pages, and Home Affairs Editor. In 1970 he entered the field of research with the Organization of Medical Care Unit, London School of Hygiene and Tropical Medicine. Until 1978, when he took up his present post, he was a Senior Fellow, Centre for Studies in Social Policy.

He has been a specialist adviser to the House of Commons, Social Services Committee, (1976–81) and a Member of the Social Science Research Council, Sociology and Social Administration Committee, (1978–80).

He is at present a member of Bath Health Authority; also a Member of SSRC, Centre/Local Government Relations Panel.

He is joint Editor of *The Political Quarterly;* and a Member of the Editorial Boards of *The British Journal of Political Science, The Journal of Public Policy* and *The Journal of Health Policy, Politics & Law.*

Private practice and public policy
Regulating the frontiers

ABSTRACT

The implications of any growth in the private sector of health care can be analysed from two very different perspectives: (1) that of the consumer sovereignty model of health care, and (2) that of the social equity model of health care. The former, it is argued, suggests developing a system of consumer protection, and the chapter examines a variety of policy options for doing so: including accreditation procedures, more information, and a machinery for dealing with consumer complaints. The latter, it is argued, suggests developing a system of positive regulation designed to shape the development of the private sector in the interests of national health care policy, and the chapter examines some of the policy options for doing so: including the development of district plans covering both sectors of health care, and the introduction of incentives to encourage desirable patterns of growth.

INTRODUCTION: MODELS OF HEALTH CARE

Polarity, perspectives, and policy options

There are two basic, polar models of health care provision. The starting point of the first is consumer sovereignty: the model is that of the market place (1). The starting point of the second is social equity: the model is that of the paternalistic rationalizers (2). The first is all about meeting the demands of consumers; the second is all about meeting needs as defined by providers. Needless to say, neither of these models actually exists in its pure form. The American health care system may reflect the rhetoric of consumer sovereignty, but the reality is more complex and less clear-cut. Britain's

97

National Health Service may be the incarnation of the principle of social equity but, again, the model does not conform neatly with an untidy reality complicated by the existence of a private sector dedicated to meeting consumer demands.

For the purposes of this chapter, however, the two models provide useful perspectives for examining the implications for public policy of continuing growth in the private sector. For the implications to be drawn for public policy from any such development are not self-evident, in the sense that they flow ineluctably from the facts. The conclusions drawn from any developments will depend on political evaluation. In turn, the political evaluation will be informed by the underlying assumptions about the desirable direction of policy: in other words, it will depend on which of the two basic, polar models dominates the assumptive worlds of the policy-makers. Self-evidently, the implications drawn by a Conservative Government (which seeks to encourage the private sector) would be different from those drawn by a Labour Government (which sees the private sector, at best, as a necessary evil), and the perspective of an Alliance Government may be different yet again (3).

To speculate about what specific governments might actually do would be a barren exercise. If it is relatively easy to identify the ideologies of the different parties, and therefore their general stance on this issue, it is very much more difficult to anticipate how they would react in unpredictable circumstances. To do so would mean making heroic assumptions not only about the future economic and political context of policy-making, but also about the role of the various interest groups involved in the health care policy arena (4). The assumptive worlds of policy makers can usefully be divided into two components (5): value judgments and reality judgments. And the former are inevitably constrained and screened by the latter: whatever the ideological imperatives driving the policy-makers, their decisions will inevitably be shaped also by the political costs—reflecting the political clout of professional organizations and trade-unions—involved in adopting various policy options.

Rather than embarking on an exercise in speculative futurology, and attempting to predict what might happen, this chapter therefore uses the perspectives offered by the two rival models to identify and discuss sets of policy options which seem to flow logically from adopting these two positions. In practice, the apparent antithesis between these two models may be blurred: if Britain remains committed to a mixed economy of health care, then public policy is likely to be informed by insights drawn from both of them. Certainly the underlying assumption of this chapter is that neither model will be pushed to its logical conclusion: i.e. that the NHS will not be scrapped in favour of a market system, and the private sector will not be abolished in order to safeguard the NHS. What, in essence, we are concerned about are the principles and practice of frontier regulation. For the purposes of analysis, however, the two models provide a useful way of identifying two approaches and specific problems for policy makers, whoever these may turn out to be in future. Before turning to an examination of policy options, this analysis therefore looks in a little more detail at the two models, to see what prescriptive implications can be drawn out from them: where their underlying logic would lead policy makers (if they were free and able to pursue it—a questionable assumption, perhaps).

The 'market' model

The market model puts the consumer in the driving seat. From this perspective, consumers are in 'the business of making economic choices about both the quantity and the quality of health care services that they desire' (6). Following on from this, the private sector of health care can be seen as a device for creating more scope for consumer choice: it measures and partially fills the gap between what, on the one hand, politicians are prepared to finance through the tax system, and what professional providers deem to be necessary and what, on the other hand, consumers want. Indeed advocates of the market model tend to assert that, given the characteristics of the political market, a tax-financed health care system will inevitably under-state the willingness of consumers to pay for health care: in Britain, if not in the

United States, the case for a market system is often put in terms of its ability to *maximize* resources devoted to health care.

The criticisms of this model are familiar (7). In summary, it is argued that it is at odds with the reality of health care, in the sense that it assumes an ability to make informed choices which in practice does not exist (—quite apart from the problems raised by inequalities of income distribution). The model, it is argued, ignores the imbalance of information as between consumers and providers: the extent to which the decisions of consumers are shaped by, and dependent on the guidance of providers. Equally, it is asserted, the model ignores the fact that the ability of consumers to shop around—i.e. to choose—may be most constrained when their need is greatest: for example, after a heart attack. Lastly, the model fails to take account of the irreversible nature of medical intervention: a faulty car can always be traded-in, but there is no equivalent redress for a patient left crippled by a botched operation.

To stress these criticisms is to suggest that the policy implications of a growth in the private sector, from the market model perspective, would be a growth also in the state's regulatory activities. It is to argue that the state would inevitably be drawn further into the business of regulating the private sector in an attempt to make reality conform with the underlying assumption of the model. To make the consumer sovereign may, paradoxically, involve a very strong dose of government intervention designed to redress the imbalances within the health care market: imbalances which are particularly marked in that market, though not necessarily unique to it. Such a conclusion is certainly consistent with the experience in other areas of public policy: note, for example, the extent of state intervention designed to make the market economy live up to its textbook claims by trying to enforce competition and to prevent monopolies. It is also consistent with the experience of the United States in the health care policy area where ironically lip-service to the market model has been accompanied by a far greater degree of government regulation than in Britain (8). The next section in this chapter examines some of the policy options for state regulation designed to protect consumer interests that would flow from the growth of the private sector in Britain.

The 'social equity' model

It is, however, the social equity model of health care which provides the dominant paradigm in Britain today, and which indeed has its institutional embodiment in the NHS. This, in effect, explicitly repudiates the market principle. Its guiding principle is that health care should be provided according to need, not in response to demand (which is why the language of consumerism sits so oddly in the context of the NHS). It is paternalistic, in a descriptive rather than perjorative sense, insofar as resources are allocated according to abstract criteria embodied in statistical formulas and judgments about the use of these resources are then made by professional providers according to their own definitions of need. Its concern is with the equitable rationing of what are seen to be inevitably scarce resources. Its aim, to exaggerate only slightly, is not so much to maximize the amount of health care that is made available as to maximize distributional social justice: indeed it can be argued that the real achievement of the NHS is to *minimize* the total expenditure on health care, while making rationing—which may, in some circumstances even mean turning away to die people who could be helped, if only temporarily, by medical intervention—socially and politically acceptable.

Using the perspective of the social equity model, the growth of the private sector raises a different set of policy questions. In particular, it raises the question of how best to safeguard the principles (if not necessarily the institutional structure) of the NHS. Once again, we come to the question of state regulation, but with a very different agenda from that discussed above, in the context of the market model. The social equity model presumes a certain set of policy aims, notably the rational pursuit of certain distributional goals. These may well be threatened by a private sector that is responsive to demand, which is bound to reflect inequalities of income and may also be distorted by the preferences of providers influencing those of the consumers. Later in this chapter I examine some of the policy options for state regulation designed to safeguard the principles of the social equity model that might come under consideration in response to the growth of the private sector.

Other telling factors

So far this discussion has deliberately sharpened up the contrast between the two polar ideological models that can be expected to influence public policy. But any realistic discussion of future policy options must also take into account other factors in the political equation, likely both to complicate and soften any government response. These are discussed elsewhere in the book, but one crucial point must be briefly stressed here. This is the interdependence of the public and private sectors of health care. On the one hand, the private sector is dependent on the NHS to provide the most expensive and most long-term care for those with the least financial resources. On the other hand, the NHS needs the private sector as a political safety valve: one reason (perceptions of social fairness apart) why rationing appears to be acceptable may in part least be that the most demanding consumers i.e. those with the most political as well as financial resources—can exit into the private sector (9).

There is a further complicating factor. This is that when we actually look at the behaviour of consumers, we find that they tend to use both the private and the public sectors: crossing the frontiers between the two systems as it suits them. Even if they use the private hospital sector, they tend to use NHS family practitioners (10). Even if they use the public hospital sector, they may use a private consultant. In this respect, the relationship between the public and private sectors is less clear-cut and more confused than in, say, education or housing. While parents may well switch a child from one sector to another, as he or she progresses through the education system, the child is unlikely to go to a private school in the morning and to a state school in the afternoon. Yet in the case of health care, a patient may well be in the equivalent of that position, receiving care from both sectors.

Indeed it is precisely this interpenetration of the two systems—if anything more evident in the case of the main professional providers, i.e. the medical profession—which poses some of the most difficult questions when it comes to state regulation, as we shall see. While we may start out with two clear-cut models, offering us very different guidelines for policy making, we shall inevitably be driven to examining policy options in the light of administrative, political and economic notions of feasibility.

PROTECTING THE CONSUMER

The consumer movement and the 1962 Report

If we assume that the market for health care is no different from other markets, it follows that the best guide to possible future action is the past history of the consumer protection movement. If buying health care in the private sector is no different from buying shoes or a refrigerator, then the obvious starting point for discussing options for policy is to look at the machinery for safeguarding the interests of the ordinary shopper.

Let us start, therefore, by looking at the 1962 Report of the Committee on Consumer Protection (11): from which flow many of today's laws and institutions. 'Consumer protection', the report pointed out

is an amorphous conception that cannot be defined. It consists of those instances where the law intervenes to impose safeguards in favour of purchasers and hire-purchasers, together with the activities of a number of organisations, variously inspired, the object or effect of which is to procure fair and satisfying treatment for the domestic buyer. From another viewpoint consumer protection may be regarded as those measures which contribute, directly or indirectly, to the consumer's assurance that he will buy goods of suitable quality appropriate to his purpose; that they will give him reasonable use, and that if he has just complaint there will be a means of redress.

From this catalogue, and the report's subsequent discussion, it is possible to identify various aspects of consumer protection. First, there is the legal protection of the consumer's rights designed to provide 'some assurance as to the quality and suitability of the goods sold'. Second, there are standards laid down by the producers themselves. Third, there is the availability of independent information, which may or may not be based on the comparative testing of the goods that are available. Lastly, there is the machinery available to consumers for seeking redress if things should go wrong or they are dissatisfied.

The evidence submitted to the Committee argued that consumer protection was inadequate on all these counts. And in doing so, the critics put forward two arguments which have obvious resonance in the context of health care:

1. Technological change

Whereas the consumer of 50 years ago needed only a reasonable modicum of skill and knowledge to recognise the composition of the goods on offer and their manner of production, and to assess their quality and fitness for his particular purpose, the consumer of today finds it difficult if not impossible to do so because of complicated production techniques ... The job of ascertaining and soundly assessing the wide range of alternative choices open to him is more, his supporters aver, than the consumer can possibly be expected to do. It is further argued that the increased sale of branded and nationally advertised goods has tended to reduce the retailer's function to that of handing over what the customer has already been persuaded to buy before entering the shop; and that partly for this reason, partly because it is almost as difficult for him as for his customer to sort out the merits and shortcomings of the goods he stocks, the retailer is far less able to perform his special and essential function of giving expert advice to the individual customer.

2. Complexity of goods

Moreover, the ordinary consumer now spends a good deal of money on appliances and equipment of types unknown, or known only to a favoured few, thirty years ago ... The quality and relative merit of each can be assessed (if at all) only by a qualified expert using special equipment ... When confronted with the need to make a choice between different models of such goods the consumer is incapable of intelligent discrimination; even price will not provide a sure signpost to the degree of satisfaction he is likely to achieve.

Relevance to medical care

The aptness of both these points to medical care is self-evident. In the case of medical care, too, 'production techniques' have become more complicated: the job of 'ascertaining and soundly assessing the wide range of alternative choices' has indeed become more difficult for the consumer. It could also be argued that the equivalent of the 'retailer'—that is, the family practitioner—may find it more difficult to give 'expert advice' about the 'merits and shortcomings' of the health care goods on offer in the private sector (and perhaps in the public sector as well). Lastly, it would probably be accepted that 'price will not provide a sure signpost to the degree of satisfaction' that the consumer is likely to achieve: conventional market signals may be difficult to interpret in the health care sector.

But before examining the implications of such arguments for public policy, in response to the growth of the private sector, it would seem essential to deal with two points. First, it may be said that the growth of the private sector has so far—in Britain, at any rate—created no demands for the strengthening of the system of consumer protection: so why assume that there will be such demands in future? Second, it may be contended that the reason why there has been no pressure for change is that the present system offers sufficient protection to the consumer: that the existing machinery is adequate. Let us examine each of these points in turn.

To assume that there will be demands for greater consumer protection is to assume also that the future will be unlike the past. The reason for doing so is partly that until recently the private sector of health care has lacked political visibility. Until the issue of pay-beds provoked political controversy in the mid-seventies, the private sector of health care was not on the active agenda of British politics (12). But it is there now, and any policies designed to encourage the private sector (such as tax concessions) are bound to give it more salience. Abortion provides a clear example of how the rapid expansion of private health care can lead to demands for more stringent public regulation (13). And although abortion is very much a special case, insofar as it is peculiarly liable to arouse strong emotions, the experience does suggest that demands for regulation increase with political visibility.

Moreover, in parallel, there has been the development of 'consumerism' in health care: there has been a subtle change in the vocabulary of discourse about health care, with the 'consumer' increasingly replacing the 'patient'—a linguistic shift which indicates a perception of users of health care services as having an active, demanding rather than a passive, recipient role. Indeed the logic of the market model, as already argued, is calculated to reinforce this trend: the real difference between the consumer of health care and the consumer of other goods is—following the logic of this model—simply that the former needs *more* protection, given the informational and other problems of making an informed choice. Significantly, perhaps, *Which?*—the journal of the Consumers' Association—has recently been paying increasing attention to health care (14).

Machinery of consumer protection in the NHS

But, it may still be argued, health care is different from other markets in that there is already an elaborate machinery of consumer protection. To return to the 1962 report of the Committee on Consumer Protection, there is in existence legislation designed to guarantee 'some assurance as to the quality and suitability of the goods sold' and, similarly, to ensure standards laid down by the producers themselves. The state already regulates the medical profession, through the institution of the General Medical Council. As the Merrison Committee put it (15), 'an instructive way of looking at regulation is to see it as a contract between public and profession, by which the public go to the profession for medical treatment because the profession has made sure that it will provide satisfactory treatment'. Lastly, consumers can seek redress 'if things should go wrong' by bringing malpractice suits.

However, it is also clear that this system has weaknesses. It does not provide independent information. And although the regulation of the medical profession through the GMC may ensure competence when doctors start out on their career, and deal with conspicuous lapses, it is doubtful whether it can guarantee 'satisfactory treatment'. This certainly appears to be the view of the medical profession itself, as reflected in its interest in other means of ensuring continuing competence, such as education and audit (16). Similarly, it can be argued that medical malpractice suits are a dubious and double-edged way of seeking redress. From the consumer's point of view, it is an expensive procedure—and legal aid is now available to only 20 per cent of the population (17). From the medical profession's point of view, it may lead to the practice of defensive medicine as in the United States (18). Not surprisingly therefore there has been considerable pressure to improve the complaints machinery within the NHS (19).

From this, it might be concluded that there has in fact been a response to a demand for more consumer protection—but expressed, paradoxically, within the context of the NHS. Indeed the various strategies for promoting 'satisfactory treatment' have been worked out on the assumption that they would be applied within the NHS. Not only is this true, self-evidently, of the complaints machinery. But it is also true of the interest in developing continuing education and medical audit. It does not therefore seem implausible to explore the implications of such developments for the private sector, particularly if this continues to grow and thus to attract more political attention.

Regulatory provision in the private sector

Indeed recognition of the fact that the private sector requires regulation is already embodied in legislation, and the requirement to register private hospitals and nursing homes under the 1975 Nursing Homes Act—the latest in a series of such acts. To quote the Department of Health and Social Security's 1981 circular (20):

> the 1975 Act covers a wide range of establishments in the private health care sector, from large acute private hospitals to small nursing homes providing long-term care . . . Given the growing roles of the private hospital and nursing home sector, registration under the 1975 Act is an increasingly important function. The main aim of the legislation is to protect the public, through ensuring that adequate standards of care and accommodation are provided. There is a need for consistency in the registration of these premises so that, without attempting to impose an unnecessary and inflexible uniformity, the procedures used by different authorities and the standards asked of proprietors do not differ significantly between authorities.

The first responsibility imposed on the registration authorities—now the District Health Authorities—is to ensure that only those private facilities are registered where the 'person-in-charge' is either a registered medical practitioner or a qualified nurse. Equally the authority is required to make certain that staffing standards are adequate, and that those employed are 'fit persons': an emphasis which goes back to the origins of the first legislation in this field, in 1927, when there was much concern about the morals (as well as competence) of those employed—and when the distinction between nursing homes and brothels appears, at times, to have got blurred (21). Lastly, the authorities are required to inspect all registered private facilities at least twice a year in order to make sure that standards are being maintained. 'In determining the staffing and accommodation standards required of premises registered under the Act', the DHSS advises, 'authorities should have regard to standards prevailing generally in the NHS'. In the last resort, the registration may be cancelled—although 'Cancellation is clearly a final resort. In most cases where problems arise they can be identified quickly through frequent and effective inspection, and resolved by discussion'.

'Standards...'—a nebulous concept

So, in effect, there is already in existence a machinery of inspection, designed to ensure that consumers of private health care get adequate treatment. The trouble is that no one knows how it works. No studies have been carried out, insofar as this author has been able to establish, to determine how different registration authorities carry out their task. The legislation and regulations certainly appear to give them wide discretion and little specific guidance on the maintenance of standards of care (in contrast to the prolific and detailed guidance about the maintenance of fire precautions). The concept of 'standards prevailing generally in the NHS' would seem to be an extremely nebulous one, capable of very different interpretations; and in the case of care for the chronically sick elderly, it would hardly appear to be a reassuring one.

Moreover, not only is the concept of 'standards prevailing generally in the NHS' nebulous, but it is also flawed by a fundamental ambiguity about the whole notion of 'standards'. Given the emphasis on levels of staffing and accommodation, it would seem that the legislation defines standards in terms of appropriate *inputs*. If this interpretation is correct, then registration and inspection would seem to have little to do with guaranteeing standards of *outputs* in terms of the quality of medical and health care delivered: the consumer's main concern, surely. In short, it would appear that the present system regulates precisely those aspects of private health care where the providers have an incentive to do better than the NHS and where consumers have least difficulty in obtaining information about what is available.

For clearly the private sector has a direct incentive to provide *better* physical facilities, such as private rooms, than the NHS: this, after all, is one of its selling points. Similarly, consumers have no special problem in assessing what might be called the 'housekeeping' aspects of private care (although it is important to remember, throughout this analysis, the special case of elderly patients: i.e. the most infirm, the most vulnerable users of the private sector, who are least able to conform to the classic 'consumer' model of behaviour). Far more problematic for consumers, as argued earlier, is assessing the quality of the treatment provided. Moreover, this is difficult not only for consumers but also for 'qualified experts': the literature on the problems of assessing quality in health care is vast, and clear conclusions are hard to find (22).

'Accreditation' as a possible requirement

One policy option for the future—if the central argument of this analysis is correct, and that a growth in the private sector will generate demands for more consumer protection—might therefore be to move towards the development of some form of accreditation procedure on the United States model. Such a procedure would involve the application of national criteria of evaluation and, presumably, the use of national teams of 'inspectors'—as in the case of the Health Advisory Service. It might also involve the systematic collection of information about the private sector, so as to provide comparative data of performance. There are obvious objections to such an approach. Criteria of evaluation are not easy to devise, and tend to be process rather than outcome based. There is a danger of creating a 'bureaucratic Frankenstein' (23); there would, inevitably, be considerable costs of administration. As against this, a system of accreditation could be introduced on a voluntary basis, (and there is, of course, no reason of principle why it should not also be extended to the NHS). That is, institutions in the private sector would be free to choose whether or not to submit themselves to the accreditation procedure, with consumers in turn being left free to come to their own judgment as to the importance they attach to such a 'seal of approval'. It could be argued after all that, following the logic of the market model, consumers might rationally prefer an unaccredited but cheaper private hospital—assuming that they are prepared to trade the possibility of extra risk against the saving involved.

A system of accreditation would, to return to the report of the Committee on Consumer Protection, provide the consumer with some basic 'independent information': i.e. that the institutions concerned met certain standards. It would not, of course, provide other kinds of information: the kind of 'value for money' information which consumers seek in other fields—see, for example, *Which?* reports on cars and other consumer durables, which scrutinize critically what customers get in return for their money, comparing the performance of Model X against that of Model Y. It is difficult to see this kind of information being generated about the clinical aspects of health care; one need only think about the difficulties involved in testing the performance of Consultant X against that of Consultant Y. But it would seem reasonable to predict increasing interest in generating such information about the hotel aspects of private care should the sector continue to grow. One way of generating more information for the consumer would, of course, be to encourage advertising by the providers of health care: the logic of the market model which, to an extent, is now being applied in the United States. But this, in turn, would invite the question of the extent to which public policy should get involved in the regulation of advertising, to ensure that the information provided to consumers did not make any false or misleading claims.

An adequate machinery of redress?

There remains the issue, also identified by the Committee on Consumer Protection, of providing an adequate machinery of redress for dissatisfied customers in the private sector of health care. One approach to this might be to make it easier, and cheaper, to bring medical malpractice suits: perhaps to devise the equivalent of a 'small claims court' in this area of policy. But, as already suggested, this might have undesirable side-effects. A more acceptable approach might therefore be to devise a private sector equivalent of the machinery that has been set up in the NHS to deal with complaints involving clinical matters. From the perspective of public policy, it might well suffice if such a machinery were set up by the private sector itself—the insurance industry provides an example—provided that consumers could be assured of an inquiry by independent experts.

All this, it may be said, ignores that health care is different from other consumer goods: that, for example, doctors have special ethical duties to their patients. But this, in turn, is to ignore that the market model of health care is based—to return to the starting point of our argument—on the assumption that buying the good of 'health care' is no different from buying any other bundle of goods or services. If, in fact, we reject this assumption—and with it the model—we are left with the social equity model of health care. And the next section examines the perspectives on public policy towards private health care offered by this model.

PROTECTING THE NATIONAL HEALTH SERVICE

An over-sharpened perception

From the perspective of the social equity model of health care, the private sector is the tempter in the Garden of Eden: a disruptive, corrupting influence. Its principles are seen as essentially antagonistic to those of the NHS: making health care available according to the capacity to pay is seen to be incompatible with distributing it according to need. Indeed it is precisely this perception of the private sector as illegitimate if perhaps inevitable—rather like original sin—which may help to explain the lack of debate about appropriate principles of regulation throughout the history of the NHS: the feeling, among the advocates of the social equity model that as long as the Church itself could be purified (24), as long as private practice could be expelled from the NHS, there need be no great concern about the private sector.

In discussing future policy options for the regulation of a growing private sector, this absolutist position is not very helpful. It offers, in effect, only one criterion for evaluating policies: whether or not they promote social equity. But, as Fishkin has argued (25), all principles of policy evaluation lead to tyranny if pushed to their logical conclusion to the exclusion of other principles: 'if applied without exception or qualification, they would all legitimize policies imposing severe deprivations when alternative policies would impose no severe deprivations on anyone'. For policy making is essentially about the trade-offs between different evaluative criteria (26). In the case of health care, for example, the equality principle has to be balanced not only against the infringements of individual liberty that might be involved in trying to abolish private practice, but also against the desirability of maximizing the amount of health care that is available to the population at large. For example, if progress towards the achievement of equality were indeed our only criterion of evaluation—as assumed, for example, in the Black Report (27)—then it might be possible to achieve this aim of policy by reducing the total amount of health care that is available: i.e. by making it more difficult for the middle-classes to get access to health care. That might well bring about more distributional equity but would surely be judged to be a perverse policy outcome.

A wider perspective leading to policy objectives

This analysis therefore concedes, without further ado, that the growth of the private sector would inevitably be at odds with the dominating principle of the social equity model, insofar as it would perpetuate and reinforce a two-class health care system. For why, after all, would anyone wish to use the private sector if it did not offer privileges or advantages, (such as more immediate access to treatment, choices of consultant, better amenities and more privacy) than the NHS? Any regulatory strategy which sought to force the private sector to conform to the social equity model would therefore be an attempt to square the circle. The regulation of the private sector should instead, we would suggest, be guided by the general criterion that its growth should 'impose no severe deprivations on anyone' expressed in two more specific objectives for public policy:

1. That the development of the private sector should not make it more difficult for the NHS to achieve its own aims (given our assumption that the NHS will continue to provide most of the health care for most of the people for the foreseeable future).

2. That the resources mobilized by the private sector should be *additional* to those of the NHS, rather than merely

representing a shift from one sector to another (on the assumption that the inevitable loss of equity implicit in the growth of the private sector can be justified only by an increase in the total amount of health care available to the population).

Existing regulation

From this perspective, the first question to be asked is how the private sector can best be regulated in order to assure the achievement of these two objectives. Here the best starting point is the 1976 Health Services Act, which created the Health Services Board. Although the main aim of this Act was to supervise the phasing out of pay beds from the NHS, it also gave the Health Services Board more general powers to regulate the growth of the private sector. Part III of the Act gave the Board power 'to control and monitor, to a certain extent, the building of new private hospitals, the conversion of other premises into private hospitals, and the extension and adaptation of existing private hospitals' (28). Specifically, the consent of the Board had to be sought for any development involving more than 100 beds in London and 75 beds in the provinces. The Board's consent could not, however, be refused unless it was satisfied that the development would 'to a significant extent' adversely affect the interests of the NHS and/or of NHS patients (a criterion which is very similar to the first of the objectives set out above).

During its short life-span, until its abolition in 1980, the Health Services Board granted 12 authorizations (29). A number of public hearings were held. In all the disputed cases, the argument revolved around the issue of whether the new developments would adversely affect the interests of the NHS and/or NHS patients by competing for scarce resources of staff, particularly nurses. In one case the Board decided to refuse permission on the grounds that the proposed development would create 'an appreciable strain upon the resources available to the NHS locally' (30).

The 1980 Health Services Act abolished the Board and transferred the responsibility for controlling new developments in the private sector to health authorities. The criteria for refusing permission—i.e. that the development would adversely and significantly affect the interests of the NHS and/or NHS patients—remained unchanged. The power to control, however, applied only to new developments with more than 120 beds. If this provision could be seen as a relaxation of controls, another section of the Act appeared to strengthen the power of District Health Authorities to regulate the private sector. A DHA may, if all existing and proposed private health facilities in its district exceed 120 beds, request the Secretary of State to designate its area for a period of up to five years. In such a 'designated' area, the DHA would have the power to control any proposed developments, whatever their size.

The Health Authority as a regulatory body

There are a number of problems about this system of regulation. The first is that any numerical cut-off point—whether it is 75 beds (as in the 1976 Act) or 120 beds (as in the 1980 Act) is bound to be arbitrary. The impact of any development in the private sector is bound to vary with the size of the district and with the nature of the proposed new facility. The significance of a private hospital of any given size will be very different in a district with a population of 200,000 from that in a district with a population of 400,000. This might suggest that the limit would be better expressed in terms of the number of beds per 1000 population. But even this fails to deal with the problem that the impact of a new development will be very different, depending on the *kind* of facilities it offers: a highly specialized, intensely staffed unit (drawing its patients from a wide, perhaps international, catchment area) has different implications from a general unit concentrating on providing elective surgery for the local population. This indicates that any size limit is bound to create anomalies, and that it might therefore be preferable to give DHAs a general power to control all developments, irrespective of size—despite the extra administrative burdens and costs (for both the public and the private sectors) that this might generate.

But this is to beg the question of whether DHAs are the most appropriate bodies to regulate the growth of the private sector. On the one hand, it may be argued that these are best placed to know whether a new local development would adversely and significantly affect the interests of the NHS and its patients. On the other hand, it could also be argued that the criterion involved is so loose and subjective (one man's significance, may be another man's irrelevance) that DHAs are likely to vary widely in their interpretation of the legislation in response to the varying nature and strength of local pressures. Hence, perhaps, the proposal—by a former Minister of Health, Dr David Owen—that the Health Services Board should be resurrected (31). This inevitably raises the question—so familiar in the context of the NHS—of how best to strike a balance between implementing national policies and avoiding centralization. The present system may make it difficult to achieve consistency across the country; resurrecting the Health Services Board would, however, reinforce centralization. One policy option might, therefore, be to reinvent the Health Services Board, but to give it an appellate function only. For example, both disappointed would-be developers and Community Health Councils might be given the right to appeal to such a Board against DHA decisions, which could thus ensure that the local criteria used are consistent.

The slenderness of the information base for criteria

More fundamentally still, perhaps, there is the question of whether the existing criteria for evaluating the desirability (or otherwise) of proposed private sector developments are adequately defined in the legislation. If not, there might be an argument either for spelling them out more specifically or for using a revived Health Services Board to develop a system/case law. The problem can be simply illustrated by considering the main issue considered by the late Board. As already noted, the Board's considerations revolved around the argument of whether private sector developments would compete with the NHS for staff resources, particularly nurses. But this raises the question of the time-scale involved, and the assumptions made about the future supply of labour. Taking a short-term view, it could be argued that the NHS and the private sector compete for a fixed pool of skilled labour (although it may be contended that, in the case of nurses, the private sector may be able to attract those who have dropped out of the NHS). Taking a longer term view, however, it could be argued that the availability of extra jobs will in itself encourage recruitment, and thus swell the total pool. So it is far from self-evident what assumptions and time-scale should be built into a system of regulation, and whether decisions about the criteria to be applied can be left to individual DHAs—each one of whom may employ different assumptions and time-scales.

Compounding complexity is the fact that the total supply of *skilled labour* is itself influenced, if not determined, by public policy. The number of skilled health service workers does not only reflect market forces but also public policy decisions about how many should be trained. Simply expanding demand does not necessarily guarantee a supply (particularly if there are restrictions on overseas immigration). This is most obviously true in the case of doctors. In the case of medical manpower, individual decisions about the effect of expanding the private sector on the availability of staff resources in the NHS can only be taken rationally within the context of a collective view about the relationship between the numbers trained and the posts required in the state sector.

The case of *medical manpower* also raises some administrative problems, particularly if it is granted that the objective of policy should be to make sure that the growth of the private sector will add to the total resources of health care that are available. This point emerges clearly from the recent report of the Working Party on Orthopaedic Services (32). Discussing the growth in the number of people covered by private insurance schemes, this argued:

> if increasingly the private surgical treatment they receive is provided in private hospitals, then of course the demand for NHS hospitals will be reduced, and waiting times for NHS surgical treatment can be expected to get

shorter. But this will only be the case if surgeons working in the NHS do not undertake fewer NHS sessions or
are not attracted to full-time private practice before
replacements for them can be found by the health
authorities with whom they have their contracts.

Precisely the same could be said, of course, about other
specialists—such as anaesthetists. But how, in fact, can
health authorities make sure that increasing opportunities for
private practice do not divert the time and energies of
consultants from their NHS commitment? The survey carried out for the Review Body in 1978 (33) showed that the
NHS was getting its money's worth from part-time consultants. Relatively, allowing for their lesser contractual commitment, they were spending more time on their NHS work
than their full-time colleagues: the whole-time equivalent of
the former was 52·3 hours per week as against 48·7 for the
latter. But in absolute terms it was, of course, much less: 29·4
hours as against 48·7. So, to put it crudely, the continuing
growth of private practice is only compatible with the interests of the NHS if it persuades consultants to spend more of
their time operating privately at the expense of cutting their
commitment to playing golf or gardening—as distinct from
switching their energies to the private sector at the expense of
reducing their commitment to the NHS. It is therefore
difficult to see how the objective of ensuring that the private
sector generates extra resources can be achieved, in the case
of medical manpower, without tighter checks on what consultants actually do and stricter limits on their ability to opt
for part-time contracts: greater freedom and opportunities to
engage in private practice, flowing from the new consultant
contract and the growth of the private sector, would also
seem to imply greater administrative oversight.

The need for more positive regulation

So far the discussion has taken as its starting point the
inherited, essentially negative system of regulation as embodied in the legislation. It is a system designed, as we have seen,
to stop developments which (according to fairly restricted

criteria) might damage the NHS. It is not a system designed to regulate the relationship between the public and private sectors of health care. At present, given the small size of the private sector, this may not matter greatly. But if the private sector continues to expand, then clearly the case for *positive regulation* will grow in strength: positive regulation being taken to mean policies for controlling the distribution and use of all health care resources, cutting across the two sectors. Thus it has been argued that 'policies, priorities and plans must be developed to include the private health care organization but at the same time allow for their development within the overall plans developed by the appropriate public bodies for the locality, the region or the nation' (34). In short, the question would seem to be whether it is possible and desirable to devise a *planning framework* which spans both the public and the private sectors.

Planning for all and public policy

Since the foundation of the NHS, one overriding aim of public policy endorsed by all political parties—has been to ensure that 'an equally good service is available everywhere', to quote Aneurin Bevan's memorandum to the Cabinet in October 1945 (35). Successive governments have committed themselves, at least since the 'seventies, to the achievement of geographical equity in the distribution of resources, and have adopted the RAWP formula in their pursuit of this objective. But, of course, this formula applies only to NHS resources. It ignores resources in the private sector. Assuming continued expansion in the latter, does this make sense? If the objective is to equalize the health care resources available to a given population, then are not private health care facilities as relevant as NHS ones?

One response to these questions could be the development of district plans which include *all* health care facilities, irrespective of ownership. There are precedents for such an approach: the French health care planning system has introduced 'cartes sanitaires', comprehensive catalogues of the available resources, which cover both the public and the private sectors (36). Similarly, the United States planning system attempts to regulate both sectors through certificate-of-need control (37). Neither system has proved conspicuously successful, but this—it could be argued—reflects the strength, complexity and heterogeneity of the private sectors in these countries, rather than inherent flaws in the approach.

How could such a system work in the UK context? One option would be to include private provision in the RAWP formula calculations (and in whatever formulas are used for sub-regional allocations). This would mean that regions or districts with a high concentration of private health care facilities would lose a proportionate slice of their entitlement to NHS resources. Clearly such calculations would have to be based on the services provided to the relevant local population, rather than the crude size of the private sector facilities (since it would be misleading to include facilities which serve patients from overseas). There would, therefore, be a need for comprehensive and detailed information about the activities about the private sector: indeed such information is essential for any attempt to co-ordinate the planning of the public and the private sectors.

Public and private sector—two different populations

One objection to this policy option might well be that the public and private sectors do not, in practice, serve the same populations. The former is all embracing; the latter is selective. If those who can afford private health care in a particular region or district are well served, then this does not necessarily mean that the rest of the population benefit in an equal degree from the lessening of the load on the NHS. Given that, as argued earlier, the private sector responds to demands, while the public sector meets needs, it does not follow that the two are substitutable in resource allocation terms. Even if it assumed that the resources in the private sector represent a net addition—rather than a diversion of energies and time by skilled staff—it may well be that the resources would be used in a different way than they would be in the NHS. As against this, however, it could be argued that the inclusion of private sector in any resource allocation formula would be to the benefit of the least well-off regions and districts. To the extent that the use of private health care is related to income, so one might expect facilities to be concentrated in the wealthiest parts of the country. Conversely, the most deprived parts of the country would tend to have the least private health care facilities. Including private resources in the RAWP calculations would thus have the effect of redistributing NHS resources to the latter.

From the point of achieving social equity, such an approach is therefore attractive. But there are obvious problems. It would mean that the health authorities in the 'surplus' resource category would have a direct incentive to veto all private developments. Conversely, however, those in the 'deficit' resource category would have an incentive to try to attract private developments. On the face of it, this would seem to represent a very desirable outcome in terms of the social equity model: in effect, it would represent a move towards 'open' and 'closed' areas for new private developers —these being defined in terms of the local balance between needs and resources. In practice, however, it may be doubted whether private developers would find the 'open' areas attractive: the very reasons that make them deprived also make them unattractive to consultants and a bad risk financially. However, to make this point is also to stress that if private resources are ignored in NHS financial planning, then the result will almost certainly be to *widen* the disparities in the total health care resources available to the populations in different parts of the country.

Incentives to private development for public policy

But the argument for regulating the private sector in a positive sense, in an endeavour to co-ordinate the two sectors in the pursuit of national policy objectives for health care, can be developed in another direction as well. If positive regulation is defined in terms of encouraging the private sector to develop in ways congruent and consistent with the policies and priorities of the NHS, then this prompts the question of what *incentives* can be offered. Present incentives to the private sectors seem to be to develop in those areas where public demand is at odds with national priorities: i.e. it largely reflects the *demand* for prompt attention by men and women of working age, whereas national priorities stress the *need* to develop services for the elderly and other deprived groups requiring long-term care (38). Not only does this mean that geographical imbalances in the total provision of health care, and the distribution of medical manpower, are likely to be accentuated, as argued above. It also means that the incentives to doctors to move into the high-prestige specialties, which offer rewards from private practice, are likely to be reinforced. If, therefore, the growth of the private sector is not to distort overall national priorities, a deliberate attempt may have to be made to steer developments into those areas where an extra investment of resources is deemed to be desirable.

Positive regulation cannot, therefore, be seen as being merely reactive. It would involve health authorities in actually inviting and encouraging private developments which fit into their own plans, and which fill gaps in their own provision (while, at the same time, using their powers of negative regulation to discourage those developments which are at odds with their own plans). The difficulty with such an approach is, of course, that it appears to run counter to the financial logic of the private sector. However, this is to ignore the fact that the health authorities also have some bargaining power. To the extent that they contract out to the private sector (39), so they can also influence its developments: if contracting out increases in scale, so the incentives to private health care developers to conform to the pattern of NHS needs would grow. Moreover, the private sector is often dependent on NHS facilities for specialized investigative procedures, so here also health authorities can exercise some leverage in influencing developments: they can offer the incentive of active co-operation for those developments which are congruent with their own plans (while, conversely, discouraging those which are not). Nor can it be assumed that the chronic care sector is irremediably unattractive to private developers (although it may be unattractive for private insurers). Of the 35,000 beds in the private and voluntary sector, four-fifths are devoted to chronic care—although obviously the number of patients is much larger in the acute sector. And there is at least some evidence that public policy contributes to the financial viability of the private and voluntary sector of long-stay health care: many patients in these beds, a study by Challis and Day has found (40), have a large part of their costs paid by the social security system. Here, too, there would appear to be scope for public policy to influence the development of the private sector by offering positive incentives.

Seeking a balance between incentives and control

So far the emphasis in this discussion of positive regulation has been on offering incentives and encouragements rather than seeking to control the operations of the private sector in detail. But the argument can be taken a step further: thus it has been contended that safeguarding the principle of na-tional policies for health care (embracing both sectors) would require the development of uniform salary and working conditions in the two sectors (41). The case for this is that, in the absence of such a system, the private sector would drain skilled manpower from the NHS by offering higher rewards.

Despite the apparent logic of such an approach, it raises some severe difficulties. In the first place, it is not clear that the appeal of the private sector is based on offering higher rewards. For doctors, its appeal is that it gives them an opportunity to supplement their NHS earnings. For nurses, the appeal may be to work in smaller, cosier units. (How, indeed, could working conditions be made uniform, given the very different physical environments in the two sectors?)

But, more important and more generally, regulation in-volves striking a fine balance between encouraging desirable developments and avoiding the imposition of rigid rules likely to stifle initiative and flexibility. The advantages of the private sector—as against the NHS—derives precisely from its flexibility and freedom from the organizational restraints which inhibit the public sector. It is made up of small units. It is diverse. It is less constricted by trade-union demarcation rules. It therefore can react to demands more immediately and sensitively than the NHS: abortion is a case in point. The dilemma of public policy is therefore how best to preserve these advantages of the private sector—for why have a private sector at all if it is to be 'de-natured' by being forced to fit into the organizational mould of the NHS?—while yet trying to steer its growth in desirable directions.

SUMMARY AND CONCLUSIONS

An exploration of policy options

This chapter has not attempted to devise a blue-print for public policy. Rather, it has sought to explore the various policy options for public policy, on the assumption of continuing growth in the private sector. Inevitably, the policies actually adopted will reflect the perceptions of the policy makers—in particular, the dominating model of health care —and the power of different pressure groups in the health care policy arena: any policy prescription which ignored, for example, the ability of the medical profession to veto change threatening its own interests (real or perceived) would be totally unrealistic.

The projection of current trends

However, certain predictions can be made with reasonable confidence. In the first place, the growth of the private sector is likely to create more demands for public regulation, whether in the interests of the individual consumer or in the collective interest of all health care consumers. In the second place, its growth is likely to promote more pressure for information about its activities, both clinical and financial. The more the private sector grows, in summary, the less likely is it to be left as a virtually self-governing, autonomous enclave: increasing political visibility will lead to demands for greater public accountability—and the demands will be all the more insistent if the growth of the private sector is encouraged by tax concessions which affect the Government's

Public Sector Borrowing Requirement just as much as actual expenditure on the NHS.

Where is the critical point?

To make this last point is also to raise a fundamental question, which can only be noted here but not resolved. To an extent at least, public policies designed to encourage the growth of the private sector are substitutable (in terms of their effect on the PSBR) for expenditure on the NHS. At what point, then, does the active encouragement of the private sector threaten the survival of the NHS as a viable institution? The same point can be made in political, as well as financial, terms. At present the private sector acts as a useful safety valve for the NHS, as argued at the beginning of this chapter. But if the private sector continues to grow, the risk is that the overflow mechanism may turn into a waste-pipe: that the exit of the most articulate, politically resourceful customers of the state sector will drain away effective political support for it. This would suggest that there is a point at which the growth of the private sector would threaten the whole balance of health care in Britain, tilting it away from the social equity model to the market model. In turn, this would imply that the aim of public policy—assuming that the social equity model remains the dominant paradigm, accepted by all political parties—would have to restrict the growth of the private sector. No attempt has been made in this chapter to define the limits of tolerable growth, to delineate precisely where the frontier between the two sectors should be—as distinct from exploring the rules for regulating the frontier. But while it would be unrealistic to suggest that we can know with precision where the line should be drawn—which would mean quantifying an abstract proposition, whose implications are contingent on political reactions to further growth in the private sector—it would be irresponsible to conclude without noting the dangers of drifting by inadvertence into a situation where the essential nature of Britain's health care system had been transformed as a result of public non-policy.

NOTES AND REFERENCES

1. See for example, RALPH HARRIS and ARTHUR SELDON, *Over-Ruled on Welfare:* Institute of Economic Affairs. (London, 1979); for a recent American restatement of the market approach, see DAVID A. STOCKMAN, 'Premises for a Medical Marketplace', *Health Affairs,* 1(1), Winter 1981, pp. 5–19.

2. HARRY ECKSTEIN, *The English Health Service.* (Harvard University Press: Cambridge, Mass., 1958); ROBERT ALFORD, *Health Care Politics.* (University of Chicago Press: Chicago, 1975).

3. SDP Discussion Papers, Health and Personal Social Services Conference, London, 6 March 1982, (mimeo).

4. RUDOLF KLEIN, *The Politics of the NHS.* (Longmans: London). (Forthcoming).

5. SIR GEOFFREY VICKERS, *The Art of Judgment.* (Chapman and Hall: London 1965).

6. Stockman, op. cit., p. 12.

7. See, for example, BRIAN ABEL-SMITH, *Value for Money in Health Services.* (Heinemann: London, 1976); and JOHN CULLIS and PETER WEST, *The Economics of Health.* (Martin Robertson: Oxford, 1979).

8. DAVID MECHANIC, *Future Issues in Health Care.* (The Free Press: New York, 1979).

9. The argument derives from ALBERT HIRSCHMAN, *Exit, Voice and Loyalty.* (Harvard University Press: Cambridge, Mass., 1970). See also, RUDOLF KLEIN, 'Models of Man and Models of Policy', *Millbank Memorial Fund Quarterly/Health and Society,* 58(3), Summer 1980, 416–30.

10. This draws on an unpublished survey of users of private hospitals by David Horne, at the University of Bath.

11. Committee on Consumer Protection, *Final Report.* (HMSO: London, 1962, Cmnd. 1781).

12. RUDOLF KLEIN, 'Ideology, Class and the National Health Service', *Journal of Health Politics, Policy and Law,* 4(3), Fall 1979, 464–90.

13. Committee on the Workings of the Abortion Act, *Report.* (HMSO: London, 1974, Cmnd. 5579).

14. See for example, the article on 'Medical Bills Insurance' in *Which?,* September 1980, 521–6.

15. Committee of Inquiry into the Regulation of the Medical Profession, *Report.* (HMSO: London, 1975, Cmnd. 6018).

16. Committee of Enquiry set up for the Medical Profession, *Competence to Practice.* (Published by the Committee: London, 1976).

17. J. LEAHY TAYLOR, 'Medical Negligence' in J. LEAHY TAYLOR (ed.) *Medical Malpractice.* (John Wright: Bristol, 1980).

18. DAVID G. WARREN, 'Medical Malpractice in the United States' in TAYLOR, op. cit.

19. See, for example, Select Committee on the Parliamentary Commissioner for Administration, *Independent Review of Hospital Complaints in the National Health Service,* First Report, Session 1977–8. (HMSO: London, 1977, H.C. 45).

20. DEPARTMENT OF HEALTH AND SOCIAL SECURITY, *Registration and Inspection of Private Nursing Homes and Mental Nursing Homes.* (DHSS: London, July 1981, H.C. (81)8).

21. BRIAN ABEL-SMITH, *The Hospitals.* (Harvard University Press: Cambridge, Mass., 1964, p. 340).

22. See, for example, the review of the literature by WILLIAM E. MCAULIFFE, 'Measuring the Quality of Medical Care: Process versus outcome', *Milbank Memorial Fund Quarterly/Health and Society,* **57**(1), Winter 1979, 118–152.

23. GEORGE DUNEA, 'Inspecting the Hospitals', *Brit. med. J.,* 20 March 1982, 890–91.

24. Barbara Castle used the ecclesiastical metaphor about the NHS: quoted in KLEIN (1979), op. cit.

25. JAMES S. FISHKIN, *Tyranny and Legitimacy.* (Johns Hopkins University Press: Baltimore, 1979).

26. RUDOLF KLEIN, 'The Evaluation of Social Policies', Paper given at the Social Administration Conference, Cambridge, 1980, (mimeo).

27. Report of a Research Working Group, *Inequalities in Health.* (DHSS: London, 1980).

28. HEALTH SERVICES BOARD, *Annual Report, 1977.* (HMSO: London, 1978, H.C. 276).

29. Ibid., 1978, 1979, H.C. 260.

30. Ibid., 1979, 1980, H.C. 354.

31. David Owen, speech given at the SDP Health and Personal Social Services Conference, London, 6 March 1982, (mimeo).

32. Working Party on Orthopaedic Services, *Report.* (HMSO: London, 1981).

33. REVIEW BODY ON DOCTORS' AND DENTISTS' REMUNERATION, *Eighth Report, 1978.* (HMSO: London, 1978, Cmnd. 7176).

34. PHILIP CHUBB, STUART HAYWOOD, and PAUL TORRENS, *Managing the Mixed Economy of Health,* Health Services Management Centre, Birmingham Occasional Paper No. 42, 1982, p. 21.

35. Quoted in MARTIN BUXTON and RUDOLF KLEIN, *Allocating Health Resources,* Royal Commission on the National Health Service Research Paper No. 3. (London, 1978).

36. VICTOR RODWIN, *The Health Planning Predicament: France, Quebec, England and the United States.* (University of California Press: Berkeley). Forthcoming.

37. DAVID S. SALKEVER and THOMAS W. BICE, *Hospital Certificate-of-Need Controls.* (American Enterprise Institute: Washington, 1979).

38. Department of Health and Social Security, *Care in Action.* (HMSO: London, 1981).

39. DAVID HORNE, 'Contractual arrangements: NHS use of the private sector', *Brit. med. J.,* 3 April 1982, 1060–61.

40. A study of the private sector of care for the elderly has been carried out at the University of Bath by my colleagues Linda Challis and Patricia Day. I am indebted to them for letting me see forthcoming publications, and I have drawn heavily in this chapter on the insights provided by their work.

41. CHUBB, HAYWOOD and TORRENS, op. cit., p. 22.

The private health care sector in Britain

ALAN MAYNARD

ALAN MAYNARD

Alan Maynard is a Reader in Health Economics at the University of York, England and Director of the Graduate Programme in Health Economics in the Department of Economics and Related Studies at York. He has been a visiting lecturer at the University Institute of European Studies, Milan, Italy, the Department of Economics, University of Otago, New Zealand, the Institute of Public Finance, University of Genoa, Italy, and the Department of Economics, University of Gothenburg, Sweden. He is an examiner for the Faculty of Community Medicine of the Royal College of Physicians of the United Kingdom and a member of the York Health Authority and the York Family Practitioner Committee. He has worked as a consultant for the Commission of the European Community, the Organization for Economic Co-operation and Development, the World Health Organization, and for governments and industry.

He has written widely in books, academic journals and elsewhere and one of his main interests for the past ten years has been the economics of the organization and regulation of health care systems. His conviction is that the nature of the health and health care policy choices, and their associated problems, are similar wherever you may go on this planet!

The private health care sector in Britain

ABSTRACT

Recent discussion in the media of the private health care industry has led to the creation of an image which bears little relation to the reality. The purpose of this chapter is to remedy this deficit in the discussion of the 'privatization' of the NHS.

The private insurance industry is very small in relation to the NHS. Although it experienced rapid growth in 1980, the indications are that it is now growing more slowly. The industry is regulated in a variety of ways by the State and its structure is very narrow: it provides largely non-emergency surgery.

The private provision of health care has expanded, in part because of the reduction in the availability of NHS pay-beds. It is shown that new private bed construction, together with the renaissance of pay-beds (post 1979) has compensated for the effects of the Labour Governments policies and that the expansion of the private bed stock in the future may be much slower. The separation of public and private hospital facilities and the new (NHS) consultant contract are departures from past policies and developments which will not necessarily lead to the efficient production of health care in the UK.

The growth of the private sector is likely to lead to increased regulation, particularly due to the growth of 'consumerism'. Attempts to get 'value for money' in the NHS are likely to lead to similar pressures in the private sector.

If regulation is defined as the manipulation of prices, quantities and quality by groups within and outside the industry, it seems unavoidable that the regulation of the private health care sector in the UK will increase. We are ignorant of the merits, both clinical and economic, of most medical practices, let alone of the relative merits of public and private provision. The managers of both the NHS and the private sector face the same problems and will inevitably seek to resolve them in the same way: with more regulation.

131

INTRODUCTION

During the last two or three years there has been a heated debate about the expansion of the private health care sector in Britain. This debate has thrown relatively little light on the true nature of the private finance and private provision of health care. Yet to get a better perspective on the issues there is a need to trace the recent history and current nature of the private health care insurance industry against facts concerning the provision of health care in both public (NHS) and private hospitals. Only then will it be possible to examine sensibly the options for expanding the activities of the private sector which will have to be set against an analysis of the implications for public policy, in particular that part which inevitably has to be concerned with the regulation of the private health care sector.

It is important to realize that the *prima facie* evidence seems to suggest that the principal objective of the bulk of the private health care market is to provide medical care for members of the working force and their families who require non-emergency ('cold') acute care. Thus the bulk of the private insurance industry's expenditure finances a narrow range of about thirty surgical activities. Generally the private sector does not provide general practitioner care, emergency care, or care for the long-term (chronic) patients (e.g. mental illness). This mould might be broken in the future, but at present those within the industry seem to think it is unlikely that radical innovations will take place. Rather they believe that the private sector will grow steadily but slowly providing much the same kind of services as at present.

PRIVATE HEALTH CARE INSURANCE

To understand the private health insurance system it is important to analyse how it is organized, to examine the elements of its recent growth, and describe the nature of its benefits to get a reasonable perspective and overview. Here are thus four basic questions about the nature of private health care insurance which must be addressed: how is it organized? how are contributions set? how fast has it grown? and what are the benefits?

How is private health care insurance organized?

The institutions in private health insurance have unusual legal characteristics and behave, in setting premiums for instance, in a rather esoteric manner. The purpose of this section is to explore the legal characteristics of the private insurers.

Although the principal carriers (or providers) of health insurance in the UK are called provident associations they are in fact ordinary insurance companies which are registered under various Insurance Companies Acts as 'pecuniary loss' insurance companies, limited by guarantee and non-profit distributing. Their prime role is to insure against losses arising from illness and health care expenditure. The companies are not limited liability institutions with shareholders but bodies guaranteed by a limited number of individuals up to some nominal amount of money. They do not distribute profits to these guarantors, whose role is indeed largely nominal apart from access to information and capacity to advise the company. All surpluses of revenues over expenditures become part of the company's reserves and are not subject to corporation tax.

Like other insurance companies, the provident associations are governed by a substantial number of statutory instruments and regulations. Insurance company legislation does not impose specific requirements as to 'working capital'. Section 21 of the Insurance Companies Act 1981 lays down the requirement for a solvency margin and regulation 4 and schedules 1 and 2 of the 1981 Insurance Companies Regulation set out the method by which such a margin must be calculated for general insurance business. There are no statutory requirements made by the Department of Trade regarding liquidity ratios, the companies appear to establish their own ratios using standard accounting practice with regard to insurance business, e.g. the ratio of cover of 'quick' (=liquid) assets to the medical insurance fund and other current liabilities is usually in excess of 1.

The private insurers are not regulated with regard to prices or the nature of their policies in a direct manner by any outside (government) or inside (industry) body. Their practices are however guided by the Statement of Insurance Practice which was introduced in 1977 following discussions between the industry and government. This Statement was made because the industry wished to be excluded from the Unfair Contract Terms Act. Amongst other things, the Statement precludes an insurer from rejecting a claim unreasonably unless fraud, negligence, or deception are involved, on the grounds that non-disclosure or misrepresentation of a material fact where knowledge of that fact would have influenced materially the insurer's judgement in providing the insurance. Thus the misrepresentation by one month of his age could not generally be used by the insurer to avoid his liability. This Statement also prevents the insurer from rejecting claims because they were made outside an overstrict time limit.

The voluntary code in the Statement is not the only limit on the insurers' behaviour. The Trade Description Acts, which made it an offence to apply a description to any goods or services which is false to a material degree, and the Fair Trading Act 1973 which amongst other things penalized any trader who used practices which have the effect of misleading consumers as to their rights and obligations affect the behaviour of the insurers. These pieces of legislation may, as Klein has indicated in his chapter, affect the insurance industry much more in the years to come as 'consumerism' grows in the public and private health care sectors.

Another constraint on the behaviour of health insurers is the Consumer Credit Act 1974. This legislation obliges insurers, if they wished to avoid the effects of this legislation, to ensure that they offered no credit by way of 'periods of grace' or payment of subscription by instalment in arrears. All subscribers must pay all their monies to the carriers in advance. Where monthly and quarterly subscription arrangements are maintained, a registration terminates automatically if payment is not received on or before the due date.

All this legislation does not differentiate between profit and non-profit making UK insurers. For 'offshore' (foreign) insurers, however, the legal requirements differ as between companies with a head office in an EEC member state and other foreign companies. The relevant legislation is the 1981 Insurance Companies Act (sections 8 and 9) and the Insurance Companies Regulations 1981 and these controls give the Trade Department the capacity to regulate and monitor foreign insurers.

How are contributions set?

Once a company has met the legal requirements, it has to design policies to sell to subscribers. The subscribers may be individual or corporate, and the insurers will seek to design different policies for particular segments of the market. This behaviour will be more apparent if for-profit firms are in the market. If a non-profit making firm sets its contributions on a community rating basis it would determine subscriptions by taking the whole population together, i.e. good and bad risks would be averaged out. A profit-making firm could then identify segments of this community who were paying in excess of their actuarial risks, in effect subsidizing in the community rating scheme the bad risks who are offered a contribution rate below their actuarial risk. If the profit making company then marketed a scheme whose contributions were related to the actuarial characteristics of the 'good risks', they could 'cream' the non-profit making market, getting the good risks and offering them similar benefits at lower contributions, leaving the non-profit making market with the 'bad' risks.

The non-profit making firm which uses community rating does so because in theory at least it can save on certain administrative costs (one general scheme rather than many individually tailored risk schemes). It however always runs the risk of being 'creamed'. It cannot offer competitive contributions unless it either has tax advantages or is more efficient than the profit-making scheme. Tax advantages are costly to the Exchequer and the incentives for efficiency in non-profit making schemes are generally muted (unlike the profit-making scheme, the directors of the non-profit-making scheme do not gain directly from increased efficiency). Thus in a competitive market, the non-profit making schemes will be forced to take the residue of the market (the poorer risks with higher costs and premiums) or they will be obliged to set their premiums in relation to their actuarial experiences. Community rating is unlikely to survive, other things being equal, if profit seeking insurers are active in the insurance market and they can identify substantial groups, or market segments, whose actuarial characteristics are good. Experience rating, by which the claims experience of particular groups are pooled to assess future contribution levels for that group, is likely to predominate in the high-growth competitive sectors of the market, e.g. group schemes. For homogeneous groups community rating will survive. In the former case the community rating will closely parallel experience rating and in the latter group no obvious market segment will exist as a base for experience rating.

Subscription contribution rates are generally offered on a yearly basis. The contributions are set usually at the beginning of the contract period and operate until its renewal. The basic subscription rate will be related to actuarial risk, either community or experience based, i.e. scale of coverage, number of people covered (single, married, or family), the age of the eldest person in the regulation, and the availability of discounts for age (e.g. young people) or size of group.

Thus contributions are set in relation to the estimate by the carrier of the likely costs of the policy. The company can estimate these costs actuarially on a community or experience-related basis. If the company is seeking to minimize its cost and maximize its market share, it will trade off the likely higher administrative costs of experience rating against administrative cost economies of community rating. Its choice will be affected by market competition and the success and vigour of its management. The choices of the market leader in the UK, the British United Provident Association are that group schemes are experience rated, and BUPACARE (for individual subscribers) and company care (for company groups of less than fifty employees) are community rated. These choices reflect current market conditions in the UK.

The principal actors and characteristics of growth of the private health care insurance industry

The private health insurance industry in Britain is dominated by three carriers, one of which, British United Provident Association (BUPA created 1947), has a market share of 70 per cent. As can be seen from Table 1, the shares of the two other carriers, Private Patients Plan (PPP created 1952) and the Western Provident Association (WPA created 1952), have increased during the 1971–80 period but remain relatively small. As a result of the developments of the 1970s, BUPA's share of the market as a percentage of total subscription income in 1980 was 70·9 per cent, and that of PPP and WPA 23·3 per cent and 3·7 per cent respectively.

There are three basic types of subscribers to private health insurance: individual, occupational, and group. Individual subscribers are those who decide alone to pay their own premium. Subscribers who enrol by individual application through a group arranged by a professional body, association, or company and pay their own subscriptions, are termed occupational group subscribers. The final category, the group subscriber covers individuals who are part of a group whose premium is paid in part or in whole by the employer.

The size in thousands and the growth-rates of each of these categories of membership for BUPA and the other two provident associations are given in Table 2. In 1980 the total number of provident subscribers was 1,636,000 (1). Of this total the majority (53 per cent) were in group schemes and 30·3 per cent and 16·5 per cent respectively were in

Table 1. *Private health insurance: market shares 1971, 1976, and 1980 (in percentages*)*

	BUPA	PPP	WPA
1971	77·9	17·8	2·3
1976	76·4	20·5	1·7
1980	70·9	23·3	3·7

*As a percentage share of total subscription income
Source. Lee Donaldson Associates (1981)

Table 2. *Market shares by size, type of subscriber, and carrier,*
1976–80

	BUPA		Individual Subscribers PPP/WPA		TOTAL	
	No. 000's	% Change	No. 000's	% Change	No. 000's	% Change
(a) individual subscribers						
1976	229	− 6·1	46	− 8·0	275	− 6·5
1977	217	− 5·2	40	− 13·0	257	− 6·5
1978	212	− 2·3	37	− 7·5	249	− 3·1
1979	218	+ 2·8	42	+ 13·5	260	+ 4·4
1980	227	+ 4·1	43	+ 2·4	270	+ 3·8
1981	235	+ 3·5				
(b) occupational subscribers						
1976	239	− 7·0	96	− 7·7	335	− 7·2
1977	225	− 5·9	95	− 1·0	320	− 4·5
1978	233	+ 3·4	100	+ 5·3	333	+ 4·0
1979	263	+ 12·9	105	+ 5·0	368	+ 10.5
1980	381	+ 44·9	116	+ 10·5	497	+ 35·0
1981	466	+ 22·3				
(c) group subscribers						
1976	356	+ 2·6	91	+ 7·1	447	+ 3·5
1977	375	+ 5·3	105	+ 15·4	480	+ 7·4
1978	409	+ 9·1	127	+ 21·0	536	+ 11·7
1979	491	+ 20·0	180	+ 41·7	671	+ 25·2
1980	639	+ 30·1	230	+ 27·0	869	+ 29·5
1981	694	+ 8·6				

Source. BUPA Internal Research Report 782

occupational groups or individual subscribers. Individual subscriptions were not only the smallest of the types of subscribers but also the slowest growing. In 1980 the group schemes growth rate was over 29 per cent for all three carriers and the rate of growth BUPA's occupational group category in that year was very large. The growth of the corporate schemes is especially noteworthy in the 1978–80 period because the economy was then relatively stagnant.

The data for 1981 are incomplete. The BUPA data do however indicate that for the market leader, the growth rates in subscriptions declined. Between 1980 and 1981 BUPA's total subscriber numbers grew from 1,247,000 to 1,395,000, i.e. by 11·8 per cent. The fastest growing group was occupa-

Table 3. *Coverage and subscribers 1950–80 (selected years)*

Year	Persons Insured (thousand)	Subscribers (thousand)	Annual net change (thousand)
1950	120	56	7
1955	585	274	52
1960	995	467	48
1965	1445	680	48
1970	1982	930	44
1975	2315	1087	− 9
1976	2251	1057	− 30
1977	2254	1057	0
1978	2388	1118	61
1979	2765	1292	174
1980	3577	1647	355

Note. The revised figure for total subscribers is 1636 (see Table 2)

Source. Lee Donaldson Associates (1981)

tional subscribers and the rate of growth of group subscriptions had fallen back substantially. It seems from this evidence that 1980 was an unusual year and the growth rate fell back considerably in 1981.

Each subscriber may mean more than one person covered. Table 3 shows the evolution of the membership coverage of the three largest provident associations over the period 1950–80. These data show that growth can be both negative (decline) and positive (rise). By 1980 the coverage of the three associations exceeded 3·5 million. This represents a substantial growth (1981 data awaited).

Generally these members are members of the working population and their dependents. By and large they are in the higher income groups, relatively well educated, and in good health. Their typical health profile is good in terms of health status and their demands for health care are usually limited to 'repairs' largely of a surgical nature.

The big three provident schemes are not the only insurance carriers. As can be seen from Table 4 however the income and expenditure of their rivals is very small indeed. This table also shows the rapidity of growth in income and expenditure in the 1976–80/1 period, the levels of activity more than doubled in monetary terms in 5/6 years.

Table 4. *UK Provident Associations, income and expenditure,*
1976–81

	BUPA	PPP	WPA	All Others*	Total
(a) Income (£m)					
1976	54·693	14·640	1·241	0·963	71·537
1977	69·129	19·899	1·696	1·299	92·023
1978	78·717	23·780	2·558	1·835	106·890
1979	90·345	27·841	3·874	2·328	124·388
1980	111·715	36·718	5·907	3·245	157·585
(b) Expenditure (£m)					
1976	41·256	10·944	0·946	0·703	53·849
1977	50·075	13·329	1·274	0·876	65·554
1978	50·685	15·019	1·973	1·112	68·789
1979	60·014	20·887	3·055	1·643	85·599
1980	92·744	30·043	4·823	2·291	129·901

*There are six other small provident associations: the Bristol Contributory Welfare Association (BCWA), the Civil Service Medical Aid Association (CSMAA), the Exeter Hospital Aid Society (EHAS), the Provincial Hospital Services Association (PHSA), Private Patients (Anglia) Limited (PPA), and the Revenue Provident Association (RPA).

Source. Lee Donaldson Associates (1981), Table 1.

In addition to the provident associations there are two main commercial carriers of private health insurance. The Crusader Insurance Company Limited and the Allied Medical Assurance Services Limited (which subinsures at Lloyds) concentrate on the provision of company insurance schemes. The premium income of these two firms is between one and two per cent of the total provident income—in 1980 about £1·5m to £3m. Mutual of Omaha, an American new (1981) entrant to this market place, also aims to provide insurance for the company market but at present its market share is quite small.

The other organizations concerned with the finance of health care are the Hospital Contributory Schemes (HCS). These are registered as non-profit making insurance companies but are separate and different from the provident associations. The HCS provide cash benefits to subscribers when they are ill regardless of whether health care treatment is offered in NHS or private institutions. Generally these cash benefits are not designed to meet the full costs of private medical treatment and pay only nominal amounts for inpatient hospital stays and for optical, dental, maternity and convalescence services. Between 1974 and 1980 the number of HCS subscribers rose from 3·3 million to 3·5 million and the premium income grew from £10·94m to £27·46m (Lee Donaldson, 1981).

The data in Table 4 put the economic role of the private sector in general and the provident associations in particular, in perspective. In 1980 the expenditure of all the provident associations was £129·9m. In 1980 total NHS expenditure was £11,875m, some 6·14 per cent of Gross National Product (GNP) (Office of Health Economics, 1981). Provident association expenditure on health care was thus 1·09 per cent of NHS expenditure and 0·06 per cent of GNP. The provident associations operations are relatively small compared to the NHS and their role should not be exaggerated.

Some of the characteristics of the data in Table 4 are of interest. The consistent and large gap between the income and expenditure of the provident associations must mean that they either have large reserves and/or have used their surpluses to finance activities other than the reimbursement of the health care costs of their subscribers. Thus BUPA appears to have financed their hospital building programme, in part at least, out of surpluses and reserves. Another fact which cannot be discerned from the data in Table 4 or from other sources is the extent of *ex gratia* payments, i.e. the degree to which reimbursement is determined by agreed tariff rates and the discretion of the associations. In 1981 BUPA, the largest carrier, made its first operating loss. This indicator of the market difficulties facing the associations after the 1980 'boom' begs clearer definition of the nature of the market 'turn round'. Better data on all these aspects of the associations would be useful to those interested in the monitoring and evaluation of the private sector: and especially to distinguish what is *not* going to private providers.

There are, no doubt, several reasons for the recent rapid growth rate of these associations. From the growth of occupational subscribers category, it is clear that the providents identified and exploited a new market. It seems that there were a variety of contributory factors to the creation of this new market. The Labour Government's Incomes Policy in 1978–9 did not regulate benefits and left employers free, if it did not positively encourage them, to pay labour in a non-pecuniary fashion, e.g. with private health care benefits. Also this Policy led to strikes in the NHS and deleterious effects on waiting lists. This Incomes Policy coincided with the approach of an election with an avowedly market-orientated option being offered to the electorate by the Conservatives. When the Conservatives entered office in May 1979 the private sector became much more aggressive in their marketing, as can be seen from the expansion of media advertising, in particular the use of television advertising for the first time.

It is likely that this market was exploited aggressively with premium-setting practices which were bold and set in relation to perhaps relatively little knowledge of the actuarial risks involved: the markets into which the industry expanded were relatively uncharted territory. Possibly this policy will be proved unwise, as actuarial knowledge improves and outlays are shown to be higher than anticipated: the 1981 results for BUPA indicate this is so. If this proves to be the case, the marketing practice can be defended as sound given the stock of information at the time of market launch, and reasonable in the light of political encouragement to expand the role of the private sector given by the Conservative Government.

The outlook for future growth seems to be 'slow but sure'. The view of Derek Damerall of BUPA (*The Times*, February 1982) is that growth has reached something of a plateau and there is no reason to believe that the very high growth rate of 1980 will be repeated. Slower growth seems inevitable unless there is a deliberate attempt by government to stimulate demand with, for example tax advantages. Such tax advantages would benefit the relatively affluent individuals who subscribed or companies and would reduce the yield of income and corporation tax. It is doubtful whether such policies are likely to be attractive to politicians either on public expenditure or distribution grounds. The health care insurance industry has grown rapidly from a very small base to a level which remains insignificant in terms of the

National Health Service: expenditure on health care by the big three Provident Associations is only just over one per cent of NHS expenditure. The indications are that the recent period of rapid growth has ended and that growth levels will be much more modest in the years to come. Despite its small size, the private insurance sector offers substantial benefits in a relatively narrow range of activities to its subscribers and their dependents, a total of some 3,577,000 people in 1980.

The benefits structure in private health care insurance

Contributions to private health care insurance schemes can give the subscriber benefits in terms of cash refunds or in kind services. Both types of benefit are always limited in extent. There is no open-ended commitment by the carrier. UK insurers provide cash benefits generally up to predetermined limits on expenditure.

Practice does however vary between the companies. The majority of benefits offered by the British United Provident Association (BUPA) are subject to cash limits of one kind or another, e.g. limits on payments to specialists for operations, per annum outpatient payments, etc. These limits vary between the different policies offered by BUPA and are clearly set out in all the contracts. Private Patients Plan (PPP) offer on their Company Masterplan 1 and Family Masterplan 1 Schemes, relatively open-ended benefits (except for outpatient treatment and hospital cash refunds), up to an annual maximum expenditure of £30,000. PPP are innovators in that they alone also market a dental scheme underwritten by Lloyds. The other substantial private carrier. Western Provident Association (WPA), have cash limits on most of their benefits. The exception is WPA's Company Supercover which provides open-ended benefits with no limit for every category of care, except accommodation, hospital cash, and maternity cash. WPA are the only private health insurance company out of the 'big three' market leaders in the UK to have any links with a company offering long term disability insurance, (this is known as Permanent Health Insurance (PHI)). If a subscriber to such a Life Assurance Company as Friends Provident is accepted as a standard life for PHI, then that person is automatically eligible for a forty per cent discount off the basic WPA subscription rate.

These provident associations and the other insurers in the private health care market provide finance for a relatively narrow range of services. It is probable that if the companies published the data, it would be seen that the majority of their expenditure (at least sixty per cent perhaps) might be seen to finance a narrow range of surgical activities. These activities are largely 'running repairs', e.g. hernias, haemorrhoids, varicose veins, and minor gynaecological procedures such as D+Cs. It is important to note that this market is largely surgical. This may account for the surgeons relative enthusiasm for and the physicians relative disinterest in, private practice.

In most respects the insurers are price-takers, i.e. they accept the bills put to them and refund those monies demanded by the medical care providers; and it is an exception for specialist claims to be questioned. The British United Provident Association have set what appears to be quite generous fees for operations. These are divided into four categories and priced (1982) between £145 and £575 per surgical procedure. The other two carriers offer full refunds on their policies. The degree, if any, of disputation over fees is a matter over which insurers and providers are reluctant to disclose. If patient demands are high and the insurers run into financial pressures, as has happened elsewhere in the western world, it is likely that the insurers will be induced to monitor the quantity and quality of work carried out and negotiate the fees paid with more vigour than hitherto. This likelihood will probably become more certain if the consumer movement develops in health care, and dissatisfied consumers have recourse to consumer protection legislation. At present, however, the insurers are price takers and generally financial intermediaries who usually pay the provider the 'accepted' (usual, customary, and reasonable) rate for the job out of subscription income.

An inevitable risk for any subscriber is that the costs of the private health care which is consumed may exceed the benefits payable by the insurer. The extent of such shortfalls varies between the different benefit types. If shortfall is defined as the difference between that claimed by, and that paid to subscribers, then one of the biggest private insurers met about 96·8 per cent of all claims, and only 5·5–6·5 per cent of subscribers to currently marketed schemes had a shortfall. However for the same firm in 1980, fifteen to twenty-two per cent of all claimants for all schemes (currently and formerly marketed) had shortfalls and on average only eighty-nine per cent of claimed costs were met. This latter outcome is produced by subscribers adhering to old policies which have not kept pace with inflation, it is hardly surprising that benefit rates adequate in 1970 are inadequate for the 1980s! Generally the impression, from the limited data that are available, is that the extent of shortfall of benefits to costs is quite small, especially for current policies which are attuned to the likely expenditure realities of the 1980s.

During the last few years the private health care market has grown rapidly. What was previously a small market in which relatively few actors, in terms of financers and providers, operated has grown into a bigger market place in which the actors are probably less informed about each others characteristics. Financial pressure, with expenditure growing more rapidly than income, may oblige the insurers, as it has in foreign health care markets, to question increasingly what is 'usual, customary, and reasonable' (UCR) in the behaviour of providers, both doctors, hospitals, and others. UCR in the United States has been found, on occasion to be an inefficient payment of monopoly rates, i.e. what is usual and customary may not be reasonable! Furthermore with UCR being paid for by the insurers, both providers and patients may be electing for inefficient use of resources. For instance it has been shown that day-case surgery for hernias is clinically, economically, and socially preferred but insurers pay for what the specialists advise (generally five-day stays), what the patients like (four days' bed rest) and what the hospital owners prefer (five days' payment for hospital beds). There is no incentive for insurer, patient, or provider to seek efficiency in the use of scarce private sector resources.

Clearly if one insurer introduces effective peer review and medical audit and the effects of this on utilization are to reduce costs, then this may be reflected in the more rapid growth of this carrier's market. Yet as long as the likely present over-payment and inefficiency is condoned by all carriers, private insurance will, like public providers (the NHS), protect inefficiency in the use of scarce resources (Maynard and Ludbrook, 1980). The decision by BUPA to discriminate against providers and seek to monitor more carefully the services given to their clients is a welcome first step on the inevitable road to greater regulation of private providers by private financiers.

Overview and perspective

The private health insurance industry has grown rapidly in the last five years but is still minute in comparison to the National Health Service. It offers to its 3·5 million members what is essentially a narrow package of medical care. Generally it does not provide long-term care for chronic cases (e.g. the elderly, the mentally ill, the terminally ill, or the handicapped). It does not provide primary care (despite private experiments most primary care remains in the public (NHS) domain) or, except for PPP, dental care. Emergency care is also catered for in the public sector.

What does the private sector provide? It provides those willing and able to pay for it with benefits which permit choice of consultant, place and time for non-emergency primarily 'cold' surgery. The choices of specialist, location (particularly with special comforts) and timing are important to many people. Waiting time for cold surgery is a fact of NHS life, although its causes are unclear; it has declined since 1978 and it could probably be reduced further by better work practices (e.g. more day-case surgery). People do not want to wait for care in pain and discomfort. They prefer to choose a well-regarded specialist in a pleasant location. While these preferences remain and the price is right, people will continue to purchase private health insurance. In a free society the exercise of such choices is perhaps unavoidable.

THE PRIVATE PROVISION OF HEALTH CARE

The last five years has seen a rapid change in the provision of private health care in the United Kingdom. One effect of the Labour Administration's seeming policy to reverse Bevan's 1948 decision to permit private practice in NIIS hospitals has been actually to encourage the rapid development of private hospitals to meet the increased demand for private care. Successive Incomes Policies and the natural propensities of the NHS to control the renumeration of doctor, nurse, and other health workers has created a ready pool of labour prepared to work in the private sector.

It is important in analysing these trends and seeking to see why private medicine has developed to try to answer two related questions about the period since 1948: why has the supply of doctor's time for private practice expanded? and why has the provision of private hospital beds changed?

Why has private practice expanded?

There is a simple answer to this question. It is that demand has risen due to rising patient incomes and increased insurance coverage. This answer however masks the pathways by which NHS doctors are permitted to work in the private sector.

In 1946 under Section 5 of the Act, Bevan conceded the establishment of private pay-beds in NHS hospitals and part-time contracts for NHS consultants because he wished to ensure that the public sector acquired the services of the best specialists. Without pay-beds and the part-time contract, his fear was that the best specialists would work in the private sector. The arrangements provided by Bevan enabled the consultant to supplement his income with the rewards of some private practice and ensured that the consultant was operating usually in the same hospital unit, i.e. travel time between his private and public roles was minimized.

As Forsyth points out the fee a surgeon might charge a private patient was limited, to between fifty and seventy-five guineas, until 1966 and this fee covered pre- and post-operative work as well as the surgical procedure. The removal of this ceiling by Kenneth Robinson meant that the insurers lost some protection but it was the price paid by the Minister in order to get consultant agreement to the reduction of pay-beds from five to one per cent of the total NHS stock. This somewhat cosmetic reduction was merited on efficiency grounds as pay-bed utilization was very low, i.e. the private health care market was stagnant in the 1960s.

At the same time there was an attempt to increase the number of people appointed to full-time consultant posts. Again, there was a compromise between the 'barons' of the medical profession and the Minister. Maximum part-time (9/11) consultants could be required to work an additional, unpaid session for the NHS and successful applicants to consultant posts were not required to specify whether they would work full-time until they were offered the post (a fudging of the original Robinson demand). The unpaid session became a bone of contention and this together with incomes policies and the generous new GP contract introduced after 1966, made the consultants' discontent grow as their real incomes relative to GPs' declined.

The recent (1981) consultant contract continued the practice of making private practice an easy option for which to elect. The proposed alteration of the consultant-junior ratio (Department of Health and Social Security, 1982) is however likely to complicate matters considerably. First, more consultant appointments will generate more competition for the available private practice work and it is a matter for speculation how this will affect fees and professional relationships. Secondly, fewer juniors will mean that consultants may have inadequate cover for their NHS patients. As a consequence their ability to do private work may be affected deleteriously. No crystal ball is needed to imagine such effects are likely to lead to disputes.

In any event the consultant, by selecting his preferred NHS contract, can work part-time or full-time for the public sector. The effects of government incomes policies has been, despite some redress in 1979, to hold back consultants pay relatively and provide an increased pecuniary incentive to undertake private practice. Clearly this practice is highly skewed geographically with more private work existing in the south and east than in the provinces, and in particular specialties (e.g. cold surgery). This unequal distribution of rewards has inevitable effects on the labour market.

How does private practice work by consultants affect the work of the NHS? The consultant is appointed and employed by the Region. The District and the Region can only guess at what sort of contract will be selected by the successful consultant. The great (and worst) tradition of the NHS is not to evaluate what happens in its hospitals so it is not clear whether the consultants have full- or part-time contracts, how much time is given to NHS. If the letter of contract were met, in reality it is likely that some part-timers may do 'too much' and some full-timers 'too little'. Thus if everything else (especially the relative efficiency of full- and part-time) was equal a part-time consultant should do less in the NHS, for one effect would be that he would treat private patients in place of NHS patients. This deleterious effect on the consultants' NHS 'output' would be worsened if the private practice was located in separate locations, access to which involved travel time costs met by the public service.

The casual tradition of the NHS not to monitor the effects of its labour contracts means it is not possible to determine whether scarce resources are used efficiently. In the interest of efficiency surely there should be a careful evaluation of the effects of contracts on the labour supply of doctors, nurses, and other workers. Unless such monitoring is carried out it will not be possible to evaluate the full costs and benefits of the part-time contract for consultants. Bevan's decision was based on the thesis that such contracts are the price to be paid to keep powerful and important elements of the medical profession in the NHS. There is a school of thought which feels the merits of this method of avoiding a split between private and public practice by doctors need to be debated more fully and evaluated carefully: a cost/benefit analysis of policy.

In summary, hospital specialists in the UK are able to work in NHS either full-time or part-time. The majority are of course full-time consultants and part-time contracts tend to exist in those specialties (especially surgery) and locations (especially the south-east) where patients are willing and able to purchase private care. The policy is clearly convenient to the medical profession: e.g. if surgeons cared for fifty private patients in the year they could augment their NHS salaries by £12,000 to £28,000 per year at existing BUPA pay rates. The effects of this work on the NHS are far from clear due to the lack of evaluation.

Private practice and hospitals: why has it changed?

As has been indicated Bevan favoured private practice in NHS pay-beds. Robinson, in 1966 reduced the supply of pay-beds because of their under-utilization, i.e. the lack of private demand. In 1975 Castle proposed and implemented to a substantial degree the policy of removing pay-beds from NHS hospitals. The logic of this policy seemed to be largely ideological, i.e. an opposition to private practice and the alleged subsidization of the pay-beds out of NHS revenues (2).

As a result of the Health Services Act 1976 the number of pay-beds was decreased considerably in the late 1970s. The figures however indicate that although the decline in the stock of pay-beds was substantial (a forty-three per cent reduction from 4444 beds in 1976 to 2533 pay-beds in 1980), the relative importance of the issue was largely symbolic; as a percentage of the NHS bed stock it was very small before the decision was taken.

The Conservative Government reversed public policy on pay-beds with the 1980 Health Services Act. This legislation abolished the statutory body which supervised the decline of the pay beds in the 1977–80 period, and delegated the power to control new private bed developments to the health authorities. The new District Health Authorities now have the power to control all new developments with more than 120 beds. Furthermore, if the District has more than 120 private beds, it can get the Secretary of State to designate it, in which case the District can control all new private developments for five years.

The effects of these policy changes on private bed provision are likely to be complex, as noted by Klein. The effect of the policy on NHS pay beds seems to be a reversal of the 1977–80 trend. By the end of 1981 the Department of Health

Table 5. *Private, surgical beds and hospitals 1975–80, Great Britain*

Year	Hospital	Beds
1975	105	2279
1976	128	2802
1977	130	3305
1978	141	2971
1979	142	3033
1980	153	3150

Source. Registered Nursing Homes in the U.K. & Republic of Ireland. BUPA
(personal communication)

had approved 95 extra pay-beds and 107 'emergency' pay-beds since the 1980 Act. Applications for another 105 new pay-beds were awaiting approval. Thus, in just over a year the NHS had responded to the new legislation by proposing increases in the pay-bed stock of over 12 per cent, (307 in addition to the 2533 stock in 1980).

The impact of Castle's pay-bed policy has however had an influence outside the NHS. Denied access to NHS pay-beds, the private sector responded by expanding the stock of beds for private patients outside the NHS (3). Table 5 sets out the details of the expansion of private, surgical beds in Great Britain in the period 1975–80. This table shows a growth in the number of private, surgical hospitals from 105 to 153 and a growth in such beds of thirty-eight per cent, from 2279 to 3150.

The projected expansion (1980–2) in the private surgical bed stock is substantial (Table 6), an addition of nearly 800 in England with significant developments in NW Thames, North Western, and the West Midlands especially. BUPA Hospitals Limited data (Table 7) indicate further that expansion plans are ambitious. Again, American for-profit involvement in this market is now substantial. The ownership of these hospitals is set out in Table 8: thirty-seven per cent of the hospitals are owned by charities, twenty-one per cent by religious orders, and forty-two per cent are owned in part by foreign, and particularly American, groups (these are set out in the footnote to the table). All these data ignore private 'special' hospitals for cancer, convalescence, day-care, maternity, the mentally ill, and other 'chronic' groups.

Table 6. *Regional distribution of projected expansion in private beds,*
1980–2, England.

NHS Region	Projected Beds Expansion
Northern	36
Yorkshire	45
Trent	25
E. Anglia	15
N.W. Thames	258
N.E. Thames	—
S.E. Thames	36
S.W. Thames	—
Wessex	—
Oxford	48
S. Western	25
W. Midlands	104
Mersey	40
N. Western	150
	782

Source. BUPA Hospitals Limited (personal communications)

The effects of this expansion in the private and public sectors will soon more than offset the decline in the number of pay-beds in the 1976–80 period (4). The nature of this expansion should be made quite clear: it is geographically uneven (Table 6), the role of the not-for-profits is significant and that of the for-profits, particularly the American, hospitals is limited, and, in terms of plans, declining (Table 7). The thrust of these developments is in a relatively narrow range of health care, surgery.

Thus the effects of the Labour Governments pay-beds policy and the expansion of private insurance has been a substantial investment in private hospital beds for surgery. The effects of the reduction in pay-beds has now been compensated for and, as can be seen by the plans of the for-profit organizations (Table 7), there are some indications that the rate of expansion of the private sector bed stock is waning.

These changes are quite slight in terms of the bed stock of the NHS: in 1980 there were 2544 NHS pay-beds and 3150 private surgical beds while in 1979 there were 296,815 non-psychiatric NHS beds (Office of Health Economics, 1981,

Table 7. *The likely expansion of private hospital beds (UK).*

	Currently Building	Planned
BUPA hospitals	148	333
Nuffield Nursing Homes Trust	32	69
Other Charitable	91	12
American profit motivated	265	188
Other profit motivated	319	254
Total	855	856

Source. BUPA Hospitals Limited (personal communication)

Table 8. *The ownership of private hospitals, 1981, UK.*

Religious	28	21%
Charitable	51	37%
Other*	58	42%
	137	100%

*Of those in the 'other' category 5 are foreign owned for profit (of which 1 is American managed), 6 are American (The Harley Street, the Princess Grace, the Wellington in London, the Princess Margaret in Windsor, the Clementine Churchill at Harrow and the Alexandra at Cheadle, Manchester) and 1 (St Anthonys at Cheam) is religious but American managed.

Source. BUPA Hospitals Limited (personal communication).

Table 3.1), i.e. the private bed stock was 1·9 per cent of that of the NHS. With the apparent reduced growth of private insurance industry and the rising number of pay-beds, it is unlikely that the surge of investment into private hospitals for surgical care will be sustained.

It is to be emphasized that the analysis hitherto has been concerned with private health care that is financed by insurance, i.e. largely acute care. There is another private sector in health care which is substantial, growing and regarded with a totally different attitude by opponents of privatization (5). This is the nursing homes market for the elderly. This market is likely to expand rapidly because of the 'greying' of the UK population. It is possible the increased number of elderly people will generate via individual and family income, social security, and other routes, resources to sustain a substantial expansion in the private nursing homes market. Indeed it is somewhat surprising that the Conservative Government has been slow to give special encouragement to this sector.

Private practice: why it has developed

Private practice has expanded because of the self interest of the actors in the market for private medical practice. The government has regulated the private sector and organized the public sector to serve rather ill-defined goals. The policies it has adopted to achieve these goals have not been evaluated carefully: a careful cost benefit analysis of the Bevan and Castle policies is noticeable by its absence. Without doubt the governments, both Labour and Conservative, by negative policies (such as phasing out pay-beds) and positive policies (such as encouraging private insurance, which rewarded providers and met patient preferences) have helped to create the present outcomes.

It has to be emphasized that these outcomes are modest. The private bed stock for surgical work is quite small and the involvement of surgeons in private work is significant but limited. The privatization of health care in Britain over the last decade has been marginal and relates to a small subset (largely surgery) of the total health care market. Extrapolation of short-term trends, as happened in 1980–81, is mischievous and is unlikely to reflect accurately the long-term growth patterns of the industry.

PRIVATE HEALTH CARE INSURANCE: WITHER OR WHITHER EXPANSION?

How can the growth of the private health care market be sustained and at what cost to whom? Whether the expansion of the private health care market withers away or continues, a variety of factors are likely to generate increased regulation, from within and from without the private sector. What are these factors and what regulation will arise?

Expansion: how and at what cost?

There are a variety of policies that a government, which is intent on encouraging the growth of private health insurance could adopt. By political statements and encouragement of NHS-private co-operation it creates an explicit policy stance. This 'moral persuasion' might not have any direct 'opportunity' costs, unlike more radical policies of a positive and negative nature.

An obvious negative approach which would favour privatization would be policies which affected the capacity of the NHS to provide health care. An extreme macro-policy would be to reduce the rate of growth of expenditure or even cut it back in real terms. Such cuts, together with demographic change (e.g. the increased number of elderly needing NHS care), would lead to the expansion of demand for private care to compensate for the contraction of the public supply of health care. Those willing and able to purchase private health care might do so if these changes led to increases in the waiting time for care in the NHS.

The Conservative Government which was elected in 1979 clearly did not wish to adopt such a radical policy. They used moral persuasion but maintained the real growth of resources available to the NHS. Pay limits (e.g. four per cent in 1982) and assumptions about increases in the retail price index (nine per cent in 1982) were unrealistic and the effects of not funding the higher pay increases out of public monies meant, in a highly labour-intensive industry in which, for example, nurse labour costs alone are in excess of forty per cent of the total NHS budget, that the pressure to cut services was present.

This pressure was increased by the Government's policy on priorities. Since the mid-1970s there has been all-party agreement that there should be a relative shift of resources from acute care into the 'Cinderella' services, i.e. care of the elderly, the mentally ill, the chronic sick, and the handicapped (see e.g. Department of Health and Social Security, 1976a). The Conservative Government, particularly since 1981, has restated this policy and announced its intention to 'monitor' developments in the constituent parts of the NHS to ensure that its priorities policy is carried out. The paradox of this redistributive policy, which in the event seems more socialist than conservative, is that unless the acute sector compensates for resource switches away from it and towards the priorities sector, by increasing the efficiency with which it uses its residual resources, waiting time will increase and the private sector will in response be able to develop its market. Thus the implementation of the priorities policy may paradoxically encourage privatization of the acute sector! The political assumption is that acute care can be made more efficient but whether it can develop in this manner at a rate sufficient to compensate resource losses is unknown. The ultimate outcome to this problem will be that, as in the past, the NHS acute care sector will be reluctant to contract. After all expenditure in acute care equals the incomes of surgeons, nurses, and other workers, not all of whom could be shifted easily into other activities if private finance does not grow rapidly enough.

The negative policy towards the NHS has not been implemented by the Conservative Government in a way which could convince any neutral observer that it meant to reduce the size of the NHS. The NHS seems to be a 'sacred cow' and if privatization is to develop, the only alternative public policy is positive encouragement of the private sector so that it supplements rather than supplants public action.

Supplementation cannot however be easily induced without reduced public revenues. For instance if the existing tax offsets to individuals earning less than £8500 per annum and receiving benefits from employers were extended so that the cost to firms and individuals of purchasing private health care insurance was reduced, this would reduce the revenue yield of the corporation and income tax system. Such offsets would make incomes policies much more difficult to manage (when they were in favour!) and would have redistributional characteristics. Essentially the benefits would accrue to the more affluent, a policy which might be politically unacceptable.

Thus further supplementation policies might not increase the resources available for health care. The typical Treasury view of user charges in the NHS has been that revenues from such charges are a substitute for taxation. This view might be extended to cover private insurance and its growth could be used as a basis for cutting NHS funding.

If private funding increased, the incidence of its growth would be geographically unequal and this would raise questions about the Government's policy of equalizing the financial capacity of the regions by using resource allocation formulae such as that devised by the Resource Allocation Working Party (RAWP) in 1976 (Department of Health and Social Security, 1976b). Klein discusses these problems in an earlier chapter: the fundamental point is that if private and public expenditures are summed and the RAWP formula applied, the London regions will lose further public resources because of the concentration of private work there, and the capacity of the London NHS services to provide services on the basis of need, as opposed to willingness and ability to pay, will be less than that of northern regions. Whether such outcomes are compatible with government objectives, let alone politically 'feasible', is not known but requires consideration.

There is no systematic evidence which demonstrates that the private provision of health care is more efficient than that in the NHS; both systems seem to have common lamentable reluctance to evaluate what they do (see Maynard, below). The expansion of the system of private health raises major problems for a distribution policy. What will happen to RAWP? What distributional goals in health and health care are we seeking as a nation to achieve? The case based on efficiency and distribution for privatization is unclear but it is apparent that such developments can only be acquired at significant costs either by giving tax rebates to encourage private consumption and/or reducing the scale of NHS operations. The latter policy and the former policy have significant hidden costs and clearly the Conservative Government is not unaware of these costs: it is pursuing neither policy with any vigour and its efforts at moral persuasion (i.e. occasional statements bordering on the platitudinous about the virtues of private enterprise in health care) are hardly vote-catchers. The costs of radical change are too great to the actors in the health care market. Marginal change may continue but unless there are major economic problems, arising from the Falklands adventure or the decline of the UK economy, the costs, in terms of dislocation to existing NHS policies and the public expenditure losses of tax offsets, of fundamental change are likely to dissuade policy makers from adopting radical innovations.

The inevitability of increased regulation

It does seem however that the rationale and form of the regulation of the private sector, both the private health care insurance industry and the private provision of care is likely to alter.

At present the private health care insurance industry acts largely as a financial intermediary: it collects contributions and spends these monies in response to billings by providers. The industry has always been aware of the need to monitor provider deviance (e.g. charging for work not done or charging in excess of usual, customary, and reasonable fees) and when the market was small this could be done in an informal manner. The growth of the market makes the amount of work involved in monitoring increase and puts pressures on the auditing system. The provident advisers no longer know all the providers and communication difficulties inevitably lead to greater resistance from providers when challenged by the auditors. Such changes may oblige the financers to develop more detailed information and monitoring capacity. It is not unreasonable that in time they will be forced to emulate the French, the Australians, and others in developing 'health care profiles' of the providers so that their decisions, and their resource implications, can be discerned, compared with their peers, and, if necessary, challenged to induce eventually coincidence with practice norms.

Another pressure which will influence the development of information and monitoring, is the consumer. The consumer protection legislation is clear in this intent and could be used by dissatisfied patients to challenge either the financers or providers of health care. For instance it could be argued that the provident companies offer a service and with that service goes a guarantee of its quality. If the quality was inadequate a patient could challenge the companies on the grounds that they had a contractual obligation to monitor and evaluate the quality of the services they financed out of their customers' contributions.

Alternatively the patient could challenge the provider directly in the courts if the services provided were apparently of poor quality. Presumably a case under the consumer protection legislation would have to be carried through by reference to detailed scrutiny of provider behaviour in the particular case and a comparison of this behaviour with established norms of medical practice. Such a comparison would necessitate the provision of a system of information generation and evaluation. If the providers did not have such a system, the defence of such legal cases would be difficult, indeed possibly embarrassing if the prosecution was well informed and aggressive. Thus the self-interest of providers may lead to the development of increased evaluation.

The pressure to develop and use information systems will be increased by other factors. At present the Department of Health and Social Security has a steering group, under the chairmanship of Mrs Körner, working on the development of health services information. This group wrote to the Department (April 1982) to ascertain its views on the information requirements for private hospitals. Clearly there would be many advantages to have an integrated (public and private) information system in health care: public policy would be easier to plan, implement and monitor.

Conflicts in the change from public/private mix

Already there is a variety of conflicts arising from the change in the public-private mix. For instance the private sector as it expands is using an increasing number of doctors and nurses who were trained at public expense. This has led to some strange demands from, *inter alia*, it is believed Conservative Ministers. One such demand is that the private sector should pay its 'share' of the cost of training these professionals and there has been discussion of the possible introduction of a levy to attain this objective. This is a novel idea. Many lawyers, architects, and accountants have large parts of their training publicly financed but there is no call for a levy on these industries. The logic of the levy proposal is not clear unless it is that private health care should be taxed on its publicly trained labour, in a way different from other sectors.

Despite the dubious logic of the levy however, the development of the private sector will have serious implications for the NHS. More doctors time will be devoted to private activity and it is possible that the renumeration of both doctors and nurses will be bid up by the private sector. Even if wages do not rise, the quality of the private environment may attract labour out of the NHS and this will contribute to its staffing problems. If these staffing problems are not resolved, NHS services will be affected. If they are resolved, the expenditure implications, in terms of training and employment, may be unattractive to the government.

If the private sector reacted to the levy proposals and criticism of their use of NHS-trained staff, this reaction might take the form of the development of private training facilities. For instance it is not inconceivable that the private University College of Buckingham might develop a medical and nursing school. The logic of such a development is not inconsiderable but if the problems were overcome the benefits would be mixed. True, the private sector would have then to shoulder, if the students were privately financed, the cost burden of training. The government would however lose control of the source of supply of doctors and nurses. This may not be a minor cost if it is accepted that doctors are the main decision-makers in a health care system and that decisions of a consultant on average in the NHS (or elsewhere more) cost £500,000 in terms of doctor, nurse, other workers, drug, and bed time (Owen, 1976, updated).

The regulation of private supply

The acceptance by the government of the argument that doctor supply does have implications for (or generate) health care expenditure would seem inevitably to bring with it a decision to regulate private supply rigorously. This regulation could take the form of a quota but clearly such regulation would be very difficult given the competing interests of the government, the professional associations (the BMA) and a regulating body such as the GMC, and the private sector.

The general thrust of current Government policy is to monitor the NHS more carefully in an effort to ensure that the taxpayer gets 'value for money'. This policy is leading to developments on many fronts: meetings with the Regions, responses by the Regions to develop a capacity to evaluate performance, the work of the Körner working groups, and the recognition by clinicians that competition for resources requires that they have to demonstrate increasingly the relative advantages of their proposals in relation to rival bids. Peer review, medical audit and budgeting, with and without rewards for the economizing clinicians and their teams, are seemingly unavoidable developments in the future.

As argued below (Maynard p.471) the health care systems of the post-war period have been characterized by the emphasis on increasing inputs (expenditure) and the failure to investigate whether these inputs led to increased outputs (in terms of improvements in health status) (see also Cochrane, 1972). It is this failure to evaluate which characterizes public and private health care throughout the world and will be challenged and reviewed in the years to come. The public and the private sectors will have to devise and implement more sophisticated and effective systems of monitoring and evaluation if the 'grand tradition' of firing money at problems and not determining whether such policies have any effects on these problems, is to be eradicated.

Thus the self-interest of the private sector and the public sector seems likely to lead to more regulation and evaluation of the private sector by itself and by the government. The problems of getting 'value for money' are the same for the Secretary of State of the Department of Health as they are for the Managing Director of BUPA or the Managing Director of Nuffield Nursing Homes. Privatization solves none of the basic health care problems, it merely sets them in new institutions which will be regulated in new ways in order to achieve efficiency and equity in the health care market.

NOTES

1. These data differ from those in the Lee Donaldson Associates (1981) Report because they incorporate revised (downwards) subscriber figures supplied to the author by BUPA.

2. If such a subsidy existed the logical policy was to identify its extent and remove it, a policy pursued vigorously since 1975 for the remaining beds. Such a policy could generate substantial revenues for the NHS.

3. This separation of private practice from NHS hospitals means that

part-time NHS consultants have increasingly to travel to practice privately.

4. Although the total private provision (pay-bed and private) of surgical beds will soon be restored to or above its 1976 level, it is likely that the changed mix (away from NHS pay-beds and towards separate private beds) will take longer to be reversed.

5. It is curious that this substantial market, or nursing care for the elderly, has not been developed by private insurance interests. With old age and dependency being a potential problem for most citizens, many consumers may wish to save during the working life to ensure the security of a good nursing home in old age.

BIBLIOGRAPHY

COCHRANE, A. L. (1972). *Effectiveness and Efficiency: Random reflections in health services.* (Nuffield Provincial Hospitals Trust: London).

DEPARTMENT OF HEALTH AND SOCIAL SECURITY (1976a). *Priorities for Health and Personal Social Services in England: a consultative document.* (HMSO: London).

— — (1976b). *Sharing Resources for Health in England.* (HMSO: London).

— — (1982). *Government Response to the Fourth Report from the Social Services Committee,* 1980–1 Session, Cmnd 8479. (HMSO: London).

LEE DONALDSON ASSOCIATES (1981). *Provident Scheme Statistics 1980.* Report for the Department of Health and Social Security.

MAYNARD, A. and LUDBROOK, A. (1980). 'What's Wrong with the National Health Service?', *Lloyds Bank Review,* October.

OFFICE OF HEALTH ECONOMICS (1981). *Compendium of Health Statistics,* 4th Edition.

OWEN, D. (1976). *In Sickness and in Health: The politics of health.* (Quartet Books: London).

PART

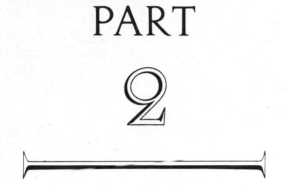

The Western European experience

The Western European experience

The Netherlands, Belgium
The Federal Republic of Germany
and France

In Europe, it must not be forgotten, governments play a large part in the health system as part of the conception of the Welfare State; each has developed using modes of compulsory insurance, the coverage of which ranges from a low of 70 per cent of the population in the Netherlands, to 90 per cent in the Federal Republic of Germany, and virtually 100 per cent in Belgium and France. It was evident in the initial reconnaissance for this study that all of these countries which covered the spectrum of experience we were seeking, were commonly concerned with closing or reducing the open-ended commitments of their systems in one way or another. In doing so, the actions being taken or discussed were inevitably likely to affect the public/private mix, above all by the introduction of regulations and controls which in some cases required new legislation, or in others imposed by fiats which virtually restrict prescriptive rights. This section, dealing with Western Europe, consists of essays by acknowledged experts with personal experience designed to provide a conspectus of experience of what is involved in current policies in the Netherlands, Belgium, Federal Republic of Germany, and France. Together they are intended to illuminate the nature of the problems currently faced by systems based on insurance schemes, and to identify the salient issues.

It is for note that while all the essays display the main concerns and features of social insurance systems, the directions shown of the present French position are perhaps different from the others. This is mainly because of the election in 1981 of a Socialist Government which was committed to retain most of the main features of the existing health system while seeking to reform them in certain particulars, to conform to broad ideological policies. Because of this we commissioned an additional essay on France by Rodwin, an American policy analyst who had been working in the CNAMTS and who has had a unique opportunity of studying the system of financing health services in France specially related to planning over recent years.

It thus also serves, because of the analytic techniques, as an introduction to the American position in the opening essay in Part 3 from McNerney—who writes authoritatively of the USA from a unique position in the world of insurance.

Health policy in the Netherlands

At the crossroads

FRANS RUTTEN AND
ALBERT VAN DER WERFF

FRANS RUTTEN

Professor Dr Frans Rutten, who was born in 1948 in The Hague. He studied econometrics at the University of Rotterdam. After graduating he was successively affiliated with the Interfaculty for Graduate Studies in Management at Rotterdam, the Economic Institute of Leyden University and the Center for Research in Public Economics of Leyden University. In 1978 he completed his dissertation on 'The Use of Health Care Facilities in the Netherlands', which comprised an empirical, econometric, analysis of patient-flows between subsectors in health care. From 1977 onwards he was deputy head of the Department of Long-Term Planning at the Ministry of Health and Environmental Protection in Leidschendam, The Netherlands. During that period he was active in several consultantships, among others for the regional office of WHO in Copenhagen, for the Council of Europe, and for the International Institute for Applied Systems Analysis. Currently he is Professor of Health Economics at the State University of Limburg at Maastricht. He is also involved in setting up an economic faculty at the same university.

ALBERT VAN DER WERFF

Professor Dr Albert van der Werff who was born in 1932 in the Hague has had considerable experience in the health field as a health systems specialist being, by discipline, a scientist and economist concerned for many years at the highest level with health policy, health economics, and health care organization.

After a career of more than fifteen years in planning and management in health affairs he was in 1977 appointed Director of the Ministry of Public Health and Environmental Protection in the Netherlands. Since then, as Head of the Staff Bureau of Health Policy Development, he is responsible for the co-ordination of health policy development, for the co-ordination of the proposed reforms of the health services system as well as the introduction of the related legislation and the co-ordination of policy-directed health services research. Dr van der Werff is also currently Professor of Health Policy Sciences at the National University of Limburg and was until 1981 Professor on the General and Medical Faculty at the University of Maastricht. He has worked as a consultant for WHO in many countries and is the author of a number of publications dealing with health policy.

Health policy in the Netherlands
At the crossroads

ABSTRACT

The administrative and financial structure of a health system largely determines the modes of regulation. Thus, in a system where most health services are financed out of general revenues, budgeting can be applied more easily than in a system which is characterized by a great variety of financiers.

The Dutch health care system is possibly unique in Europe in the sense that although social insurance legislation is of considerable importance, there still exists a large private sector providing twenty-five per cent of the resources for health services. As far as personal health care is concerned, the majority of services in Holland are rendered by legally independent corporate bodies, administered by independent private boards. This is the case both in ambulatory care as well as in hospital care. The Sickness Funds which carry out the social insurance legislation are also legally independent corporate bodies.

The subject is introduced by a description of the health services and the regulation to which these are subject in the Netherlands. A number of problems, such as a disproportionate cost increase, the unbalanced growth in the system, and the lack of cohesion between services are identified. The current regulatory measures are evaluated, and future developments are discussed.

The need to solve the problems is enforcing the Dutch Government to more regulation and intervention. This situation raises the question of selecting the proper balance between market mechanisms and government control. In this respect budgeting is considered as a regulatory instrument to set limits to disproportionate growth and to allow at the same time sufficient freedom to private enterprise to solve their own problems within certain limits.

One of the key issues in future health policy is believed to be the tension between increasing demands on the health care sector, due to the high expectations of people living in a welfare state and government regulation aimed at reduction of supply. This might even prejudice the effective use of regulatory instruments even when these are legislated.

INTRODUCTION

Health policy in the Netherlands is at the crossroads. Traditionally personal curative care has in principle been regulated by the market mechanism and government intervention has been limited, in particular, to quality control. The development of the welfare state which recognized health as a social right for all residents, and the related increase of health expenditures, which is exceeding the economic potential of the country, is forcing the Dutch Government now to more regulation and intervention. This situation raises the question of selecting the proper balance between market mechanisms and government control. In this essay an attempt is made to illuminate this question.

First, we present a picture of the history of government regulation and intervention and a characterization of the Dutch health services system in this respect.

Then the major problems observed in the Dutch health services system are listed in the next section. Following this the objectives and nature of the present regulations are evaluated as well as the effectiveness and efficiency of the regulations in solving the identified problems. In this respect consideration is specially given to volume regulation, price regulation, cost regulation, and financing regulation. In 1982 the existing regulation will be replaced and extended by new regulations introducing much more government control and intervention. In the penultimate section the objectives, nature, and expected effects of the future regulation will be explored. Again, attention will be given specially to volume regulation, price regulation, cost regulation, and financing regulation. Attention will also be paid to quality regulation.

The essay is concluded by an evaluation statement with respect to the balance between market mechanisms and government control as are currently being developed in the Netherlands.

HISTORY OF GOVERNMENT REGULATION
AND INTERVENTION

Traditionally in health care, private enterprise has always been important in the Netherlands. In general, the government restricted its engagement in health to controlling only those factors within society which were outside the control of individuals. This was primarily concerned with the role of government to organize and finance preventive care which directly involves the population as a whole. In principle personal care, both preventive and curative, has invariably been left to the private sector. In this respect the Dutch government has limited its involvement to a policy of creating the conditions which allowed the private sector to organize services and to provide care. Tariffs and prices for services were regulated by the market mechanism and were established through a process of bargaining between the providers on one side and the Sickness Funds on the other. Government did not however stand completely aside. Quality of care has always been subject to control of government. Quality control by government which was initiated in the nineteenth century has traditionally been a corner-stone of the Dutch health service, and it has received considerable emphasis over the years. For this purpose independent and well equipped inspectorates were established, operating from national and regional offices and supervising medical care, mental care, drugs, food, and veterinary products. This division of labour between the government and private sector, monitored by government control on the quality of care provided by the private sector has dominated the Dutch services for more than 100 years. It has still great influence today. In general, environmental protection is provided by government and all costs involved are covered by general taxation and special levies. But as far as personal health care is concerned the majority of services in Holland are operated by legally independent corporate bodies, administered by private boards.

The Sickness Funds too are legally independent corporate bodies.

Table 1. *The financing of health care services in the period 1975–80 in millions of Dutch guilders.*

	1975	1976	1977	1978	1979	1980	1975	1976	1977	1978	1979	1980
Total costs	17·038	19·300	21·379	23·509	25·568	27·774	100	100	100	100	100	100
Sickness Funds Insurance Act	7·248	8·216	9·160	10·123	10·995	11·955	42·5	42·6	42·7	43·1	43·0	43·0
Special Sickness Expenses Act	4·088	4·664	5·223	5·806	6·324	7·438	24·0	24·1	24·4	24·7	24·7	26·8
Private resources	4·477	5·002	5·441	5·887	6·379	6·717	26·3	25·9	25·5	25·0	24·9	24·2
Government	1·135	1·267	1·380	1·587	1·698	1·523	6·7	6·6	6·5	6·7	6·7	5·5
Other categories	90	151	172	106	172	141	0·5	0·8	0·7	0·5	0·7	0·5

CHARACTERISTICS OF THE DUTCH HEALTH SERVICES AND ITS REGULATION

The financing of health services

Health care services in the Netherlands are financed from various sources. From Table 1 it can be inferred that public resources finance more than seventy-five per cent of total health care expenditure. The total cost of the health care sector amounted to 8·75 per cent of GNP in 1980. When considering these figures it should be noted that these represent direct payments from financing agencies to health care facilities. Subsidies from general revenues into social insurance funds, which are quite substantial, are not taken into account (if these are counted as government subsidies the share of this item would increase to 18 per cent). The same goes for private payments, which are made under the social insurance regime. In the public sector two Acts are important with respect to financing: the Sickness Funds Insurance Act (Ziekenfondswet, ZFW, 1964) which replaced the Sickness Funds Decree of 1941, and the General Special Sickness Expenses Act (Algemene Wet Bijzondere Ziektekosten, AWBZ, 1967). In the private sector numerous private insurance companies offer a large variety of insurance policies.

About seventy per cent of the population is insured with the Sickness Funds, which operate the social insurance system of the Sickness Funds Insurance Act. The activities of these Funds are under the supervision of the Sickness Funds Council. Individuals with an income above a certain income level (approximately Dfl. 43,000, in 1982) have to acquire private insurance against health care expenditure, while employees with an annual family income under that income level are compulsorily insured by Sickness Fund Insurance. Others (like the self-employed) may acquire membership of the public insurance scheme on a voluntary basis. The premium of the compulsory public insurance is a uniformly fixed percentage of personal income (in 1982: 9·2 per cent with a maximum of approximately Dfl. 3,400) and is met jointly by the insured employee and by the employer. All members of the family are covered at no extra cost. Privately insured and voluntarily insured pay a nominal premium. The privately insured, of course, pay this premium for each person insured. Retired, elderly people with an income below a certain level (approximately Dfl. 24,000, in 1982) are entitled to participate in the Sickness Fund insurance scheme at reduced premium rates. Finally, civil servants are not compulsorily insured under the public scheme, but may buy private or public insurance, or enter their own insurance scheme.

The premium for old people's insurance schemes does not cover the actual cost of treatment and is supplemented by substantial amounts from the General Fund of the compulsory insurance scheme and the government. The Sickness Funds Council administers both the General Fund, into which compulsory Sickness Funds' insurance contributions are paid, and the Fund for Elderly Person's Insurance. The premium for the voluntary public insurance scheme is met by the policyholder and varies from one region to another. Special reductions may be granted to persons in the lower income brackets. Medical care is provided by medical and paramedical practitioners, hospitals, and other institutions on a contract basis.

Insurance for the heavier risks, i.e. for exceptional expenses is governed by the General Special Sickness Expenses Act. The purpose of the Act is to insure the entire population against the risk of exceptional expenses, such as those incurred by patients at institutions which care for long-stay patients and the physically and/or mentally handicapped. A recent development is also to finance different ambulatory services from this general fund, such as home nursing services (from 1980 onwards) and ambulatory mental health services (from 1982 onwards). This scheme is a national insurance scheme applying in principle to all residents of the Netherlands. The premium is a percentage of a person's wage or income (3.3 per cent in 1982), and is paid by the employer.

The independent practising professionals as well as the ambulatory services and hospitals acquire their income by means of a system of tariffs, a system of budget-financing, or a mixed system of tariffs and budget-financing. The reimbursement of physicians' services is dependent on whether the treatment concerns a publicly or privately insured person. Furthermore, the renumeration system differs with respect to general practitioners and specialists. In the public sector the following payment mechanisms exist:

The general practitioner is paid through a capitation system: he gets a fixed amount of money per year for each publicly insured person in his practice regardless of the quantity of care provided during that year. The fees are uniformly determined for the whole of the Netherlands;

The specialist gets a fixed amount of money for each publicly insured patient referred to him by the general practitioner (who issues a so-called referral card), which in effect entitles him to one month of outpatient treatment. If continuation of outpatient treatment is necessary after one month an additional amount of money per month is given to the specialist. For major operations (both therapeutic and diagnostic) in an inpatient or outpatient setting, the specialist receives a fee for service. Some specialists may also receive a fixed amount for each day a patient of theirs is occupying a hospital bed. These fees are the same for the whole of the country.

In the private sector, physicians demand a fee for each service to their private patients. Because private fees are considerably higher than those charged in the public sector, this form of price discrimination implies a subsidy from the private sector to the public sector. In 1980, 1·8 billion Dutch guilders were spent on the services provided by physicians (free entrepreneurs), of which 52 per cent was paid by Sickness Funds. Although still small in number, the percentage of physicians who are employed by a hospital or municipality and work on a salary is increasing.

Ambulatory facilities acquire their income on the basis of budget-financing. Hospitals are dependent on a tariff system.

Community health services

Broadly speaking the ambulatory subsector is divided into *community health* services, *general practitioner* services, *home nursing* and *ambulatory mental health care* services.

Community health services provide preventive services directed towards the community as a whole and include control of communicable diseases and quarantine, collection and analysis of epidemiological data, school health care, ambulance services, advising municipal and other official bodies on public health, sanitary supervision and disinfection (in large ports). There is no complete coverage of the entire country as yet. Although 'municipal' health services are in operation in the cities and 'district' health services in some rural areas, elsewhere there are still shortcomings. These services are made available by the municipalities. Finance is provided by government from general taxation.

General practitioner services

Personal curative care for predominantly minor and chronic disorders is provided by general practitioners. Practically all of these physicians operate in private practices either in solo or in group practices. The number of general practitioners per 1000 inhabitants amounts to 0·36. The average size of a practice of a family practitioner is 2800 (1980). There is a complete coverage, although the geographical distribution of the general practitioners is still in need of improvement. The number of integrated primary health care centres in which general practitioners participate, is still limited and shows a slow development. The remuneration system has already been discussed above. General practitioners are paid through a capitation system for publicly insured patients and on a fee-for-service basis for privately insured patients.

Home nursing services

Home nursing services are provided by the 'Cross Organizations', which are private corporations as well. Almost three million families are members of one of these Cross Organizations. Before 1970, each Cross Organization was linked to a religious movement: protestant, catholic, or non-denominational. During the seventies a process of 'uncolouring' or integration has taken place. Today each Cross Organization consists of one or more basic units which cover geographically equal target populations. There is now complete coverage. The work of the Cross Organizations was initially financed by contributions and payments by their members. Over the years, adjustment by the State, provinces, and municipalities became necessary, and the share of private contributions gradually decreased to 40 per cent. The disadvantages of this mixed system were that every subsidizing authority applied its own standards and that the total income is derived from contributions the amount of which the various bodies decide independently of one another. For these reasons this financing system was replaced by membership fees, supplemented by payments from one single source, as provided by the General Special Sickness Expenses Act.

Ambulatory mental health services

In ambulant mental health care, in addition to privately practising psychiatrists, a large number of institutions such as socio-psychiatric units, medical educational bureaux, institutions for (medical) psychotherapy, consultative bureaux for alcohol and drugs, youth psychiatric services, etc. are active. Besides these institutions there are other bodies operating locally or regionally in this field under somewhat different names, and sometimes with a somewhat different set-up. A number of agencies in the field of social service also do work that is closely related to mental health care. The size of the institutions and the nature and extent of their activities display considerable variation and are at the same time subject to considerable change. Duplication and overlap with regard to both the package of services and the field of operations of each institution are the rule rather than the exception. The whole field is at present in a state of great flux. Mental health care is the responsibility of various ministries, each of which is responsible, for historical reasons, for part of that care.

Consequently the financing of ambulatory mental health services is fragmented. Main sources are the General Special Sickness Expenses Act (socio-psychiatric services, medical educational bureaux, and institutions for (medical) psychotherapy), government funding by the Ministry of Public Health and Environmental Hygiene (Consultative bureaux for alcohol and drugs) and the Ministry of Cultural, Recreational and Social Services (youth psychiatrist services). Privately practising psychiatrists are paid on the basis of fee for service for which the clients concerned may be insured by the scheme of the Sickness Funds Insurance Act, or by a private insurance scheme. Sickness Funds limit their payments to privately practising psychiatrists up to a maximum of 90 days.

From 1982 onwards the ambulatory mental health services will be financed on the basis of the General Special Sickness Expenses Act. This financing however is made dependent on the condition that the ambulatory mental health services have to be integrated into 'Regional Institutes of Ambulatory Mental Health Care'. These regional institutes are offering a co-ordinated intake to patients and are operated by one single management.

Hospital care

In 1980 short-term hospital care was provided by 250 institutions (5·5 beds per 1000 capita): 90 per cent of these hospitals are private. Long-term nursing care is provided by about three hundred hospitals including nursing homes for mentally retarded old people (3·0 per 1000 capita); 60 per cent of these hospitals are private. In the Netherlands there are about seventy psychiatric hospitals (2·0 beds per 1000 capita) of which ninety per cent are private. The mentally handicapped are treated in a total number of 130 institutions (2·0 beds). Almost all of these hospitals are private. The total hospital sector consists of 750 institutions (12·5 beds per 1000 capita).

Traditionally these institutions have their religious 'colours' i.e. protestant, catholic, or non-denominational. As far as short-term care is concerned, and in particular in urban areas, there are three main hospitals, each with its own specialist units and the associated technical equipment, operating next to each other and in a competitive relationship. This situation which still exists in many areas accounts for the relatively large number of beds in use (5·5 beds per 1000 capita). Although the distribution of the hospitals could be improved, accessibility is not a problem in this densely populated country. Almost all hospitals can be reached easily. Outpatient facilities are very well developed and adequately used. All short-stay general hospitals provide outpatient care. Long-stay hospitals are developing day-care centres. Psychiatric hospitals usually provide outpatient services to their clients. In general, waiting lists do not exist. The majority of specialists still practise privately within the context of the (short-stay, general) hospitals.

In 1980, approximately 40 per cent of total resources allocated to institutions providing inpatient care were comprised of payments under the Sickness Funds Insurance Act, while 40 per cent of payments were made under the provisions of the Special Sickness Expenses Act. Another 15 per cent of total resources for inpatient care came from private sources (mainly private health insurance companies), the remaining 5 per cent consisting of government subsidies and internal financing.

Short-stay general hospitals charge a bed-day price. The inpatient and outpatient services of specialists are charged separately on a fee-for-service basis. Financing of acute hospital care, is derived principally from the Sickness Funds (for those patients who are insured by the compulsory scheme) or from private insurance companies. The cost involved in nursing in long-stay hospitals is covered for all patients whatever their income level, on the basis of the General Special Sickness Expenses Act. Psychiatric outpatient and inpatient care is paid for by Sickness Funds or by private insurance companies depending on the insurance scheme the clients concerned have to adopt. Payments for clients who need long-stay psychiatric care extending a period of one year are taken over by payments on the basis of the General Special Sickness Expenses Act. The cost of the care provided to mentally handicapped persons is fully covered by the same Act.

Regulation with respect to the volume and with respect to the organization of the services has been initiated in the beginning of the seventies on the basis of the Hospital Facilities Act (1972). From the date of enforcement of this Act, it was not any longer permitted to build or extend a facility which requires an investment of more than 500,000

Dutch guilders without a licence granted by the Minister of Health. From 1979 the Hospital Facilities Act was replaced by the Amended Hospital Facilities Act. This new Act was designed to be much more flexible, and provided for drawing up regional hospital plans for certain categories of facilities on the basis of an instruction of the Ministry of Health. These plans which have to be developed by the Provincial Governments need the approval of the Minister of Health. The Council of Hospital Facilities advises in this respect. On the basis of the approved plans, licences may be granted for constructing or reconstructing hospital facilities. A new element introduced by the Amended Hospital Facilities Act was the provision for closing down facilities.

Diagnosis, treatment, and referral of an individual patient is a joint responsibility of the individual physician and the patient. Privately practising professionals or hospital boards are free to decide which activities they wish to perform. In this respect, however, there are exceptions. Specialized clinical functions requiring large investment such as heart surgery, high voltage radiation therapy, neuro- and whole-body scanners, etc., cannot be offered without government permission. In addition, since 1976, hospital boards have not been allowed to extend the number of specialties. This regulation was achieved by using the Sickness Funds Insurance Act on the basis of which Sickness Funds can refuse contracts for new specialties.

The referral process

In The Netherlands there is now a complete division of labour between the general practitioners and specialists in hospitals. This is regarded as necessary for efficient functioning of the referral system. This division between general practitioners and specialists has enabled front-line services at primary care level and specialist services in the outpatient departments of hospitals at the secondary care level to be fully developed. Compulsorily or voluntarily insured individuals seeking care can only gain access to the health services via the family doctor, who is always a general practitioner.

Specialists work in the hospitals, where the diagnostic and

treatment facilities are concentrated. Consultation with a specialist can only take place after referral by the family doctor. Otherwise the health insurance schemes will refuse to pay the bill. In this way the referral system can be made to work efficiently.

MAJOR PROBLEMS OBSERVED IN THE DUTCH HEALTH SERVICES SYSTEM

The effect of the Dutch health services on the health of the people is generally accepted as excellent. The state of medical science and technology in the Netherlands ensures a high level of extensive services and assistance.

Nevertheless, Dutch health care is confronted by serious problems, although it is not unique in this respect. In most industrialized countries health care has developed into one of the most important and extensive sectors of the economy, requiring up to 8 to 10 per cent of the national income and employing 4 to 6 per cent of the total working population. In other countries one finds a similar acceleration of costs in recent years, which exceeds the rise in expenditure on other communal services and which is caused by the ever-increasing demand for therapeutic services in hospital care.

The major problems may be grouped together as follows:

Unbalanced growth

The system of health services is still out of balance at various points. As a consequence of medico-technical developments, together with the major elements making up cost including remuneration, the hospital sector has become subject to a disproportionately large part of the strain. Until the beginning of the seventies, this sector was able to expand almost unchecked. On the other hand, preventive care and ambulatory health services have not developed as greatly as they might, while the mental health services have lagged behind in their development.

Insufficient cohesion

The complex of health services displays poor cohesion. Functional cohesion is lacking, both horizontally and vertically, resulting in independent functioning of services alongside one another. Co-operation between the executive institutions of health care and the other welfare services is often absent, as indeed is co-ordination of policy.

Disproportionate cost increase

Health expenditures are growing disproportionately in comparison with other sectors and exceeding the economic potential of the country. Instruments for the control of cost development, both with respect to the whole and to the individual sectors, are still inadequate, and indeed partly lacking. The structure of the financing of health care is too fragmented, and in certain respects it does not foster the necessary collaboration between the services. Because the financial mechanism adapts too passively to existing organizational situations, it fails to exert corrective influences on the co-ordination of the various services. At the same time, the burden of health care expenditures on different population groups is unequally distributed.

EVALUATION OF THE OBJECTIVES, NATURE AND EFFECTS OF PRESENT REGULATION

Fields of attention for regulation

The main problems threatening the effectiveness and efficiency of the Dutch health services have been recognized for many years. In 1974, the Dutch government defended the 'Memorandum on the Structure of the Health Services' in Parliament in which document these problems were listed and a clear statement was made with respect to the basic policies and strategies necessary for the future. The basic policies were directed to correct the imbalance of growth by strengthening primary health care, to improve the coherence of the health services on the basis of the concept of regionalization, and to remedy the disproportionate increase of health expenditures by introducing much more governmental control. This document has to be considered as a salient point in the development of the health services in the Netherlands and as a first step on the road to a government-controlled system. A coherent system of legislation is now under development for the whole of the health services in order to provide a basis for the realization of what are now generally agreed as strategies to be adopted for Holland.

This system comprises legislation with respect to:

the patients (patients' rights),

the individual health care workers and their professional work,

the volume and quality of the services, as well as the organization of the services,

tariffs (and prices and salaries) of the services rendered,

the financing of the health services system.

This paper will concentrate on regulation with respect to the volume and quality of care, the organization of the health services, tariffs (and prices and salaries), the cost of the health service, and its financing, since these are the items relating to cost which should be subject to control.

This section will accordingly deal with the objectives, nature and effects of the current regulation.

Volume regulation

Volume regulation, based on the Hospital Facilities Acts (1971 and later 1979), aimed in particular at a reduction of the bed capacity of hospitals. The political target, launched in 1975, to bring the number of beds of acute general hospitals down to four per cent (actual 5·5 per cent) was not achieved.

The first Hospital Facilities Act (1971) was, however, inadequate as an instrument in this respect as the Act did not provide the legal basis for closing down facilities. At the same time the amending Act of 1979 has not really been used for this purpose since the process takes time. Because of the introduction of a regional hospital planning system which needs a lengthy preparatory phase in which the national guidelines for planning have to be developed, a decentralized planning machinery has to be built up, and plans have to be drawn-up and approved. Again, it has to be recognized that there is invariably resistance against closing down a facility. In most cases a reduction of beds was achieved by way of a fusion of two or more hospitals and their replacement by one newly built facility. In this way the growth of acute beds was slowed down a bit. But the regulation was certainly effective with respect to the organization of long-term nursing homes, as the aim in this case was to extend the existing capacity. A particular problem is that relating to psychiatric hospitals. It is accepted that the bed capacity has, however, to be carried out in combination with a redistribution of the facilities over the country. This reorientation in institutional care, cannot be initiated separately from the reorganization which is planned to take place in the ambulatory mental health services. Similar problems arise with respect to institutional care for the mentally handicapped and physically handicapped.

Regulations affecting the hospital sector have also caused side effects which were not foreseen, and perhaps not even recognized today. Because of the pressure on this sector, hospitals organized themselves far more efficiently and effectively than they would have done without regulation. This is particularly true for the short-stay general hospitals. Management in these hospitals has improved considerably because of the appointment of professional managers. The attention paid to hospitals also has attracted all types of experts. The National Board of Hospitals, which represents the interests of the hospitals, as well as the hospitals themselves, were able to strengthen their staffs and to develop the expertise needed to make full use of the freedoms not restricted by the prevailing regulations. As a consequence the services for preventive care and ambulatory care have lagged even more behind their relative positions in the health sector, before the introduction of the regulations. This lack of balance was aggravated by the methods of financing, since financing on the basis of social .security legislation has allowed more growth to the hospitals than the financing of preventive care and ambulatory care, which traditionally derives from general taxation (see paragraph 'Financing' below). As a result the imbalance of growth in the Dutch health system has continued. Thus, the Hospital Facilities Act failed with respect to the *first* policy goal. But the Act also failed with respect to the *second* policy goal as it did not provide an instrument to remedy the lack of coherence in the system. It was expected that a restructuring of the hospital sector would initiate a process of restructuring throughout the whole health services system. This did not occur however, as the hospitals defended their own interests rather than taking the lead in the process of reorientation in collaboration with the other services. With respect to the *third* policy goal, costs certainly were influenced favourably, as the increase of the number of beds as well as the increase of highly specialized clinical functions came under control. This effect was, however, almost nullified because of the circumstances in which the reduction of beds was achieved by replacement of two or more hospitals by one newly built facility. Old, relatively cheap beds were replaced by a smaller number of expensive beds. Consequently in those cases the bed price per day increased considerably.

The main source of disproportionate growth, however, viz. the volume of services in terms of outputs such as the number of consultations, and the nature and number of diagnostic and therapeutic procedures, remained out of range. The volume and growth of these activities were (and still are) largely determined by the specialists. Since these professionals are paid on a fee-for-service basis, it may hardly be expected that the volume and growth of the medical activities can be kept between certain limits without government intervention. In addition the Hospital Facilities Act does not provide for regulation with respect to manpower. In principle, all professionals are free to settle down wherever they like and to start a new practice or enter into an existing partnership in a hospital. This lack of regulation, both with respect to the volume of medical activities and to manpower makes the implementation of a policy of cost containment illusionary.

Price regulation

Price regulation based on the Hospital Tariffs Act aimed at control of hospital costs. As explained earlier, hospital boards and managers have to prove that the tariffs they charge meet the actual cost before they secure approval by the Hospital Tariffs Agency. The tariffs are used by both Sickness Funds and Private Insurers when reimbursing hospitals.

The costs have to be calculated on the basis of guidelines. In addition, guidelines are provided to determine the tariffs. In particular, in the recent past a restrictive tariff policy has been in effect which enforces hospital managers to operate their facility more efficiently. If difficulties arise, experts of the Central Organization for Hospital Tariffs (Centraal Orgaan Ziekenhuis Tarieven) check the actual costs, taking advantage of the opportunity to discuss the efficiency of the operation. This instrument has proved to be effective in the Netherlands since it puts a ceiling to hospital costs without much interference in the responsibilities of management. The instrument, however, is only partly effective with respect to overall expenditures as the volume in terms of outputs is not brought under control (see 'Volume regulation' above).

The present financing system of hospitals, based on the reimbursement of a fixed price per bed-day, provides clear incentives towards full utilization of hospital capacity. This follows from the fact that marginal costs in hospitals are considerably lower than marginal benefits, the last reflecting more or less *mean* costs of hospital operation. Furthermore, because the number of bed-days is the key variable for reimbursement, the development of such policies as the substitution of inpatient care by outpatient care, or the establishment of day-care units within hospitals are not encouraged. Moreover, the system is frustrating to the management of institutions because of the degree of detail of norms related to the tariff built-up. These norms are related for example to the number of nurses per occupied hospital bed. As the length of stay decreases, nursing becomes more intensive. As a result the pressures experienced on the hospital with respect to cost containment are to a certain extent reflected in a high workload of the nursing staff, and a relatively low income level. On the other hand the privately practising specialists within the hospitals are still free to increase their throughput and the hospital boards and managers allow them to do so. In this way, the pressure on the hospital staff is continuously increasing. Yet in contrast with hospital staff, most categories of specialists are earning extraordinarily high incomes. Until 1982 price regulation was restricted to hospitals only, and consequently this regulation had no effect with respect to the hoped-for improvement of cohesion between services. The effect, too, with respect to a more balanced growth was negligible.

The cost of health care

The previous paragraphs have dealt with the regulation of volume- and price-components. It was observed that regulation is as yet incomplete and consequently containment of all costs of health care is not yet within reach. As has been pointed out, nearly one-quarter of all costs is paid for out of private means. In the early 1970s concern grew about the development of the costs of health care provision. Calculations at that time, which were based on extrapolations of trends in cost development, pointed to a frightening 12 per cent share of GNP for health care expenditure in the 1980s if the then, current health policies were unchanged. The government therefore felt the need for control of all health care costs and sought to introduce the concept of budgeting in health care.

At that time detailed information on cost development, however, was lacking and attempts were made to fill this gap. This resulted in the construction of the first so-called 'Financial Survey' by the government in 1977. This survey, which is published each year with the annual budget of the Ministry of Health and Environmental Protection, provides detailed information on the total cost of health care provision in the Netherlands, including the costs in the private sector. It contains seven chapters, referring to *total health services costs, hospital services, specialist services, medicines* and *medical aids and appliances, ambulatory health services, community health services*, as well as *management and administration*. It does not only provide a financial analysis of past developments, but it also gives a forecast for the coming five-year period, based on predictions of wage- and price-indices of the Dutch Central Planning Bureau. The forecast for the coming budget year is thus gradually being turned into an instrument for indicating the financial ceiling for cost development in that particular budget year. This 'macro-budget' is discussed and decided on in the Council of Ministers and provides a basis for issuing governmental guidelines for price/tariff policy on the basis of the Health Tariffs Act, for setting growth targets (limits) for ambulatory health care and, in the near future, for formulating budget-restrictions for decentralized planning on the basis of the Health Services Act (see paragraphs on 'Volume and quality' and 'Cost containment through Budgeting' below). The Financial Survey has proved to constitute a powerful tool for government policy indeed, because it provides the essential insight in developments in both public and private sectors in health care.

Financing

As has been indicated the main sources of finance in health care are social insurance funds, government subsidies, and private resources. The first and the last are mainly earmarked for curative medical treatment and the provision of care to the sick and disabled, while prevention and other community health services are largely financed out of government subsidies. Health care provision, financed from government funds, is subject to heavy pressure because of the existing and increasing competition between alternative priority areas for allocating government funds. Social insurance funds are a more secure basis of finance, as premiums are set and collected according to previous cost-development, and resources are exclusively earmarked for allocation to health care. This has led to a continuous relative growth of the advanced, especially inpatient, medical treatment at the cost of prevention and base-line services. In spite of explicit government policy statements about a planned enforcement of preventive and primary health services, the percentage of resources allocated to institutional health care increased from

57 per cent in 1975 to almost 59 per cent in 1980. This illustrates the predominance of the financing structure in guiding health care developments.

The regulatory activities of such financing agencies as the Sickness Funds, apart from price and wage bargaining, are of a limited nature. Each Sickness Fund employs one or more physicians who give advice on the medical treatment of patients belonging to a particular Sickness Fund and who may object against excessive or otherwise undesirable forms of medical treatment. In 1973 an extensive national information system was created by the Sickness Funds in order to stimulate utilization review. Nowadays, systematic statistical analysis of variation in treatment patterns is carried out in order to increase the potential for control.

Private insurance companies have somewhat different incentives for investing in controlling activities. Because they use the price level of insurance premiums as an instrument for competition, they may increase their market share as a consequence of lower insurance benefits payments, which result from a tight control policy. With the increasing tendency towards market segmentation and competition in the private insurance sector (discussed more thoroughly below) it is almost certain that private insurance companies will increasingly invest in a system for the control of payments of insurance benefits. Some insurance companies are known to be successful in containing costs by carefully reviewing hospital and medical care provided to their insured. In several instances in the last decade attempts have been made to introduce cost-sharing in the public insurance system: the introduction of deductibles in relation to the consumption of medicines has been suggested as well as patients' contributions to the cost of referral. These attempts all failed because of political pressure against the supposed interference with firmly established rights of citizens to free care. It seems obvious that cost-sharing in the case of the consumption of pharmaceutical products may contribute considerably to the effective distribution of benefits in this field. Figures show that a great amount of medicines purchased are actually not consumed, and thrown away. Nevertheless, the Netherlands remains one of the very few countries in Europe where medicines can be acquired completely free under the public scheme.

The division of the health care sector into public and private sectors has important consequences for the distribution of health care costs over population groups. There seems to be a continuous divergence of the public and private sectors, the public sector for low income-earners being based on mutual solidarity, while the private insurance market tends to balance premium and risk. In the last decade, competition in the private health care insurance market has grown considerably; market segmentation through the introduction of age-specific premiums and special insurance policies with large deductibles became more important. This resulted in the near bankruptcy of voluntary public insurance funds because of the transition of healthy people representing relatively good risks from voluntary public insurance to the private insurance sector, where they pay less by way of premium. (*Note* that in the case of voluntary public insurance funds, the inflow of money from premiums should equal total insurance benefits paid.) But, more importantly, it made for a still larger gulf between the two sectors with respect to the personal distribution of health care expenses. Depending on income level and occupational factors the percentage of family income spent on health care insurance for a married couple with two children may vary from less than 4 per cent to almost 15 per cent. This unequal distribution of health care expenses provoked an attempt in 1975 to introduce a public insurance system for the entire population offering full coverage. This failed because the government feared this would have a negative influence on the already weak economic situation, and subsequently did not bring an act before Parliament. Furthermore, some government circles claimed that introduction of this general insurance act would involve redistribution of income for certain population groups, which was thought to be unacceptable—a strange argument given the current, somewhat unequal, distribution of personal expenditures. Recently, fresh discussions on the insurance- and finance-structure of the health care system were opened as a consequence of the financial problems of the public sector. Thoughts in government circles are now directed towards a simplification of the public insurance-structure and a tight regulation of the private insurance market, ensuring the calculation of fair premiums and constraining market-segmentation. *In summary*, it can be stated that the personal distribution of health care expenses is rather skewed and that developments in the private insurance market tend to make this distribution even more so.

In other countries, many studies on the distribution of public expenditure benefits including health care have been carried out. These are often based on evidence from household surveys. In the Netherlands, until recently no large surveys on health care consumption have been done, so limited information on the distribution of health care benefits over income groups is available. There are, however, detailed data on the differences in consumption between the publicly and privately insured, which can be considered as two global income groups, viz. low- and high-income earners respectively.

Recently, data have been published on the differences in health care consumption between these groups. Most important are the differences in the number of hospital-days between both groups: in 1977 the publicly insured consumed 1600 hospital-days per insured against consumption by the privately insured of 1000 hospital-days, which indicates a difference of 56 per cent. This enormous difference in consumption patterns, which to a less degree can also be found in other subsectors of the health care system, can be partly explained by the fact that those publicly insured show higher morbidity rates than those privately insured. This, however, cannot be the whole story. It has been shown that the *supply elasticity* of hospital consumption is half as large for privately insured than for publicly insured, suggesting that admission and discharge policies in hospitals depend on the relative number of hospital beds in the particular region, and discriminate between the publicly and privately insured. In this patients study it was suggested that privately insured, who face higher *inconvenience costs* of illness, are better capable of resisting pressures towards having more extensive clinical treatment (see previous discussion on financial incentives) than the publicly insured. 'The better off ... are better able to work the system'. There may also be an influence in the different control activities of Sickness Funds on the one hand and private insurance companies on the other hand, the latter having greater incentive to exercise control. Finally, the existence of private insurance policies with considerable cost-sharing by the insured may also have a dampening effect on the health care consumption of this particular group. The tentative conclusion is that observed differences in the distribution of health care benefits between publicly and privately insured do not necessarily reflect differences in need, but may point to a greater efficiency in the provision of health care to the privately insured.

OBJECTIVES, NATURE, AND EXPECTED EFFECTS OF FUTURE REGULATION

Towards more government regulation and intervention

While there is confirmation of the recognition of health care as a social right for all residents, the Dutch Government is moving now in the direction of recognizing a like necessity to control costs through government regulation, involving a higher degree of intervention with respect to the whole of the health sector.

In the preceding section, it has been observed that the present regulation is inadequate in order to balance the growth of the different services within the system. Current legislation is designed primarily for the hospital sector and is therefore of little value in making the total system more coherent.

In addition, there is no legal basis for the co-ordination of the health services with the social welfare services; and finally, the present regulations do not provide an adequate instrument to the health authorities to cope with the problem of disproportionate growth of costs. In the current economic circumstances, the government is paying particular attention to the latter problem. In this alteration from an emphasis on private practice, towards greater government control, a milestone of significance is the acceptance by

Parliament that legislation is needed to carry out the already agreed basic policies and strategies.

In 1982 provision is being made for the passage through Parliament of the Health Services Act which will replace the Hospital Facilities Act. The new Act will cover regulation with respect to the whole of the health services and it will embrace both institutions as well as privately practising professionals. This act will probably be effective from 1984 onwards.

At the same time the Specific Social Welfare Act (Kaderwet Specifiek Welzijn) has been passed by Parliament. This act provides a framework for planning of health services and social services in one single system. The Health Services Act, along with the Specific Social Welfare Act are designed to introduce the decentralization of administrative responsibilities, to the level of provinces and municipalities. This new legislation also comprises regulations to enable patients or clients to participate in the decision-making process. The Health Services Act is introducing a major change concerning government regulation and intervention. For the first time in the history of the Dutch health services, the final decisions with respect to volume, quality, and organization of the services will be taken by the government, albeit that the providers of care will be involved in the decision-making process. For this purpose the Act provides an advisory structure at all three levels of administration. At the National Level a National Health Council will be formed by a merger of the Central Health Council and the Hospital Facilities Council. In addition a grievance procedure has been introduced: and in accordance with Dutch traditions health care itself will continue to be rendered by the private sector.

From 1982 onwards, the Health Tariffs Act has come into force. This act replaces the Hospital Tariffs Act and extends price regulation to the whole of the health services. Control with respect to tariffs will be carried out by the Central Organization for Health Tariffs. In contrast with the Health Services Act, the regulations of the Health Tariffs Act will be applied nationally.

Thus to *summarize* the present position, as explained above, the existing financing system is based on the Sickness Fund

Insurance Act (1964) and the General Special Sickness Expenses Act (1967). In accordance with the development of legislation concerning volume, quality, and organization of services, and tariffs, an attempt to promote a General Act of Health Insurance failed. The present Administration is investigating now to what extent a revision of the financing system is technically and financially feasible. For the time being, this will mean that the Health Services Act and the Health Tariffs Act will have to be made effective within the context of the existing social security system.

Volume and quality regulation

Regulation on the basis of the Health Services Act is directed to the structural build up of health services, the objective being to organize these services effectively and efficiently and in mutual relationship so that they are functioning as a coherent whole. It is not necessary to apply this regulation to all services and at the same time. If required, different categories of services may be brought under the regime of the act, step by step.

The Minister of Health will indicate which services will come under the jurisdiction of the national, provincial, or local authorities. As a rule, the decisions with respect to volume, quality, and organization, as well as the allocation of resources will have to be made at those administrative levels where the authorities concerned can exercise the best judgment.

The Minister of Health is preparing the implementation of the act on the basis of a plan of introduction which has to be discussed in Parliament. Reports on progress will require to be submitted to Parliament periodically.

To guarantee adequate care the Act provides for the possibility of making demands upon institutions with respect to quality. For this purpose, quality standards will be developed. These requirements concern personnel and facilities, hygiene and safety, as well as the effective and efficient functioning of an institution. Moreover, quality standards will be developed and applied to the legal form of the institution, such as the composition of the board, the articles of association and the organizational structure, as well as the way the institution has to render account of its operations. In addition, quality regulation comprises guarantees with respect to the users.

The Health Services Act provides quality regulation for institutions only. Quality regulation for physicians, nursing and other paramedical professionals—concerning the individual execution of their professions—will be provided by a separate Act, i.e. the 'Act on the Health Care Professions'.

With respect to services rendered by institutions, the Health Services Act introduces a four-year plan, which will have to be revised every four years or earlier if the actual situation or the expected long-term development makes this unavoidable. The national government will draw up national plans for those services which relate to more than one province. Taking into account the recommendations of the National Council for Health, the Minister of Health has to establish guidelines which have to be considered by the provinces and municipalities in their planning efforts. These guidelines include 'global' indications with respect to the volume, distribution, and organization of health services, the nature and degree of co-ordination between the health services as well as between health services and social services. Part of these guidelines are indications for the planning period concerned, with respect to the permitted upper limit in terms of manpower, facilities, cost, and financing which may have to be allocated to carry out the plans. Municipal plans need approval by the provincial authorities and financial plans need approval by the Crown on the advice of the Ministry of Health. An approved plan is the basis for issuing certificates and licences. An institution cannot receive payments on the basis of the Sickness Fund Insurance Act or the General Special Sickness Expenses Act, unless a request for a certificate has been allowed by the authority concerned. In this respect, recommendations of the Sickness Fund Council have to be taken into account. The certifications comprise regulations regarding the volume, quality, and organization of the services. An institution cannot be built, rebuilt, or extended without a licence, which is only allowed by the Minister of Health after consultation with Provincial

Authorities and the National Health Council. If the approved plan indicates it should be so, a facility may partially or completely be closed down, or the volume of its activities be reduced.

In addition to volume regulation with respect to institutions the Health Services Act provides for volume regulation with respect to individually (and privately) practising professions. On the basis of the Act the Minister of Health may issue, if necessary, a prohibition to practice in some areas or in the whole of the country without a licence. Provinces and municipalities will be authorized to allow licences on request to open a new practice. To this end specific norms will be issued per category of profession. In addition to the settlement itself, regulation may come into force with respect to the volume of activities of those professionals who have already set up practice. In this connection provinces and municipalities will be authorized to indicate how the volume of existing practices *may be reduced*. In all these matters the authorities have to consult committees on which the profession concerned, related professions, the users, the sickness funds, and private insurers are represented. Priority areas for a settlement policy are specialists, family practitioners, dentists, and physiotherapists. Volume regulation with respect to manpower is subject to planning so that the number of posts which may become available in the planning period have to be brought into agreement with the number of candidates for these posts. In the Netherlands, the general right of people to education is recognized. Today all residents are free to choose to study what they wish and there are no financial barriers. The limitation to this freedom of choice may be the existing capacity of the facilities of education. Up till now a *numerus fixus* for students has been applied in case the number of candidates was in excess of the capacity of education. If however, a strict volume regulation with respect to individually practising professionals is introduced, the number of students will have to be brought in line with the future labour market situation, or it will have to be accepted that there may be unemployment among medical professionals.

Volume regulation with respect to individually (and privately) practising professionals is not part of the four-year planning process. The advantage of this arrangement is that the regulation may be initiated immediately after the Health Services Act comes into force. This does not mean however that volume regulation with respect to institutions will be effected independent of volume regulation with respect to individually (and privately) practising professionals. The Act, therefore, stipulates that the planning of institutions will be closely linked up with manpower planning related to professionals practising on their own.

Price regulation

Regulation on the basis of the Health Tariffs Act has to be applied both to institutions as well as to individually (and privately) practising professionals, and stipulates that without approval of the Health Tariff Agency no new or higher tariffs may be charged. The tariffs will be the outcome of a bargaining process between the institutions and individually practising professionals or their representative bodies on one side and the Sickness Funds and the Private Insurers on the other. The Health Tariff Agency (the Central Organization for Health Tariffs) has to approve the agreed tariffs. In case no agreement is achieved, one or eventually both parties may request the agency to fix a tariff. The Health Tariff Agency will judge the proposed tariffs on the basis of guidelines which refer both to the level and the specification of the tariff build-up and to the method of calculation. The guidelines are to be developed by the agency but need the approval of the Minister of Health, who together with the Minister of Economic Affairs may give instructions to the Health Tariffs Agency, if this may prove to be necessary. If the Agency appears to be unable to set a tariff the Minister is authorized by law to take over. The Health Tariffs Act provides also the legal basis to government to give indications with respect to the level of incomes earned by privately practising professionals as well as with respect to the cost elements resulting from this income, which should be considered in calculating the tariff.

The procedures which have to be followed with respect to 'norm incomes' of privately practising professionals have been elaborated in the 'Temporary Act for the Establishment of Norm Incomes of Privately Practising Professionals'.

The regulation opens up the possibility of gaining a clearer insight into the way available resources are allocated, so that in particular a more effective control of the number of posts and the employment of manpower in institutions becomes feasible.

Cost containment through budgeting

In a previous section the development and use of the Financial Survey as a form of macro-budget was discussed. There is also the possibility of introducing budgeting at different levels of decision-making in the health care sector in the near future. There are however problems in applying this concept in a health care structure in which there are many financiers and a large private sector.

At the national level there are several circumstances reacting with the development of the Financial Survey towards a macro-budget for the health care sector. A budget can be considered as a means to delegate a certain task, together with the authority to use a defined set of resources in order to perform that task. This implies the possibility of imposing a tight financial restriction while conferring freedom of resource allocation within this restriction. A number of observations on the current health care financing structure in the Netherlands and its relation to the opportunity of imposing budgets, have to be made. First, the government does not yet possess all the necessary legal instruments to contain fully the costs of health care provision since it cannot control the growth of diagnostic and therapeutic activities. Furthermore the financing of a large part of health services still has an 'open-ended' character. There is also the social insurance character of the system, which prevents the imposition of a tight macro-budget, if this endangers the opportunities of those publicly insured to exercise their legal and clearly described rights to health care provision. Under the Public Health Insurance Acts, health care supply should be adjusted in order to be able to meet health care demand, which may increase due to exogenous factors like the ageing of the population or medical technological development. Finally, an important share of health care provision is financed out of private means (24 per cent in 1980. See Table 1). The direction in which such means are spent obviously cannot be fully controlled by the government.

An even more important factor hampering the introduction of budgeting is the fact that the potentialities for reallocation between subsectors of the health care system are limited. Because these subsectors are financed out of different funds and by different financiers, most of the separate flows of finance towards health care facilities are earmarked for specific purposes.

For instance, it would be fruitless to come to a decision to invest more into arrangements for prevention at the expense of resource allocation to curative care in the context of a macro-budget, as long as social insurance money cannot be transferred to the budget of the Ministry of Health and Environmental Protection, from which resources are allocated to prevention (Social insurance funds are largely earmarked for purposes of curative treatment). Similarly, private insurance benefit payments cannot be made available, of course, for general preventive programmes.

It is clear that budgeting on a national level assumes a large degree of control on the health care sector by central government, as, for instance, is the case with the National Health Service in the United Kingdom. The Dutch government does not exercise such a degree of control and may not even do that in the future unless major changes in the financial and administrative structure are made. The relevance of the Financial Survey will depend on the present and future legislation on health care regulation in the Netherlands. It may eventually provide a threefold framework; one for infrastructural developments (Health Services Act), one for prices and wages (Sickness Funds Insurance Act and General Sickness Expenses Act).

With respect to the Financial Survey providing a financial framework for infrastructural developments it may again be pointed out that the Hospital Facilities Act and, more particularly, the Health Services Act, propose a decentralization of planning power to regional and local public authorities (provinces and municipalities) without changing the financing structure of the health care system. Especially in a period of economic recession this can only be done if clear, *a priori*, limits are set to the growth of health care expenditure in a regional area. Therefore, both laws allow for the formulation of central guidelines regarding the maximum quantity of resources to be allocated to health care in a given period for a given area (province). As was suggested above, this 'regional budget' has to be derived from the national financial framework, provided by the annual Financial Survey.

The same observations made with respect to the viability of introducing a macro-budget for the health care sector apply here with respect to regional budgeting. The opportunities to reallocate resources for local authorities should be improved in order to make the concept of decentralized planning work. Again, limits are posed by the intricate financing structure which appears in Holland. Further, in the new legislation, planning authority will be delegated to the local government agencies, while the actual allocation of resources and the operational control within health care institutions will remain with the local financiers. This may make for inefficiency in those cases where lack of co-operation between the two local organizations prevents feedback of information necessary to balance planning, financing and control. Finally, there is a discrepancy between resource allocating power at decentralized level and the social insurance character of the public part of the health care sector which implies nationally prevailing uniform rights to health care provision. It is more than an impression that the concept of decentralized planning combined with tight budget controls does not easily fit in with the present administrative and financial structure.

With regard to the possible introduction of budgeting at the institutional level there are undoubtedly problems associated with the present hospital financing system. An acknowledgement of the disadvantages of this system has led to an experiment with hospital budgeting. From 1982 onwards, four Dutch hospitals are on a three-year contract, which incorporates the provision of a fixed budget for that period, based on historical costs *plus* additions for price and wage increases, for the costs of the experiment, and for the mean increase in other financial allowances made to Dutch hospitals. Because of the many financiers involved in reimbursing hospital services, a great deal of time and energy was involved in setting up this experiment and extra administrative arrangements (e.g. for the final financial settlement) are needed to run it. During parliamentary discussions over the 1981/82 budget a majority in parliament favoured a rapid introduction of hospital budgeting in the whole of the Netherlands. Apart from the fact that an objective way of fixing a hospital budget has yet to be found, it will be clear that there are administrative and technical difficulties, related to the involvement of so many organizations concerned in hospital reimbursement, which will prevent an early realization of this policy.

Future trends in financing

Given the current problems associated with the fact that a large variety of financiers operate in the health care sector, it can be assumed that attempts will be made to simplify the finance structure of the health care sector. In a recent report (1981) made by civil servants at the request of the Prime Minister, suggestions were made to abolish the voluntary public insurance scheme and the special public insurance scheme for the aged in an attempt to unify the public insurance scheme. These suggestions are now the basis for firm governmental plans to be issued at the end of 1982. According to the report this should be accompanied by regulating measures concerning price-setting and unification of insurance policies in the private sector. In this way some of the disadvantages which arise from the current system could disappear. Another approach, which appears to have substantial political support, would be more or less gradually to extend the general public insurance scheme (cf. the General Special Sickness Expenses Act). This can be done either by raising the income level, under which employees are compulsorily insured, or by extending the working area of this law toward primary care or hospital care. Our estimate would be that in the long run, all basic health care facilities will be financed out of public resources, most probably under the regime of one single general health insurance act. It is acknowledged, however, that finance from general revenues would be more in accordance with the planning system of the Health Services Act and the concept of regional budgeting that goes along with it.

The financing of physician services will be one of the key issues in future discussions on cost containment. The possibility of containing the costs of physician treatment may be illustrated by considering the way in which physicians and, in particular, specialists may maintain or increase their income under the current remuneration structure. Their opportunities to realize this, depends on a number of exogenous variables. *First*, the number of referrals per specialist, representing the patient flow to a specialist is, of course, the most important variable in this respect. The total number of referrals to specialists increased in the period 1968–77 by about 22 per cent. At the same time the number of specialists increased by about 38 per cent in spite of collective action by specialists to establish 'closed-shops'. As a consequence, the number of patients per specialist decreased for several specialties. *Secondly*, government intervention to contain the level of fees has been successful as can be inferred from the fact that mean fees decreased in real terms by more than 6 per cent in the period 1968–77.

The only possibility for specialists to compensate for this decrease is to increase 'productivity' in terms of patients. The figures show that specialists in several specialities were successful in maintaining or even increasing their incomes. These are specialists in surgery, internal medicine, cardiology, urology, and gynaecology. The increase in number of 'operations' per specialist varied in the period 1968–77 in these cases from 13 per cent (urology) to 67 per cent (internal medicine). The most recent data show that the total number of both therapeutic and diagnostic activities increased by about 13 per cent yearly (Financial Survey, 1981).

The potentiality of controlling the development of physicians' services is limited within the present structure. Financing agencies in both the public and the private sector are involved in review activities with respect to the utilization of physicians' services, but the impact of their actions is still rather small. The formation of 'medical audit' and 'hospital audit' groups within health care institutes is stimulated by the government, and financial arrangements for the promotion of utilization review are being set up. Finally, a national committee has been installed to investigate the causes of current developments and to recommend policies toward the more efficient use of diagnostic facilities.

When considering the development of total cost for physicians' services, another possible course of action besides manpower planning, which is dealt with elsewhere in the chapter, is of course to adjust fee levels downwards. Such a policy can be supported by the fact that a survey on incomes of medical specialists showed that the incomes of specialists in several specialties were considerably higher than the income agreed on earlier by the government and specialist organizations, which is used to determine the level of fees for referral and specialists' 'operations'. Currently, policies are aiming at reducing these differences in a few years to *zero*. In 1980, the moderation of fees as a consequence of this policy led to a decrease of costs by 65 million Dutch guilders. The dangers of such a policy in this open-ended structure, however, are obvious.

In *summary*, it can be stated that given the present remuneration structure, it is difficult to contain the costs of physicians' services. There is considerable pressure in parliament towards getting all physicians to work on a salary basis. The government has agreed to promote a salary system. One of the impediments, however, is the fact that physicians who work as free entrepreneurs have paid considerable sums of money to 'buy their practices' and expect to get back a fair amount of money when selling theirs to their successors. To find a settlement for buying-off physicians in free practices, which can be financed and is acceptable for all physicians, is extremely difficult, as can be inferred from the slow progress made by the committee dealing with this problem. Another committee officially set up by the government, is considering a restructuring of physician remuneration, but has not yet come to a conclusion. One of the alternatives considered is the introductuion of a regressive fee structure. This can only be a temporary solution and ultimately a salary system is probably more suitable in the situation in which most resources come from the public sector, and adequate monitoring is lacking.

HEALTH POLICY IN THE NETHERLANDS:
AT THE CROSSROADS

The experience in Holland has shown, as elsewhere, that the problems of unbalanced growth, insufficient cohesion between services and rising costs which have been identified, cannot be solved without a certain amount of government regulation and intervention. But how far should this go? The experience also shows that government regulation and intervention results in attempts to get around the rules. It also frequently actually discourages responsibility, leadership and initiatives in the private sector. Again, as we have seen, regulation has side-effects too. Usually this provokes further and even more detailed regulation. In the Netherlands, parliament has moved a long way in the direction of a government controlled health services system. In the very near future, the final decisions with respect to the volume, quality, prices, costs, and financing of the services rendered will be made by the government. There are, however, still many dilemmas remaining.

The dilemmas with which Dutch health policy making and health planning will be confronted, are problems of rising demand. These dilemmas are mainly the same problems which are faced by the Dutch welfare state as a whole. People are well educated. They understand their rights and they are more articulate in their demands. Because of this, health care is caught up in the 'revolution of higher expectation'. Being able to do more, means that more is expected, and indeed demanded. Pressure groups are playing their several roles in this development. The Welfare State also takes care of illness. Lack of income is no constraint and being ill means more attention and consideration. The behaviour of people with respect to their own health leaves much to be desired too: and in addition people are not caring for each other any longer, since the State has taken over the responsibility. Elderly people are making a large demand on the health services. In spite of the efforts to improve the working environment, labour absenteeism has increased considerably over the years. Chronic labour unfitness has grown out of proportion and has reached an alarming level.

Regulation and government intervention are principally affecting health and the health services via the supply side. Governments are better equipped to regulate supply than to regulate demand, as so many 'cultural' factors are involved which are out of reach of government control.

The newly designed instruments of volume, quality, price, cost, and financing regulation also have some limitations. These instruments in particular influence demand only via the supply side. If however, a limitation of supply does not result in a decrease of demand, tensions will arise. These tensions may grow to such an extent, that under political pressure the demand will have to be met.

This indeed is likely to become the major dilemma of health policy in the Netherlands, in particular because volume regulation planned for the future does not include such outputs as number of consultations, nature and number of diagnostic procedures, prescriptions of drugs, and treatments. Thus, there is no control on the volume of activities and therefore these cannot be budgeted for. This situation may cause discrepancies within the system. Clinical specialists, working in the environment of short-stay general hospitals, will make use of technological development and consumer expectations to attract a disproportionate share of the limited resources. As a consequence, health policies directed to a strict control of health expenditures will be implemented at the expense of the weaker sectors such as preventive care, ambulatory services, care of the elderly, mental health care, and care of the handicapped. This effect cannot fully be corrected by financial regulations as the financing system will continue to remain pluralistic for the years to come. It will not be unlikely, therefore, that the Dutch Government may decide at a later phase of development to interfere also in the freedom of health professionals in their professional practice and to seek to assess the benefits of related technology.

Striking a balance between the market mechanism and government control in the Dutch situation will probably entail, therefore, the introduction of a budgeting system throughout the health services. Not only on the basis of 'investment limits' but also on the basis of 'cash limits'. These limits will necessarily be subjected to strict governmental control. At the same time the basic package of health care services to which all insured families or individuals are entitled, should be guaranteed. But within these limits maximum freedom should be left to private enterprise to solve their own problems within the context of their own responsibilities. The regulation based on the Health Services Act, in combination with the Health Tariffs Act provides a first step to achieve such a goal. Volume regulation on the basis of the former Act, however, which is limited in its present form only to the infrastructure, may have to be extended to control the volume of health activities as well. In addition, the present financing system will have to be reviewed.

Cost containment in
health insurance
The case of Belgium

ROBERT VAN DEN HEUVEL
AND ANDRÉE SACREZ

ROBERT VAN DEN HEUVEL

Robert van den Heuvel who was born in 1926, is a Doctor of Law and Master of Financial and Business Sciences (University of Louvain). After a short training at the bar of Antwerp, he became Private Secretary to the Minister of Transport and Communications. In 1954, he joined the Alliance Nationale des Mutualités Chrétiennes (ANMC) and became its President in 1976. He is currently Chairman of the European Association of Mutualities and also President of the Board of Governors of the National Institute of Health Insurance. He is also a member of the Board of Governors of the University of Antwerp and member of the Council of the International Federation of Voluntary Health Service Funds.

ANDRÉE SACREZ

Andrée Sacrez was born in Moustier-sur-Sambre in 1935, she is a Master of Economic Sciences and of Business and Administration. From 1958 to 1965 she was assistant at the 'Institut des Sciences économiques' of the University of Louvain. In 1965 she became a member of the research department of the ANMC (Alliance Nationale des Mutualités Chrétiennes) and was appointed head of the department in 1973. Besides various publications on health insurance and health policy, she also plays an active role within the AIM (European Association of Mutualities) as general reporter for the commission dealing with the study of the relationship between health insurance and the medical profession, as well as with the problems of fee tariffs.

Cost containment in health insurance
The case of Belgium

ABSTRACT

A compulsory Health Insurance system has been operating in Belgium since the end of the Second World War, through five national non-profit (and one public) sickness funds. While largely regulated by law and by decrees it operates with a fair degree of autonomy and although under government supervision and control, much of its operation is accomplished by means of consultation between the main partners, that is; sickness funds, the medical profession, hospitals, and both sides of industry.

The escalation of health expenditure in the sixties and early seventies which progressed virtually uncontrolled, eventually provoked a number of measures to contain costs, the end result of which, now, is that in real terms, expenditure has levelled off and there is effectively 'zero growth'. This has been achieved largely as a consequence of negotiation and mutual persuasion, mainly between the sickness funds and the different medical and paramedical professions, with the government a powerful policy influence, but remaining in the background in the direct negotiations.

INTRODUCTION

Health insurance has been compulsory in Belgium since the end of the second world war. It operates under the supervision of the National Sickness and Invalidity Insurance Institute but is carried out by five national non-profit sickness funds and one public fund (1).

When compulsory insurance came into force on 1 January 1945, it proved necessary to call on the private sickness funds which had contributed so much to the extension of voluntary

209

health care insurance for more than half a century. Those organizations were and still are more than insurers. Most of the sickness funds were and still are a part of the social movement. They do not only execute the compulsory health insurance according to the legal regulations: they also aim at defending and protecting the health care consumers—individually and/or collectively. They also contribute to the development of health policy. Besides the compulsory insurance, they offer some complementary services such as convalescence, appliances and aids for the handicapped, home nursing and domestic aid, health education and information. Some also operate their own facilities: hospitals, medical centres and pharmacies, but without limiting the freedom of choice of their members. Lastly but not least they pay special attention to the underprivileged among their members: the elderly, the disabled and the invalids, for whom they organize social guidance, welfare services, and social activities.

The development of these activities is based largely on a decentralized system a feature of which is co-operation between volunteers and professionals. The volunteers play an important part in the sickness funds, not only in contributing to some specific activities but also in participating in the definition of the sickness funds policy. The Christian sickness funds underlined the role of the volunteers in their 1976 Convention.

The development of complementary activities and services is a part of the competition between the five private sickness funds. It has to be noted that while *membership* of a sickness fund *is compulsory*, the *choice* of a sickness fund *is free*.

The Belgian medical care system is liberal in concept and practice. Thus, the physician has total therapeutic freedom and he is generally paid on a fee-for-service basis. On the other hand, there is for the patient unlimited freedom of choice of doctor and hospital. There is no separate listing for general practice, nor a mandatory reference system for patients. Finally, no distinction is made between private and public hospitals either for health insurance benefits or for the way in which general regulations are applied.

It will thus be evident that the framework of the Belgian

health care and insurance system encloses a comprehensive package of health care, including maternity, dental care, and drugs which covers 99 per cent of the population (2).

Expenditure on the scheme increased rapidly during the seventies (Appendices I and II) but a degree of stabilization has been achieved since 1979 (Appendix III).

This recent stabilization is the result of a progressively more efficient containment of health expenditure. It is important to note that the savings resulting from all the measures taken since 1978 amounted in 1981 to 19,550m BF (total expected expenditure: 159,686m BF). It is interesting to point out however that at the same time the Belgian population is ageing. The elderly (over 65) represented 13·43 per cent of the total population in 1961 and 14·23 per cent in 1980. It is manifest that this group need much more health care than that of the rest of the population.

The trends in cost are not the same for the different types of services (Appendix IV). There has been a significant growth in the expenditure of hospital stay (3) (Appendix V). It has been much lower however for drugs. The main measures taken are analysed later in this paper.

The health insurance system has two major sources of finance: contributions and State subsidies. The contributions of the workers and employers (c. 60 per cent of the total resources) are based on a percentage of the wages: now 5·55 per cent (1·80 per cent supported by the employees and 3·75 per cent supported by the employers). From 1963 till 1981, the State subsidies (c. 40 per cent of the total resources) were of two types: (a) a main subsidy allocated according to the total cost of care; and (b) a further subsidy to compensate for the loss of contributions of the unemployed, who are not required to pay any contribution for social security.

Because of the uncertainties of public finance, the government has since 1978 continually reduced its grants for social security. Indeed the subsidies for health insurance are no longer allocated according to the legal prescriptions. A new law of 26 June 1981 considerably modified the system and abolished the compensation of the contributions of the unemployed. It involves *de facto,* a reduction in this source of finance which effectively means an added burden to be borne

Table 1. *Reduction of the state subsidies.*

Year	Amount (millions BF)	Health Insurance profits (millions BF)
1978	1·393	−1·403
1979	836	5·979
1980	1·270	2·930
1981	7·621	6·771*
1982	8·420	9·180*

*Estimated

by the insurance system, which has still to cover the health care of the unemployed and their families (4) (Table 1). These reductions increased the deficits, particularly during the last two years. Further, the poor economic outlook is not only responsible for the crisis in public finance but also for a lower growth (indeed negative at constant prices in 1982) of the contributions. There is however a general feeling that in the present economic situation the level of contributions cannot be raised.

OBJECTIVES OF REGULATION

General objectives

First of all, the *State* aims at cutting down the subsidies. The economic depression has led to a massive increase in unemployment, which means supplementary costs for the social security and for the government.

Given that the state subsidies for health insurance are now exclusively based on the expenditure on the elderly and invalid people—80 per cent of their cost—the government will more than ever limit its part in the financing of the compulsory health insurance system. The subsidy to the health insurance cannot grow faster than the national income, since at present, the Belgian Government is pledged not to introduce any new taxation.

For 1982, however, the present Minister of Social Affairs is prepared to make some transfers of contributions within the social security in favour of the health insurance system. The new Minister has openly admitted that new means were needed in order to maintain essential services within the package of health insurance.

The goals of the *sickness funds* are both to safeguard and improve the efficiency in the health care insurance system without an unjustified increase of the contributions, as well as to guarantee the accessibility of health care to all their members. The role of the funds is crucial. They do not want a collapse of the basis of the social insurance—the principle of 'solidarity' (risk-pooling)—and they cannot accept a money barrier which would discourage the underpriviliged from getting necessary medical care.

Hitherto the Belgian health insurance system has been comprehensive and the sickness funds are currently opposing any proposals which tend to limit the health care coverage. Some people want, for instance, to exclude primary care from compulsory insurance and to leave the so-called 'small risks' to private insurance. The funds do not agree with such moves. In these cases the profit-making private insurance companies will tend to select the 'better risks' and the contracts offered will thus often be too expensive for the underprivileged. Further, it is believed it will in time lead to two sorts of health care systems: one for the lower classes of the population, the other more luxurious for the wealthy. Finally, it would curtail the results of recent efforts to promote primary health care.

Particular objectives

More specifically, the objectives of the measures concerning *hospitals* are to avoid undue expenditure by containing the growth of the daily hospital rates as well as the frequency and the length of stays. Apart from this financial objective, the regulations aim at developing a more appropriate policy concerning the care and lodging of elderly and chronic sick people. More generally, it can be said that all these measures are aimed at putting 'the right person in the right bed' which involves at once limits on the extent as well as probably a requirement for the reorganization of the hospital network.

In Belgium, there is neither a *numerus clausus* for medical students nor a direct regulation regarding the *supply of doctors*. The only regulations are indirect. The conditions required for the qualification as specialist do *de facto* limit the supply of specialists. There is also a compulsory planning regulation for sophisticated medical equipment as well as for highly specialized services like coronary units.

Until now, there has been *no limitation on the supply of general practitioners*. Nevertheless, the number of first year medical of undergraduates has decreased over the last five years.

As far as *the quantity of medical services* supplied is concerned both the representatives of the medical profession and of the funds have agreed to the setting up of an ambitious system to prevent unnecessary multiplication of medical services.

The Belgians are large *drug* consumers. The objectives of drug regulations are to discourage high consumption not only to lighten the cost for the insurance system but also to avoid the kind of over-consumption which might not of itself be healthy for the consumer. Again, some regulations are aimed at limiting the prices of drugs.

Belgium is a small country and has a very good road network. There is consequently less need for a *'distributional'* *regulation* of health care facilities and providers, perhaps with some rare exceptions in the south-east.

NATURE OF THE REGULATIONS

The common responsibility of both sides of industry (unions and employers), of health care providers and of sickness funds is the basic characteristic of the Belgian health insurance system. They are all represented on the Board of Governors of the National Health Insurance Institute, which has a regulatory capacity whereby the government has a right to veto the decisions of the Board. This however is exercised extremely rarely. The tariffs (of fees and prices) of health care are determined by negotiations between the health care providers and the sickness funds. Further, they have to be approved by the government. Consultation and co-ordination are the main characteristics of this system. The search for better use of insurance resources, and for a financial balance cannot be achieved without a fair degree of consensus between groups concerned.

All regulations are made centrally, some applying as macro-controls, some on a micro-scale.

Hospital care regulations

Regulation of the *supply of hospital facilities* has a relatively long history. A 1966 law raised the first norms of hospital planning and set out the number of beds allowed for specific services (for instance surgery) per 1000 inhabitants. This regulation was not made mandatory until 1973. Theoretically, the building of new hospitals is not allowed, neither is it allowed to increase the capacity of a hospital, or to renew a hospital, without the authorization of a special committee which takes its decisions according to the criteria laid down by regulation.

A proposition that there should be a 5 per cent reduction in the number of general hospital beds failed last year. The present government, however, has given notice of its intention to achieve this aim. Special state grants for reconversion of a hospital (or of a part of it) into a nursing home for elderly disabled people are forecast.

Finally, there is a special limitation of the number of university hospital beds.

As far as the *daily hospital prices* (5) are concerned, some rules are fixed yearly in order to control the increase in hospital expenditure. Price limits have been introduced for various expenses such as staff, food, laundry, etc.

In fact, the present daily hospital price system does however indirectly contain an incentive to retain the patients longer than necessary by prolonging the duration of *hospital stays* since the income of the hospitals is fixed according to the number of patient days. Some measures are being taken this year to reduce the effect of this incentive to inefficient management and alternative ways of paying hospitals are now being discussed. It seems likely that, in the future, length of stays will be monitored by means of profiles, according to the type of hospital and to diagnoses.

In order to shorten the over-long stays, patients who remain in hospital for more than six or twelve months and whose health state does no longer require medical care but only nursing, could well have to pay a larger portion of the daily price. Alternative care will be made available for them in nursing homes or through home care. In such cases the health insurance arrangements will provide for a flat amount covering the costs of nursing and domestic aid. The objective is to assure equal treatment of all chronic sick and elderly people whether they stay in hospital, or in an old people's home, or with their family.

Doctors' services

As has been already indicated, there is no direct regulation regarding the supply of doctors in Belgium.

With regard *to practice* there is a utilization review scheme by means of 'profiles' which is now operational for some specialities.

The *total number of services and of prescriptions* of each doctor are registered and after a statistical selection, the apparently abnormal profiles are examined by an evaluation committee. This committee is composed of an equal number of doctors representing the profession and of doctors chosen by the Board of Governors of the National Health Insurance Institute. If necessary, the case is transmitted to the Medical Society for disciplinary action, or in case of fraud to the Board of Medical Audit of the National Health Insurance Institute.

Some micro-regulations have been introduced designed to reduce *the quantity* of some technical services (i.e. biochemical pathology and radiology). For instance, there are some restrictions which apply to the freedom of the pathologist or the radiologist to prescribe services.

Furthermore, *the provision of sophisticated services* (e.g. coronary units) or of very expensive technologies like CAT scanners is limited by the national planning arrangements.

As far as the *quality* of care is concerned, there are as yet no rules, but it is hoped that the profiles of medical practices will finally allow better quality control.

With regard to *prices* and *fees*, restrictions on the increase of fees and actual reductions of specific medical fees (e.g. for biochemical pathology), were approved as a result of negotiations between the profession and the sickness funds.

Drugs

Regulation on the *prices of drugs* is relatively severe in Belgium. There are two different levels. *First*, a special price committee for drugs advises the Minister of Economic Affairs who fixes the prices of all drugs, those that are reimbursed by the health insurance system as well as those that are excluded from the insurance.

Secondly, the prices of the drugs that are to be reimbursed through the health insurance system are discussed again in a special committee of the National Sickness and Invalidity Insurance Institute composed of representatives from the health insurance system and from the pharmaceutical industry. These discussions usually have a positive result.

On a proposal of the Sickness Funds, the *reimbursement system* for drugs was totally modified in 1980. The former system in which the personal fraction was a fixed amount was not satisfactory.

Neither the practitioners nor the patients were interested in the price of drugs. The health insurance system could not take advantage of any price competition between the pharmaceutical firms since the latter were not stimulated to sell cheaper products because the patients' fraction was a flat amount and therefore the real cost was not known to him. The drugs are now *classified* according to their *therapeutic and social utility* and divided into *four classes*.

The health insurance coverage—which is now expressed as a percentage of the price varies from one category to another. It is total for the first class (so-called life-savers) and reduced to zero for the last one. This new system aims at influencing *the behaviour of both new consumers and prescribers* as well as discouraging the use of drugs, the utility of which is not proved. But it cannot entirely succeed without an adequate information source which encourages the doctors to prescribe more economically, e.g. by indicating comparative prices of similar products. Such information is not yet readily available. Currently the patents of a certain number of drugs are expiring and therefore some regulations are being prepared to promote *'generics'*. It requires, among others, new calculations for the retail margins of the chemist as well as reliable information for both prescribers and consumers.

Finally, the opening of new *pharmacies* has been controlled since 1974.

Cost-sharing

The effect of co-payments for the cost of health services for which the patient is responsible has changed over the last few years. In principle, *cost-sharing* is only applied when the patient himself decides to use medical services or when he can influence the prescriber, for instance, for drugs, physiotherapy and in some cases for hospitalization.

The new system of drugs reimbursement can, if the consumption remains the same, result in a *higher personal contribution* for the patient, especially for elderly people (an average of 25 per cent).

Patients pay 25 per cent of the fees for doctors home and office visits. Since 1 April 1982, they also pay 40 per cent of the fees of physiotherapists, with exceptions for traumatology, intensive care, orthopaedic surgery, for which the cost-sharing is reduced to 20 per cent.

The patient also has to pay a *fixed amount per hospitalization day*. This daily payment is a contribution towards the cost of the accommodation provided by the hospital.

Retired persons, widows and invalids with low incomes generally pay less (6).

EFFECTS OF THE REGULATIONS

It is not very easy to evaluate the effects of the several measures that have been taken during the last years. Unfortunately, they are not taken in a closed world where everything remains the same. Nevertheless, it is possible perhaps to analyse some major facts and changes.

Financial regulations

The regulations to support a policy designed to contain the disposable income of the health insurance system have failed. The policy resulted in a compulsory health insurance system receiving less by way of subsidy from the government but the reduction was not sufficiently counterbalanced by receipts from other resources or as a result of cutbacks of the expenditure. The deficit of the insurance scheme as a whole was thus grave, despite the large amount of economies achieved during recent years. At the end of 1980, it had accumulated to 14·2 billion BF which the State has undertaken to amortize in 12 years.

The main reason for the failure of this policy can probably be attributed to the lack of political determination of recent governments, who hesitated to raise new contributions to compensate for the abolition of important subsidies, even though the contribution level for health insurance in Belgium is the lowest of the EEC countries (Table 2).

Mandatory planning and geriatric beds

The regulations *regarding mandatory planning for hospital beds* also partly failed. First of all, it has to be remarked that the

Table 2. *Contributions for Health Care Insurance: EEC 1.7.81.*

Country	Employee %	Employer %	Total %	Wage Ceiling %
Belgium	1·80	3·75	5·55	—[1]
France	4·95	11·00	15·95[1]	79·080 FF[2]
Germany	4·90	4·90	9·80[1]	42·300 DM[3]
The Netherlands	4·30	7·35	11·65	48·750 fl.[4]

1. Revised contribution figures for health care insurance only, excluding disablement benefits insurance.

2. This ceiling only applies for a part (4·5 per cent) of the contribution of the employer. No ceiling for the worker.

3. In Germany, this wage-ceiling only applies to employees. The employees whose wages exceed this ceiling are not compulsory insured. Nevertheless, the employer has to support a part of the private insurance premium paid by the employees, whose wages exceed this ceiling.

4. The contribution will increase in 1982 (from 11·65 to 12·88 per cent).

Table 3. *Evolution of the number of hospital beds.*

Year	Short-stay beds	Psychiatric beds	Long-stay (geriatric) beds	Total
1971	45·828	26·553	3·285	80·392
1975	50·417	26·337	6·788	87·164
1979	52·827	24·637	9·884	90·201
1980	53·477	24·506	11·072	91·889
1981	53·889	24·182	11·674	92·436

decision to extend or rebuild some hospitals taken in the 'golden sixties' are only now coming to fruition. It partly explains why the number of hospital beds is still growing (Table 3).

Theoretically, Belgium has an efficient regulation system to contain the development of the supply of hospital beds. But the legal criteria are not respected. One of the reasons is once again the lack of real political will, especially under the influence of local interests. At the same time mechanisms are not efficient. The criteria are fixed by a national Commission but they are in effect applied by three regional Commissions. The investment costs are subsidized by the regions, but the working costs are supported through the national health insurance system. This complicated structure does not promote the sense of responsibility of the regions and explains a great deal of the failure of the hospital regulations regarding the bed supply. Yet regionalization will go on further for general political reasons.

Another cause of this failure is *the lack* of alternative solutions such *as nursing homes for invalid elderly people.* If the decision of the present government to reduce the number of beds by 5 per cent succeeds, there is some prospect it will be possible to release the necessary funds to start such nursing homes.

Regulations which affect the *daily hospital cost* charged have been much more successful, particularly in 1979 and in 1981 (Table 4).

The 1982 costs will probably be influenced by the shortening of the working week and increases in the salaries of the staff during 1980/1.

It is interesting to notice that the daily hospital prices are

Table 4. *Average daily hospital prices.*

Year	Average cost charged BF	Annual growth %	Retail prices index annual growth %
1977	1·575	+6·7	+7·1
1978	1·698	+8·0	+4·5
1979	1·689	−0·5	+4·5
1980	1·825	+8·0	+6·6
1981	1·845	+1·1	+7·6

fixed by the Minister of Public Health (7), who is advised by a special committee. The sickness funds are represented in this committee.

Containment of the cost of doctors' services

The introduction of utilization review and medical necessity tests (profiles) will undoubtedly have some preventive effects (avoiding over-utilization).

Other measures have also had a positive result. The total expenditure per insured person for medical care (general practitioners, specialists, etc.) has grown more slowly over recent years (Table 5).

This relatively favourable trend results from negotiations and co-ordinated policies between the health care providers and the sickness funds. Another positive effect of negotiated arrangements is the decrease of the rate of growth of the expenditures for biochemical pathology, radiology and nuclear medicine *(in vitro)* (Appendix VI). Fees for biochemical

Table 5. *Medical fees per insured person.*

Year	In BF at the prices of 1970	Annual growth %
1975	2·454	+ 7·8
1976	2·626	+ 7·2
1977	2·814	+ 6·7
1978	3·098	+ 10·7
1979	3·177	+ 2·9
1980	3·156	− 0·6

pathology and nuclear medicine procedures were reduced and the regulations regarding radiological and clinical biological investigations were strengthened.

Drug regulations

An international comparison of the average ex-factory price of drugs (Table 6) shows that the position of Belgium in 1979 compared favourably with other countries.

Table 6. *Average ex-factory price of drugs (1980)[1],*
(for the 30 per cent of drugs sold most in Belgium).

Country	Belgium = 100
Italy	66
France	79
Belgium	100
Great Britain	115
The Netherlands	118

1. For reimburseable drugs only.

Despite the fact it is difficult to control prices because of the cost structure of pharmaceutical products, Belgium has succeeded reasonably well in containing the prices of drugs (Table 7). Nevertheless, the industry is now asking for price increases which are not always justified by recent devaluation of the Belgian franc.

The action of the *Special Price Committee of the National Health Insurance Institute* has certainly something to do with

Table 7. *Drug prices (9), (reimbursable drugs only).*

Year	Average price of drugs BF	Annual growth %	Retail prices index annual growth %
1975	243	—	—
1976	260	+7·0	+9·2
1977	275	−5·1	+7·1
1978	286	+4·1	+4·5
1979	291	+1·9	+4·5
1980	294	+0·9	+6·6

the control shown by this trend. Once more, it is worth noting that the concerted action of responsible people from the health insurance system and the pharmaceutical industry is the basis of this committee's success.

After only nine months' experience, the new *reimbursement system* shows a very positive result for the health insurance scheme. The expenditure of the health insurance scheme in current prices shows a reduction of about 4 per cent. It will of course also be necessary to look at the consequences for patients, to ensure that the co-payment for necessary drugs did not increase out of proportion.

The new system however will only be really efficient for the health insurance system and for the patients if adequate information—'*transparence list*' (8)—is given to the doctors. In addition there should be a *better mechanism for reviewing prescriptions*. The regulation concerning the *opening of pharmacies* has not hitherto been very successful. From 1974 (the date of the law on the opening of pharmacies) until 1980, the number of chemists' shops increased by more than 10 per cent. There is now one chemist's shop for 1790 inhabitants. This situation is due to the fact that the law of 1974 has not been complemented by a regulation concerning the taking over of pharmacies. There is, for example, no regulation which obliges a pharmacy to close when the chemist retires and the facility provided in the area is unnecessary. The difficulty of the problem is indicated by the fact that there are no financial measures to compensate the owner.

Cost-sharing

Until now, cost-sharing is more often seen as one of the means to finance health insurance rather than a real deterrent to utilization.

It is relatively easy to reduce the health insurance deficit by introducing or increasing a *personal co-payment* of the patients. Most people are more resistant to new taxes or contributions than to certain cost-sharing. But if cost-sharing is intended to influence the behaviour of the health care consumers, it has to be recognized it will only be applicable to a few; otherwise it can be a barrier to the use of necessary medical services, which is a situation which cannot in principle be accepted by the sickness funds. The present system of co-payments seems to be acceptable, but an inquiry among sick people should be undertaken to measure the effect of such payments on personal budgets, to ensure that the insurance coverage is still satisfactory, particularly for the underprivileged.

Cost-sharing can also influence *the behaviour of the health care providers*, for instance the physiotherapists. It will be very interesting to follow the evolution of physiotherapy after 1 April 1982, when the patients will have to pay higher personal charges. Above all, to be both acceptable and efficient, therapeutic priorities have to be respected, as is generally accepted for medicine and physiotherapy.

CONCLUSION

The Belgian compulsory insurance scheme, although largely regulated by law and by decrees, operates with an important degree of automony and consultation between the most important partners involved: sickness funds, medical professions, and hospitals as well as both sides of industry, while the government supervises and controls.

None of the partners can decide alone; therefore there is a constant search for a balance of power, and acute conflicts arise when one of the partners does neglect that basic rule (such as happened in 1964 and 1980 when we had doctors' strikes in Belgium).

One has to have in mind the important role that the sickness funds in Belgium do not only play in operating the compulsory health insurance system but also in research, in policy making, in offering complementary benefits and taking new initiatives in both the health and social fields.

Because of the decentralization of the system and because of the fact that the insured people enjoy a total freedom of choice of sickness fund, and can change every three months, the funds are particularly sensitive to their members' opinions and wants.

When one looks at the evolution of the health insurance

expenditure during the last decade, one notices that after the nearly uncontrolled growth of the '60s and of the beginning of the '70s, there has been impressive cost containment, so that 'zero growth' in real terms has actually been reached (9). Due to its ageing population, Belgium cannot however in the long term hold on a 'zero growth' of health expenditure.

Meanwhile it is interesting to observe that the cost containment achieved is very often the consequence of negotiations and mutual persuasion, mainly between the sickness funds and the different medical and paramedical professions. One can even say that these common agreements have, in many cases, been more sucessful than authoritarian regulations.

This might show that even in a compulsory scheme covering practically the entire population, there is space for flexibility and private initiative as long as all the partners involved respect the basic rules of democracy, *inter alia* to face realities and to assume their own responsibilities.

This will be even more true in the immediate future as we will be facing further progress in medical technology, and the consequences of our unfavourable demography, while the economic situation is not likely to improve. This situation will require a better cost-effectiveness analysis and more cost-consciousness, by information and education of both health care providers and health care consumers.

NOTES

1. The membership of the public fund is very small, only 1 per cent of the total insured people.

2. The compulsory insurance for self-employed (14 per cent of the population) has a less comprehensive coverage. In this contribution, we only refer to the general scheme.

3. In Belgium, the daily hospital rate only includes the cost of accommodation and nursing; the other expenditures: medical fees, drugs . . . are not included.

4. At present, there are about 500,000 unemployed workers.

5. See note 2.

6. e.g. 10 per cent for doctors' visits and 20 per cent or 10 per cent for physiotherapy and a lower maximum for drugs.

7. In the present Government (1982) the same Minister is in charge of social affairs and social security (health insurance) and public health.

8. i.e. List of comparative prices of similar products.

9. For the Alliance Nationale des Mutualités Chrétiennes the first figures for 1981 show a zero growth (at constant prices).

APPENDIX I

Health care, expenses per insured

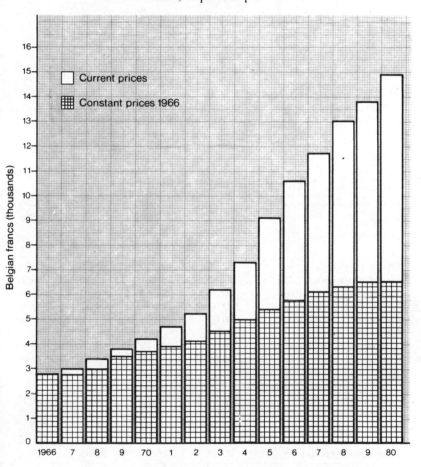

APPENDIX II

Some general data

	1970–80 %
Index of retail prices	102·70
Average hourly wages (industry)	139·90
Number of doctors	
general practitioners	+ 92·60
specialists	+ 34·40
Insured people	+ 9·80

Health insurance expenditure

	Volume[1] 1970–80 %	Average cost price 1970–80 %	Part in the total expenses 1970 %	1980 %
Office visits GPs	32·04	191·36	3·92	3·91
Home visits GPs	17·83	139·67	5·54	3·99
Office visits psychiatrists	86·35	99·47	0·49	0·48
Office visits pediatricians	29·93	145·35	0·57	0·48
Office visits specialists	30·65	109·59	3·18	2·40
Office visits specialists for internal diseases	30·65	109·59	3·18	2·40
Surgery	58·98	184·98	4·08	4·79
Biochemical pathology Art. 24 (without personal fraction)	292·51	32·18	5·92	7·97
X-rays	176·92	54·79	5·15	5·73
Magistral preparations	−9·74	99·00	6·06	2·82
Specialities	21·16	127·74	16·73	11·97
Hospitalization day	30·68	326·49	18·83	27·07

1. Number of medical acts, supplies or hospitalization days.

APPENDIX III

Trends in the health expenditure per insured person

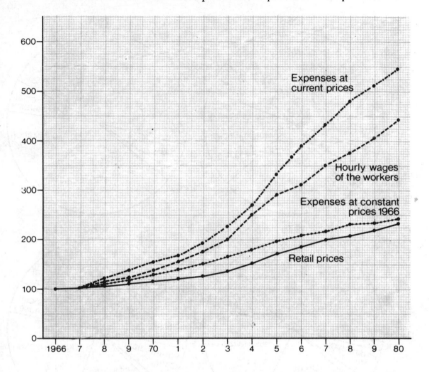

APPENDIX IV

Proportionate expenses per service, 1960–80

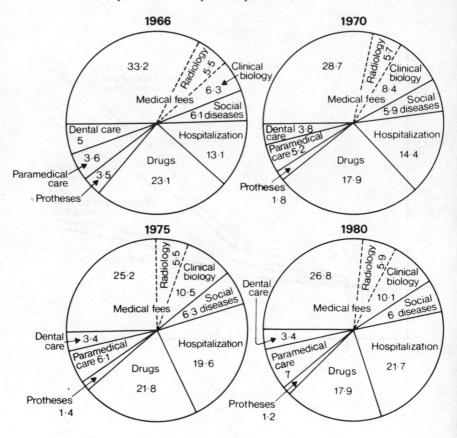

APPENDIX V

Hospitalization

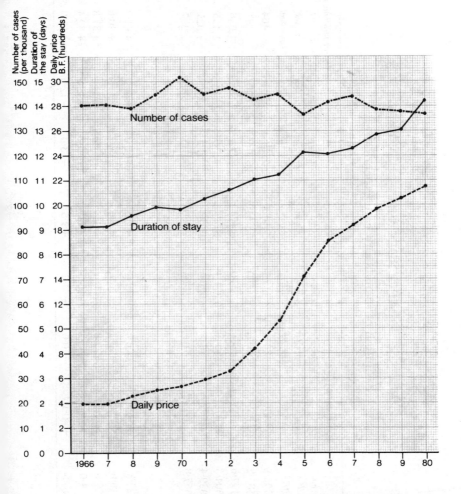

APPENDIX VI

Evolution of some health care expenditure

Year	Biochemical pathology						Radiology						Nuclear medicine in vitro					
	Amount million BF	%	Cases (thousands)	%	Average price per case BF	%	Amount million BF	%	Cases (thousands)	%	Average price per case BF	%	Amount million BF	%	Cases (thousands)	%	Average price per case BF	%
1975	7,775·9		59,436		130·8		4,112·7		7,182		572·6		504·7		464		1,088·0	
1976	9,585·2		67,869		141·2		4,930·0		7,814		630·9		820·9		751		1,092·5	
1977	11,177·6		76,613		145·9		5,723·0		8,474		675·4		1,185·4		1,056		1,122·4	
1978	13,504·3		90,018		150·0		6,271·4		8,627		727·0		1,554·1		1,455		1,068·1	
1979	14,039·4		95,772		146·7		6,929·3		9,184		754·5		1,860·4		1,927		965·2	
1980	12,567·8		95,869		131·1		7,217·4		9,866		731·6		1,627·2		2,217		733·9	
Yearly evolution																		
75–76		+23·3		+14·2		+ 8·0		+19·9		+8·8		+10·2		+62·7		+61·9		+ 0·4
76–77		+16·6		+12·9		+ 3·3		+16·1		+8·4		+ 7·1		+44·4		+40·6		+ 2·7
77–78		+20·8		+17·5		+ 2·8		+ 9·6		+1·8		+ 7·6		+31·1		+37·8		− 4·8
78–79		+ 4·0		+ 6·4		− 2·2		+10·5		+6·5		+ 3·8		+19·7		+32·4		− 9·6
79–80		+10·5		+ 0·1		−10·6		+ 4·2		+7·5		− 3·0		−12·5		+15·0		−24·0

Expenditures and attempts of cost containment in the statutory health insurance system of the Federal Republic of Germany

FRITZ BESKE

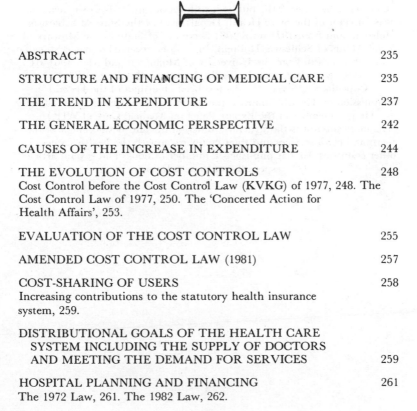

FRITZ BESKE

Dr Fritz Beske is Director of the Institute of Health Systems Research in Kiel (Federal Republic of Germany) and Professor of Public Health and Social Medicine. He qualified in medicine in 1951 at Keil University. After some years of research at the Institute of Hygiene at Kiel University he entered the public health service in 1958. For 6 years he was Director of the State Health Department of the State of Schleswig-Holstein, and from 1971 until 1981 Secretary of State in the Ministry of Social Affairs of Schleswig-Holstein. In 1955 he received a master's degree in public health from the University of Michigan, and from 1961-64 served as a medical officer in the European Bureau of WHO in Copenhagen. Since 1972 he has been chairman of the Federal Commission on Health Affairs of the Christian Democratic Party (CDU). He is a member of the Expert Panel on Medical Care of WHO.

His main interest is the structure, functioning, and development of the German health services and their comparison with the health services in other countries. He has published a number of books and several articles especially on these subjects.

Expenditures and attempts of cost containment in the statutory health insurance system of the Federal Republic of Germany

ABSTRACT

The rising costs of medical care and, as a result, the problem of expenditures and cost containment especially in the statutory health insurance system which covers about 90 per cent of the population, is of major concern in the Federal Republic of Germany. The trends in expenditures as well as causes for this development are described for the period 1960–80.

Cost control started in 1975 with voluntary agreements between physicians and the sickness funds. From 1977 onward a number of laws were passed in order to reduce expenditures, including a law on cost control in hospitals. On the Federal level a Standing Conference, the 'Concerted Action for Health Affairs', has been convened, whose 60 members are representatives from all the main bodies concerned in health matters, and its main objective is cost control.

There is wide and controversial debate over whether cost containment should and can be achieved mainly through legislation or through the operation of the various mechanisms of self-government which apply in the statutory health insurance system. This is largely a political issue. There are, however, good reasons for less bureaucracy and more freedom in matters related to health.

STRUCTURE AND FINANCING OF MEDICAL CARE

In the Federal Republic of Germany medical care is financed mainly through the *statutory health insurance system* which covers 90·3 per cent of the population.

The latest data concerning *membership* of the statutory health insurance system are for 1978. According to these data 57 per cent of the members of the statutory health insurance system are compulsorily insured, 13 per cent are voluntary members, and 30 per cent are retired. The figures include family members (Mitversicherte) and persons who are insured in the statutory health insurance system by the state e.g. handicapped persons.

7·5 per cent of the population belong to private health insurance. 6·7 per cent of those covered by the statutory system have additional private insurance e.g. for choice of physician in hospital or for a single room in hospital (private 'luxury' expenditures). 1·9 per cent of the population have some kind of other coverage e.g. welfare recipients or veterans. 0·3 per cent of the population have no coverage. Those are exclusively well-to-do people.

State employees (Beamte) get a refund for medical expenses of about 50 per cent to 70 per cent according to their family status and certain services such as dental services, hospital care, and drugs. Most of them have private insurance for the difference in making up 100 per cent of their expenses.

For those who are privately insured the amount of coverage of expenses for medical services is defined by their contract of insurance. All the others, the members of the statutory system, veterans and those covered by welfare, have full coverage of medical care including physician services, dental services, hospital services, drugs, medical appliances, and preventive services. There is only a minimum of cost-sharing, mainly for drugs, dentures, and transport.

The contribution rates to the statutory system are calculated as a percentage of the basic income. Fifty per cent are paid for by the employees and 50 per cent by the employers up to a certain income level. The income level is adjusted every year.

The system and the functioning of the *statutory health insurance system* is extraordinarily complex and complicated. In essence it is regulated by law, the 'State Insurance Regulations' (Reichsversicherungsordnung, RVO), and governed through self-government. In general according to their types of employment, employees belong to different types of individual sickness funds (Krankenkassen). There are altogether 1296 sickness funds (1981).

White-collar workers have different funds from those of blue-collar workers and to some extent other regulations.

The individual funds are self-governed and are organized at both state and federal levels.

All *physicians and dentists* who work for the statutory system belong compulsorily to the Association of Sickness Funds/ Dental Physicians (Kassenärztliche Vereinigung, KV; Kassenzahnärztliche Vereinigung, KZV).

The Organization of Sickness Funds negotiate with the Organization of Physicians and Dentists concerning details of the provision of medical and dental care and the remuneration for services. The funds negotiate also with the hospitals concerning *per diem* charges.

The public health service with very few exemptions does not provide curative medical care.

In 1981 the rate per population was: one practising physician for 442 inhabitants, and one practising dental physician for 1855 inhabitants.

In 1980 in Germany there were 77·3 beds in acute hospitals per 10,000 inhabitants.

THE TREND IN EXPENDITURE

After the Second World War the statutory health insurance system was at a low level. Funds and provisions of medical care were limited. As the economy in Germany grew, so contributions to the sickness funds increased. In combination with legislation by which more and more services were made available to the members of the statutory system the amount of services expanded. This expansion required a continual increase of contributions by employees and employers.

In the period 1956–60 the expenditures of the statutory system increased at an annual rate of about 15 per cent. Many warnings about the ultimate effect of this went unheeded, mainly because of the general economic situation. During the 1960s health expenditures increased at an annual rate of about 10 per cent, moving up to some 20 per cent between 1971 and 1975. This 'cost explosion' now became a major public and political concern.

At this time possible future trends of health expenditures were published. The most important forecast came from the

Minister of Social Affairs in the state of Rhineland-Palati-
nate *Geissler.* He forecasted that *ceteris paribus* in the year
2000, half of the GNP would be absorbed by the expenditures of the statutory health insurance system and he called
for remedies. This was the beginning of a debate about cost
containment in the statutory health insurance system.

It is of course true that the expenditures of the statutory
system are only part of the overall expenditures for health. It
is usual to indicate health expenditures as a proportion of
GNP, in order to show the development in a given country,
and for international comparisons. There is however, some
uncertainty of what constitutes health expenditures, and
different elements of health expenditures are used in different
countries. Since in Germany 90·3 per cent of the population
belong to the statutory system and since the data of expenditures of this system are valid and comparable over the years,
only the statutory system will be dealt with here. There has
moreover never been much concern about either the increase
in public, in private health insurance, or in private expenditures for health.

It is certainly true that public expenditures for health have
been frequently the subject of discussion and some adapta-
tions have been made. This has not however, been other than
a minor issue. Private health insurance companies were also
concerned with the increase in health expenditures, and this
caused and is still stimulating some discussion. It should
however, be noted that the private sector is not regulated by
the State with the exception of some kind of formal control
over and responsibility for the fee-schedule for medical services in private *praxis,* which is the responsibility of the
Federal Government. An amendment of this fee-schedule is
at the moment under discussion. By far the major constant
concern however, is still the situation in the statutory health
insurance system.

Another major problem is the payment for the construction and maintenance of hospitals which is not the duty of
the statutory system but paid for by federal, state and—partially—community money. This problem will be considered
later.

The expenditures for different kinds of health services

increased at a different rate. Table 1 shows the expenditures for the major categories of health from 1960–80.

Altogether expenditures have increased in the period from 1960–80 from 9·5 billions to almost 90 billions. Compared with 1960 the major increase has been for dentures (1969 = 1; 1980 = 27·3), followed by drugs, dressings, bandages, and medical appliances from other sources than from pharmacies (1969 = 1; 1980 = 22·6) and hospital care, which increased from 1 in 1960 to 16·2 in 1980. It should be noted that the increase for dental care apart from dentures (1980 = 11·8), for drugs, dressings, bandages, etc. out of pharmacies (1980 = 11.5) and for ambulatory medical care (1980 = 8·2) is below these figures.

During this period from 1960–80 the average contribution per member of the statutory health insurance system, which is paid 50 per cent by the employee and 50 per cent by the employer, increased from DM292 to DM2530.

Table 2 indicates the expenditures for the major categories of health by the statutory system in per cent of the total expenditures for the period 1960–80.

In 1960 the greatest share of the expenditures was 30 per cent for *cash benefits granted for sickness leave.* This was followed by expenditures for *ambulatory medical care* (20·9 per cent), *hospital care* (17·5 per cent), and for *drugs, dressings, bandages, etc. out of pharmacies.* At the beginning of 1970 cash benefits for sickness leave were transferred from the sickness funds to the employers for the first six weeks of sickness leave for blue-collar workers. For white-collar workers this arrangement dates from 1931. Accordingly the share of expenditures for sickness leave paid for by the statutory system dropped to 10·4 per cent in 1970, and further to 7·8 per cent in 1980.

In 1980 the highest share of the expenditure, 29·6 per cent, went to *hospital care.* Hospital care now constitutes by far the greatest expenditure for health, in absolute as well as in relative figures. It is perhaps remarkable that 8·5 per cent of the total expenditures go on dentures.

Considering the particular role of the *physician in ambulatory care* (each patient has firstly to contact a physician working in an ambulatory *praxis:* he is not allowed to go to hospital directly without being referred by a physician except in case

Table 1. Expenditures for the major categories of health of the statutory health insurance system 1960–80. Total in billions and as index of 1960.

Year	Ambulatory medical care		Dental care without denture		Drugs, dressings, bandages, etc. out of pharmacies		Drugs, dressings, bandages, medical appliances, etc. from other sources		Denture		Hospital care		Cash benefits	
	Total	Index	Total	Index	Total	Index	Total	Index	Total	Index	Total	Index	Total	Index
1960	1·9	1	0·5	1	1·1	1	0·2	1	0·2	1	1·6	1	2·7	1
1965	3·2	1·7	0·9	2	2	1·6	0·4	1·6	0·4	1·5	2·9	1·9	3·7	1·4
1970	5·4	2·9	1·7	3·7	4·2	3·9	0·7	3·1	0·8	3·1	6·0	3·8	2·4	0·9
1975	11·2	6	4·1	8·8	8·9	8·1	2·6	12·2	4·1	15·6	17·5	11·2	4·6	1·7
1980	15·3	8·2	5·5	11·8	12·5	11·5	4·8	22·6	7·3	27·3	25·3	16·2	6·6	2·5

Table 2. Expenditures for the major categories of health of the statutory health insurance system as a percentage of the total expenditures 1960–80.

Year	Ambulatory medical care	Dental care without denture	Drugs, dressings, bandages, etc. out of pharmacies	Drugs, dressings, bandages, medical appliances, etc. from other sources	Denture	Hospital care	Cash benefits
1960	20·9	5·2	12·2	2·4	3	17·5	30
1965	21·4	6·4	13·6	2·5	2·7	19·8	24·8
1970	22·9	7·2	17·7	2·8	3·5	25·2	10·4
1975	19·4	7·1	15·3	4·4	7·2	30·1	8
1980	17·9	6·5	14·7	5·6	8·5	29·6	7·8

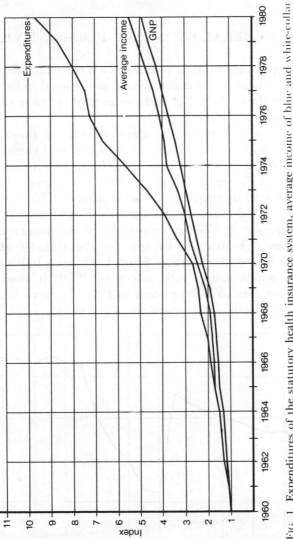
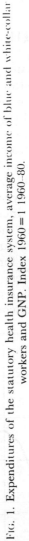

Fig. 1. Expenditures of the statutory health insurance system, average income of blue and white-collar workers and GNP. Index 1960 = 1 1960–80.

of emergency), his share at 17·9 per cent seems fairly moderate. It has decreased from 20·9 per cent in 1960 to 17·9 per cent in 1980.

THE GENERAL ECONOMIC PERSPECTIVE

The dates given above gain importance if the expenditures of the statutory health insurance system are related to two sorts of economic data: the GNP and the average income of blue- and white-collar workers.

Figure 1 demonstrates the development of these three items from 1960 to 1980. Whereas the GNP and the average income of blue and white-collar workers increased from 1960 to 1980 by a factor of about 5, the expenditures for the statutory system increased by a factor of about 10.

The increasing expenditures for health resulted in a continuous increase of the contributions of employers to the sickness funds (Figure 2). In spite of the transfer of cash benefits for blue-collar workers from the sickness funds to the employers which came into effect in 1970, it rose from roughly 8 per cent to 11·6 per cent in 1981. By April 1982 the average contribution amounted to 12 per cent.

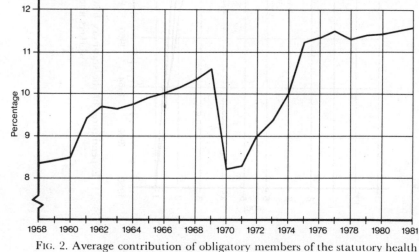

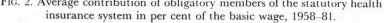

FIG. 2. Average contribution of obligatory members of the statutory health insurance system in per cent of the basic wage, 1958–81.

The increasing contribution to the statutory health insurance system gains even more in importance if seen as part of the overall contributions to the social security system. Figure 3 indicates the maximum contributions of employees and employers (actually the contribution of the employer constitutes a part of the income of the employee) for medical care, unemployment, and retirement and disability. Whereas in 1960 the contributions for these three parts of social security were DM189 per month, the contributions increased to DM1328 in 1981.

The total of contributions being made to social security, including health, is now a major factor in the overall cost of industry as well as for the individual employee. It is likely, if no checks are instituted, that the contribution mainly for

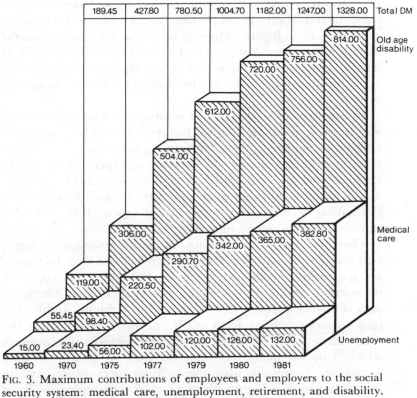

FIG. 3. Maximum contributions of employees and employers to the social security system: medical care, unemployment, retirement, and disability, 1960–81.

health as well as for retirement and disability will continue to rise. This situation has in combination with an economic recession in Germany led to the generally accepted conclusion, that the economic limit of contributions to social security, especially to the statutory health insurance system, has been reached.

CAUSES OF THE INCREASE IN EXPENDITURE

There has been considerable discussion about the causes that have given rise to the increase of expenditures for health to the present level. Some of the contributions to this question are of a political nature. Thus such items as the profits of the drug industry and the income of doctors and dentists have been talked about as important causes of the increase in expenditures in health. There is of course no single cause for this development. A number of factors could be quoted as having contributed in one way or another to the increase in expenditures, especially in the statutory health insurance system.

Irrespective of what kind of remedy for cost containment will be prescribed, or whether the remedy will be political or based on scientific judgement and expert advice, it is necessary that the reasons for the increase of expenditures should be identified and explored. There is however no doubt that at this point politics enter the picture. It is evident that the evaluation of causes for the increase of expenditures in health cannot be made purely on scientific grounds.

There are causes extraneous to health insurance systems and have to do with life-styles which involve such factors as an increasing consumption of alcohol and tobacco, with overweight, and with inadequate physical exercise. There are also the consequences which flow from a highly industrialized society, such as road traffic accidents, and from the demands of a fairly wealthy society interested in the comforts which can be made available as part of health services provision. There are also the consequences of an ageing population with a higher proportion of old people who have both a greater need and demand for health services. Still on more general grounds, but with consequences for the health insurance system, is the increase in hospital beds and in hospital manpower. The ratio of *acute hospital beds* per 10,000 population has increased from 73 in 1960 to 77 in 1980. It is notable that there is a wide discrepancy in the scale of hospital beds per 10,000 population, which are financially supported through the hospital law, between the different States in Germany, with 53 at the bottom of the scale and 146 at the top. Some of these differences can of course be explained, such as the urban/rural differences, in the proportion of old people, and the existence of medical faculties for teaching. On the other hand such a wide discrepancy indicates that there is a considerable surplus of acute hospital beds, a view supported by the fact that States with fewer acute hospital beds do not complain about deficiencies in hospital care.

The *number of practising physicians* has increased from 69,350 in 1960 to 139,430 in 1980. During this period the number of physicians working in hospitals has almost doubled. In 1980 some 47 per cent of all physicians worked in hospitals, 44·5 per cent in ambulatory medical care practising on their own, with a continuous trend to more specialists and less general practitioners. It is forecast that in the year 2000 there will be about 216,000 practising physicians in Germany, which is an increase of more than 70,000 physicians over 20 years. At the same time it is estimated the population will decrease. In 2000 it is estimated there will be one practising physician for about 220 inhabitants.

In 1960 there were 15,800 *pharmacists,* in 1980 some 29,000. An increase is expected of up to 46,000 pharmacists by the year 2000.

The number of practising *dentists* is relatively stable at some 31,000. Shortly however a policy for a marked extension of dental faculties will be completed, and it would seem the number of dental physicians will increase considerably.

The same development as for instance with physicians and pharmacists can be observed with *paramedical personnel.* The number of nurses, physical therapists, masseurs, and others has increased continuously. Other ancillary professions have tended to emerge.

Of considerable influence on the expenditure of the statutory system was the *Hospital Law of 1972*. Until then the construction of a hospital was the responsibility of the hospital owner—public, private, or voluntary—supported through State money the amount of which differed considerably from State to State since it was decided by the individual State. The *per diem* paid was the result of negotiations between the hospital and the sickness funds. It never covered the actual costs. The hospital had to pay the difference.

With the new Hospital Law of 1972 the construction of hospitals became a public affair. The States had to develop hospital plans. Construction and reconstruction of hospitals were paid almost up to 100 per cent from public funds according to the hospital plan. There is some limitation now in the amount of money available for hospitals.

According to the Hospital Law of 1972 the *per diem* paid for by the sickness funds had to cover all running costs of a hospital which fulfilled the requirements of the hospital plan and which was estimated as being administered economically. The construction of a considerable number of modern hospitals, which involved a greater number of beds and provision of the latest technical equipment, caused a further increase in the *per diem*. As a result the *per diem* agreed rose from an average of DM42 in 1970 to DM180 in 1980. In combination with some other factors (e.g. increase in hospitals personnel) this was the cause of the considerable increase of expenditures of the statutory system for hospital care. As mentioned above, the expenditures for hospital care constitute now about 30 per cent of all expenditures.

The financing of the costs of medical care for *retired people* within the statutory health insurance system is a problem which has led to continual discussions and sometimes changes. Almost every change increased the financial burden of the active worker mainly because the amount of money which had to be paid through the old age insurance system to the statutory health insurance system was reduced in order to relieve the old age insurance system and to avoid a further increase of the contribution to it. At present the old age insurance system pays a contribution which amounts to 11·7 per cent to the statutory system. In 1980 the total *contribution* of the old age pension fund to the statutory health insurance system was DM14·5 billions whereas the *expenditure* for those who received old age pension was DM29·3 billions. This is partly due to the increasing proportion of retired people as well as to the fact that retired people get the same benefits as every member of the statutory system. Indeed, under certain circumstances retired people gain by getting exemption from the need to meet co-payments, as in the case of drugs because of the chronicity of their illness.

By law the statutory health insurance system has been given the responsibility to provide care for certain groups of the population (as for instance *handicapped persons and students*) without recouping the full expenditure for these groups from public funds. Other responsibilities have been given for purely social reasons e.g. *cash benefits for leave from work* for the mother or father of a sick child; *sterilization* on social grounds; and cash benefits in the case of *maternity*, again without full remuneration of expenditures by the public. These are some of the reasons for the increase in the overall expenditures of the statutory system.

An almost unique situation is the fact that in spite of the resistance from the sickness funds, certain benefits have been given to the members of the statutory system by court decisions. These include the treatment of alcoholism, the provision of dentures, orthognathia, and psychotherapy. As will be appreciated, the cost of these benefits are considerable.

The most important factor, however, is the *constant enlargement of benefits* of the insured by law up to a point where virtually everything which is possible in medicine and for any length of time including hospital care is granted to members of the statutory system. Only with the last two laws (Krankenversicherungs-Kostendämpfungsgesetz) and (Krankenversicherungs-Kostendämpfungsergänzungsgesetz 1981) has some kind of co-payment been introduced.

Above all, according to the official policy of the Federal Government, each advance in medicine should be immediately at the disposal of all members of the statutory health insurance system.

THE EVOLUTION OF COST CONTROLS

Cost control before the Cost Control Law (KVKG) of 1977

According to the provisions of the 'State Insurance Regulations' (Reichsversicherungsordnung, RVO) patients are entitled to 'adequate effective and economically sound medical attention'. The term 'economically sound' indicates that there have always been attempts to achieve cost effectiveness. In order to achieve this goal 'Review Boards' and 'Appeal Boards' have been established. In these boards the Association of Sickness Fund Physicians (KV) and the sickness funds are represented in equal numbers. Until the Cost Control Law of 1977 only the KV chaired the boards. Under the Cost Control Law, representatives of the KV and the sickness funds chair the boards in alternate years.

The purpose of the Review Board, which is being broadened under the Cost Control Law, has mainly been to identify individual member physicians whose cost pattern is exceptional as compared with other physicians of the same specialty; to inform these physicians about their cost pattern; to advise them how to deliver services more economically and finally to ask for a refund. The same procedure applies for dentists.

For both physicians and dentists the review of their work is mainly concentrated on quantity and less on quality although, especially in the advisory phase, questions of quality are discussed in relation to quantity.

The work of the Review Boards had and still has a twofold effect. On the one hand every physician and dental physician is cautioned to deliver his services on economically sound grounds. On the other hand individual physicians who cause relatively high expenditures are liable to be picked out and subjected to enquiry.

The result of the work of the Review Boards cannot be quantified. The Boards are a necessary element of any insurance system. Their strength is based upon the fact that they are part of the self-government of the Association of Sickness Fund Physicians as well as part of the combined self-government of Fund Physicians and sickness funds without public control. The effectiveness of these Review Boards however, is limited. They can contribute to cost control, but they cannot solve the problem of escalating costs.

After discussion in the early 1970s about the increasing expenditures of the statutory system and the necessity to constrain costs, the Federal Association of Sickness Fund Physicians (Kassenärztliche Bundesvereinigung, KBV) took action in 1975. Together with the Federal representatives of the sickness funds a recommendation was made to the Associations of Sickness Fund Physicians on the State level, which have the duty of negotiating with the sickness funds on the State level increases in the global compensation for medical ambulatory care, in order to limit the global increase. This resulted in a reduction of the global compensation for ambulatory medical care in 1976. This action thus came before the Cost Control Law.

The increase in 1974 and 1975 of the global compensation for ambulatory medical care from the statutory system, amounted to 13·4 per cent. It is notable that it dropped to 5·9 per cent in 1976 as compared with 1975, and to 4·8 per cent in 1977 as compared with 1976.

This result indicated that it was possible to constrain expenditures for ambulatory medical care on a voluntary basis by the self-government of physicians and the sick funds. There was, however, no doubt that results of this magnitude were limited and that in the long run other additional measures were necessary for long-range cost control. It was requested by both the Association of Sickness Fund Physicians and the Associations of Sickness Funds that some priority should be given to supporting independent action through the self-government of physicians and sickness funds and that public intervention through regulations by law should be avoided as far as possible.

The principle that appropriate increases in global compensation could be recommended by the Sickness Fund became part of the Cost Control Law for physicians as well as for dentists and with some modification also in respect of the global expenditure for drugs.

The Cost Control Law of 1977

The general concern about the increase of expenditures especially of the statutory health insurance system eventually however caused legislative action. On 1 July 1977 the Cost Control Law (Krankenversicherungs-Kostendämpfungsgesetz, KVKG) came into effect. The main discussion before passing the Law was on the question whether priority should be given to more self-government or to more regulatory influence by the Federal Government. The Law itself was in the event a kind of compromise although it has the effect of strengthening the position of the Federal Government. This Law can be considered as the most important statute since the Law of 1911 on which the basic foundations of the statutory health insurance system were constituted.

Until the Cost Control Law the statutory health insurance system was an 'insurance' in the real sense of this word. This meant in effect, that the expenditure had to be covered by contributions to the statutory system. The level of contributions was therefore determined by expenditures, as in any other kind of insurance. With the Cost Control Law the insurance system has in fact been abandoned, at least as far as the philosophy of the Law is concerned. By this Law the first steps have been taken toward a system in which the contributions of the members of the statutory system, fixed at a certain level, define the amount of expenditure. This is in fact hardly an insurance system.

The goals of the Cost Control Law can be briefly described:

1. The burden to the German economy caused by the expenditures of the statutory health insurance system and consequently by the contributions of employees and employers to the statutory system should be limited.

2. This limitation of expenditures should not result in limitation of necessary services to the patient. On the contrary, the results from advances in medicine should be made available to the insured.

3. The control mechanisms should enable arrangements for the self-government of the statutory system to control the

expenditures and to keep the contributions to the system in some sort of gearing with the increase of income of the members of the statutory system.

To achieve this particular goal the intention is to link the increase of expenditures of the statutory system with the increase of the so-called 'Grundlohnsumme', which is the basic income level of employees, or in other words, the average insurable wage from which the contribution to the statutory system is calculated. In short the expenditures for health should be linked with appropriate economic data.

Those who criticize the KVKG Law and especially the linkage of the expenditures for health with economic data claim that there is no relation whatsoever between the need for health services and the increase of the 'Grundlohnsumme' which is actually the result of the bargaining between employers and labour unions.

In order to implement the limitation of the increase of expenditures of the statutory system, recommendations at the Federal level of the Association of Sickness Fund Physicians and the Association of Sickness Fund Dental Physicians in connection with the Federal Associations of Sickness Funds for the size of the global sum that goes from the sickness funds to physicians and dentists, have been introduced by the Cost Control Law. These recommendations are addressed to the negotiations of physicians and dentists with the sick funds at the level of the States, because it is at this level that the global sum which the sickness funds have to pay to physicians and dentists is fixed.

Defining the rate of increase of the global sum for physicians and dental physicians, besides the increase of the 'Grundlohnsumme', some other factors have to be taken into consideration: office costs; the working time of the physician, and the amount of extension of services justified by medical reasons such as those arising from the progress in medical care, or epidemics.

More complicated than the limitation of expenditures for ambulatory medical care and for dental care, is the limitation of the expenditure on *drugs*. There has been so far no contract between contracting parties as to the expenditure on drugs. The plain fact is that drugs have been prescribed by physicians and paid for by the sickness funds without any limitation.

The Cost Control Law now requires that the Federal Association of Sickness Fund Physicians and the Federal Associations of the Sickness Funds recommend a maximum global sum for prescriptions, in fact a limited increase of the global sum for prescriptions—taking into consideration the development of prices of prescriptions, the number of patients, and—again—the 'Grundlohnsumme'. The Law also stated that in a case where the maximum global sum is exceeded 'significantly', steps have to be taken in order to find the causes of the increase of expenditure. If it should be that this did not arise from an unpredictable increase in morbidity, there should be reviews of the pattern of physicians' prescribing with the aim of seeking appropriate refunds.

In addition to the recommendation of a global sum for drugs and mechanisms, to enforce the recommendation two further steps have been taken in order to limit expenditure on drugs.

Firstly, the Federal Joint Commission of Physicians and Sickness Funds as part of the joint self-government of the statutory system is required to publish guidelines which enable the physicians to make price comparisons and facilitate the selection of quantities of therapeutically adequate prescriptions.

Secondly the Joint Commission is required to establish a list of prescriptions which are generally used for minor ailments (Bagatellerkrankungen) and which will in general not be paid for by the sickness funds. Because of the difficulty of defining the term 'minor ailments' and for other not too obvious reasons, the Joint Commission has so far not succeeded in establishing such a list. In a law of 1981 which enlarges mechanisms of cost control (Krankenversicherungs-Kostendämpfungsergänzungsgesetz, KVEG) the duty to establish this list has been given to the Ministry of Labour and Social Affairs. The list has however still not been published.

In concluding the subject of drugs, it should be mentioned that in the meantime there are several lists available to physicians in which information is given on price, composition, quality, etc. These are published by the pharmaceutical industry, by private persons, and by researchers. In addition the Federal Government has created the so called 'Transparency Commission' (Transparenzkommission) in order to give detailed information on drugs.

Again there has been an interesting development concerning information available to physicians concerning drugs in the State of Lower Saxony. The State Association of Sickness Fund Physicians (KV) has now accumulated detailed information on more than 1000 drugs (the number is continuously increasing) and computerized the information in such a way that the individual doctor in his office can have this information available at any time through a terminal. For the time being this information is mainly for general practitioners and for internists. It is, however, intended to expand the service to other medical specialties.

The increase in the number of different lists with detailed information on drugs is producing confusion and is provoking many complaints. The final question which has to be answered politically will be: 'Should there be more regulations or more free market?'

The Cost Control Law also introduced some other regulations intended to dampen down costs. They concern the provision of household help; of home nursing care; the restriction of rest and recuperation in spas; linkage of ambulatory and stationary care; and cost sharing. The question of cost sharing will be dealt with later. Generally it could be said that undoubtedly those changes may influence the expenditures of sickness funds, especially the restrictions of rest and recuperation in spas. The importance of these regulations can, however, be summarized as marginal.

The 'Concerted Action for Health Affairs'

In order to discuss and to agree upon the recommendations concerning the increase of the global sum for ambulatory medical care, dental care, and drugs, and in addition to discuss major problems of health connected with the provision of medical care and to make recommendations as to the

efficacy and efficiency of medical care, a Standing Conference on the Federal level has been created by the Cost
Control Law; The Concerted Action for Health Affairs
(Konzertierte Aktion im Gesundheitswesen). This Conference
has sixty members and consists of representatives of the main
associations concerned: sickness funds, private health insurance, physicians, dentists, hospitals, pharmacists, pharmaceutical industry, trade-unions, and employers. The States, the
municipalities, and counties are also represented in this
conference. The Concerted Action for Health Affairs is convened by the Minister for Labour and Social Affairs. This
Ministry is on the Federal level responsible for the statutory
health insurance system. Other Federal Ministries are represented without having votes.

The Concerted Action meets twice a year. The meetings
are prepared by a committee composed of members of the
Concerted Action. In the first meeting every year, which has
to be held before 31 March, the recommendations concerning the increase of the global compensations for physicians
and dental physicians, and for the global sum to be spent on
prescriptions have to be passed. In the second meeting, which
takes place in the autumn, matters concerning the effectiveness, the efficiency, and the rationalization of the health care
system are discussed as well as matters concerning the development of basic medical and economic data in order to
direct the policy. If appropriate, recommendations are made.

According to the Cost Control Law the situation of hospitals including cost control has to be discussed in the Concerted Action but without the right for the Concerted Action
to make recommendations. The results of the discussions
should however be published, including some kind of agreement on how the Concerted Action thought the expenditures
for hospitals should develop. This particular point was however changed later.

The problem of hospitals will be dealt with in a separate
section of this paper.

The recommendations of the Concerted Action have not
been without effect. Below are the recommendations of the
Concerted Action concerning ambulatory medical care, dental care and drugs for the years 1978–81, together with the

real increase of expenditures of the sickness funds. The time interval does not cover exactly a year but rather the proposed time period of the recommendations.

Ambulatory medical care (in percentages).

	Recommended increase	Real increase
1978	5·5	4·0
1979	5·5	5·6
1980	6·0	7·0
1981	4·0	7·2

Dental care (in percentages).

	Recommended increase	Real increase
1978	No recommendation	6·1
1979	5·5	3·7
1980	6·0	4·0
1981	4·0	6·4

Drugs (in percentages).

	Recommended increase	Real increase
1978	3·5	6·4
1979	5·7	5·4
1980	5·9	8·8
1981	4·5	8·3

As seen from the figures above, especially for dental care and for ambulatory medical care, the real increase of expenditures is not far in excess of the recommendations; sometimes it is even below. The situation concerning drugs is somewhat different. Here the real expenditure exceeded the recommendations especially in 1980 and in 1981 by about 3 per cent.

EVALUATION OF THE COST CONTROL LAW

As stated above the philosophy of the Cost Control Law can be seen as a tendency to change the character of the statutory health insurance system from a system which is based on the principles of insurance towards a system where the global sum of expenditures is determined by central decisions. The end result of this would undoubtedly be a global budget system. It will be a political decision whether or not this way should be followed, based on political convictions about the structure of society and the form a health care system should take.

In detail there is much criticism concerning the global recommendations and their effect in the long run. Already physicians and dental physicians claim that their income is decreasing. It must in this respect be questioned how far the income level can be reduced without endangering the economic situation of physicians and dentists working in private practice. The question arises as to how global recommendations about the yearly increase of expenditures can be put into practice in a situation where some 90,000 physicians and dental physicians work as private practitioners in their own practice. How can a recommendation on the increase of expenditures of drugs be put into effect in a situation where some 1000 pharmaceutical firms work in a free market system, and where each firm has to make its own calculation? How should the cost for medical progress, for the development of new drugs, etc. be incorporated in a system with fixed expenditures?

The crucial point of the Cost Control Law however, is the fact that with very few exceptions, services have not been limited. The members of the statutory health insurance system have unlimited access to the whole range of medical and dental care.

The principles of the Cost Control Law are:

The increase of the overall expenditures of the statutory health insurance system should not exceed the increase in the basic wages of the insured.

The contributions of employees and employers to the statutory system should be stable.

The rights already granted to all members of the statutory system for services should not in general (or with very few exemptions) be reduced.

All members of the statutory system shall be entitled to have access through the statutory system to all new advances in medical care.

In every insurance system there are, generally speaking, only two possibilities if expenditures increase:

1. If the option is for unchanged services the *premiums or contributions* have to be adapted to expenditures.

2. If the option is for stable premiums or contributions the *services* have to be adapted to the fixed income of the insurance.

All other measures, as for instance rationalization of services, etc., lowering of income, review boards, and detailed information about costs and prices, are helpful and to some extent necessary, but they will never solve the problem of equating supply with demand.

AMENDED COST CONTROL LAW (1981)

The Cost Control Law of 1977 was a compromise. Actually the discussions on the draft of the Law before its passing indicated that certain politicians, political parties or parts of the Federal Government were in favour of more centralized regulations and of more control. Besides the question of control, it also contained a compromise concerning hospitals. As a result there were complaints from the physicians, dentists, pharmacists, the pharmaceutical industry, and the sickness funds that the hospitals which caused the relatively highest expenditures of the sickness funds were not bound by recommendations as to the increase of expenditures.

Two further laws have been passed as a consequence: the Amended Cost Control Law (1981) and the Hospital Control Law (1981).

Again the Amended Cost Control Law was a compromise. The draft of the Law included more regulations concerning the structure of the sickness funds as well as the provision of care including drugs. The Federal Government however, has asked the Minister of Labour and Social Affairs to prepare a further Law concerning the statutory health insurance system. This Law shall be mainly concerned with principles and basic structures of the statutory system and is therefore likely to be called 'Statutory Health Insurance System Reform Law' (Krankenversicherungs-Strukturreformgesetz).

The principles of the Cost Control Law have not been changed by the Amended Cost Control Law. Important new provisions are:

A central list for dentures has to be established.

The fees for dentures are for a period of 12 months and reduced by 5 per cent (court decision pending).

The Federal Ministry for Labour and Social Affairs is empowered to publish a list of drugs for minor ailments that are not to be the responsibility of the statutory system.

The agreements between sickness funds and the producers of bandages, medical appliances etc. as well as of spectacles are prolonged, without increase (most probably, the producers will go to court).

Provisions were incorporated for cost-sharing of users (see below).

COST-SHARING OF USERS

Until the Cost Control Law all expenditures for health of the statutory health insurance system covered all costs without any co-payment from the users. The Cost Control Law introduced some kind of cost sharing by the users:

DM1 for each medicament
Up to 20 per cent for dentures
Up to 20 per cent for orthognathia
Limitation of subsidy for rest and recuperation in spas.

The Amended Cost Control Law introduced the following changes or amendments:

DM1·50 for each medicament instead of DM1,
DM4 for bandages, medical appliances, massages etc.
Spectacles with entitlement for vision test only every
third year
40 per cent for dentures

There are exemptions for children, mothers, and for social reasons.

There has been much discussion about the value of co-payments. Educational aspects have been claimed as well as financial aspects. There is however, not much scientific evidence for either. Apparently the demand for services for which cost-sharing by the users is required has decreased. A final judgement is not however possible as yet.

Increasing contributions to the statutory health insurance system

In addition to efforts to control costs and expenditure attempts are being made through legislative and administrative action to increase contributions to the statutory health insurance system. This concerns, for example, those who with a low insurable income, yet with additional income from other sources, pay a low contribution to the statutory system, yet have all services available. It is intended to include the additional income into the calculation base for the contribution to the statutory system. This concerns, however, mainly retired people. From the beginning of 1984 retired people with additional resources shall be included into the calculation base for contributions to the statutory scheme.

Attempts to increase contributions to the statutory health insurance system are legitimate. In cases where without adequate reasons there is an imbalance between contributions and rights to services, it should probably be mandatory to safeguard the 'normal' member of the system and adjust contributions. These attempts have, however, no relation to cost control.

DISTRIBUTIONAL GOALS OF THE HEALTH CARE SYSTEM INCLUDING THE SUPPLY OF DOCTORS AND MEETING THE DEMAND FOR SERVICES

There is no state planning of health care services in Germany except for hospitals. The distribution goal of the government and all political parties and relevant groups is to ensure that there is equal distribution in such a way that every citizen has access to all services within a reasonable distance. This goal has been fulfilled with very few exceptions.

The statutory health insurance system has a special obligation to provide the members of the system with adequate services. Until 1960 the statutory system incorporated a definition for ambulatory medical services of a fixed ratio of physician per so many insured persons. This ratio had been constantly adjusted to meet the demand for services and advances in medicine. In 1959 this ratio was one physician per five hundred insured persons. By decision of the Supreme Court on Constitutional Affairs (Bundesverfassungsgericht) in 1960 it was decided that to set a ratio was unconstitutional and that every physician who fulfilled the requirements of the statutory system should have the right to work for the statutory health insurance system. This is still the situation of today.

In the early 1970's there was some discussion concerning the distribution of some specialties in ambulatory medical care and especially of the distribution of general practitioners. The major complaints concentrated on a shortage of certain specialties and of general practitioners in rural, and particularly in suburban areas. In some respect this also concerned dentists.

As a consequence the Law on the further Development of the Statutory Health Insurance System in 1976 (Krankenversicherungs-Weiterentwicklungsgesetz, KVWG) introduced an obligation for all State Associations of Sickness Fund Physicians/Dental Physicians to develop plans for an even distribution of physicians and of dentists. In the case of a shortage of physicians or dentists in certain areas, incentives should be given in order to fill the gap. As a last resort, the State Associations were allowed to stop the opening of a new *praxis* in areas with normal coverage or with a surplus of doctors until the area which was not fully covered had been sufficiently supplied with doctors.

Since then, all State Associations have developed plans of supply with physicians and dentists. Only in very few cases have they taken advantage of their right to close certain areas. In general the problems have been solved through advice and through financial incentives.

Under the statutory system, access to ambulatory medical and dental care is free including the free choice of physician. Whenever a member of the statutory system wishes to see a physician he is entitled to do so. There are no barriers whatsoever. In general he must however choose a physician in his neighbourhood. Should he be prepared to pay the transport himself, he is entitled to see any physician in Germany.

For hospital care, a referral certificate of the doctor working in ambulatory *praxis* is necessary, except in emergencies.

HOSPITAL PLANNING AND FINANCING

The 1972 Law

In 1972 for the first time in Germany a Federal Law concerning hospital planning and hospital financing was passed (Krankenhausfinanzierungsgesetz, KHG). This law has three major elements:

1. The States are obliged to develop a hospital plan. The purpose of the hospital plan is defined as securing for the population the provision of efficient hospital care including an equal distribution of hospitals over the State. Only those hospitals that are according to their efficiency part of the hospital plan are entitled to financial support as provided in the Law for construction and for certain kinds of permanent investment.

2. Hospital investment is a public responsibility. The Federal Government pays one-third of the permanent investment in hospitals and a fixed sum which covers one-third of hospital construction cost. Two-thirds of the investment cost has to be paid for by the States. The States are allowed to transfer one-third of the investment cost to the municipalities and counties.

3. Hospitals that are part of the hospital plan are entitled to a *per diem* repayment that meets the costs of a hospital administered on economic grounds.

The Law includes a number of restricting regulations for the hospitals, as well as regulations about how to proceed in order to negotiate a *per diem* between hospitals and sickness funds. It has guidance on how to secure a *per diem* set by the State if the negotiations between the hospitals and funds about the *per diem* are without results, and about hospital planning. Details for the *per diem* are part of a Federal regulation (Bundespflegesatzverordnung).

As a result of this Law many new, modern and well equipped hospitals have been built in all States of Germany and include the latest technical equipment. In general they have more beds than the older ones, and in certain instances a big hospital has replaced some small ones. The running costs of new hospitals are in general higher than before but these running costs are guaranteed through the hospital Law. Motivation to run a hospital as economically as possible has probably decreased. As a consequence the expenditure of hospitals in the statutory system has continually been rising. The expenditure now represents 30 per cent of the overall expenditure of the sickness funds.

It is almost generally accepted that the number of acute hospital beds exceeds the need, although it has to be conceded there is no scientific proof about the required number of acute hospital beds. Any reduction in hospital beds however, meets strong local opposition. Some thousand hospital beds have been closed, but almost exclusively through closing small hospitals.

Very soon after passing the hospital Law more discussions about hospital planning and hospital financing took place, mainly caused by the constant increase in construction and running costs and by the increasing difficulties of cutting down the number of acute beds. The participants in the Concerted Action continued to complain that the hospitals were not included in the recommendations of the Concerted Action.

The expenditure on hospital care became also a major concern of the sickness funds.

The 1982 Law

In December 1981 a Federal law especially for the purpose of controlling costs in hospitals was passed (Krankenhaus-Kostendämpfungsgesetz, KH-KG). It was enforced on 1 July 1982.

This law includes regulations concerning hospital planning, hospital investment, and the *per diem* payable. Three of the new provisions of the new law are specially notable.

1. On the State level joint committees of sickness funds and hospitals are to be created, mainly in order to examine the economic operation of hospitals. This special monitoring is added to those actions already in existence.

2. On the Federal level the German Hospital Association and Federal Associations of the Sickness Funds have to develop recommendations concerning principles for the economic management of affairs and the efficiency with special regard for the manpower required, as well as for other expenses in hospitals. Should the Joint Committee not be able to issue these recommendations within one year the Federal Government is entitled to decree these principles itself.

3. Recommendations concerning expenditure on hospital care are now to be included in the provision of the Concerted Action. Since however, the right of each single hospital to a *per diem* payment that meets the running costs has not been changed nobody quite knows how recommendations of the Concerted Action are to be pursued.

It is impossible to evaluate a new Law that will only be enforced in the future. There is however, at the moment in Germany some scepticism on the part of experts that this Law will have much effect. On the contrary, there is more urging for a completely new system of hospital planning and hospital financing. So far, nobody knows what kind of system this could be. But there is a tendency to ask for a system with fewer regulations, with less Federal influence and with more responsibility for the single hospitals. Above all there is pressure for some kind of free market even for hospitals, with the possibility of profit, and of course with the risk of loss.

The French health care system

J.-F. LACRONIQUE

J.-F. LACRONIQUE

Jean-François Lacronique is a professor in Public Health at the University of Créteil, near Paris. Formerly trained as a radiologist, he became interested in the use of computers in medicine. This experience led him to health services research, and most particularly to health economics.

In 1977, he graduated from M.I.T. (Cambridge, USA) in business administration. Back to France, he spent a year as a medical columnist at the newspaper *Le Monde*, before entering the Cabinet of the Minister of Health in 1979.

He became Deputy Director of Health and Hospitals in the Ministry of Health in July 1980 and is currently still in the same position.

The French health care system

ABSTRACT

The French health care system seeks to reconcile two major ideological objectives which in essence are contradictory; namely, equity towards the population at large and freedom on the part of the doctor. There is a compulsory insurance scheme covering virtually all the population which had a built-in provision to enable it to be part of an income redistribution mechanism. It was also intended there would be a single comprehensive Plan, but the tradition of a number of independent bodies prevented the intended unification of 'Funds'. This essay describes the history of regulation of health services in France with particular reference to the planning and management of hospitals as well as more recent efforts in the monitoring of utilization of services. In particular it comments on the search for a closer relationship between the public and private sectors and the moves for a closer control to check the growth of expenditure which is alarmingly high. Among other things this has led to a check to the production of doctors. The essay concludes with a reference to the likely effects on the health care system of recent political changes in France, particularly with the advent of a Socialist Government.

INTRODUCTION: THE SPIRIT OF COMPROMISE

The French health care system is characterized by its ambition to reconcile two major ideological orientations, that are classically considered as contradictory:

the first one is egalitarianism, as it is expressed in the preamble of the French Constitution 'The nation guarantees to all, protection of health . . .'

the second one is liberalism, since the vast majority of the physicians still work in private practice.

267

In order to achieve what may appear as an impossible compromise, the financing of health expenditures is assured through a mandatory health insurance scheme, which now covers in principle the whole of the French population.

It was however stated in 1945 when this system was created, that the Social Security in France will not merely work as an insurance for health related risks, but also as a redistribution of income mechanism aimed at serving solidarity principles. This last objective was supposed to be achieved by the fusion of the various regimes applicable to the different professional categories, into a large and comprehensive insurance plan for every citizen. But this unification was not even attempted, thus leaving a very complex situation where traditional structures survive, mixed together with more modern conceptions of health care organization.

THE REGULATION OF HEALTH SERVICES IN FRANCE

In 1981 the French population spent 7·8 per cent of the Gross National Product on health care. Six years before, health expenditures represented only 6·7 per cent of the GNP. This rise signifies an average annual increase in health care expenditure of 16·8 per cent. Understandably, such a sharp increase in expenditure has caused considerable concern in the government, and has stimulated efforts to identify the causes, and control the rate of growth.

One of the most apparent reasons for the rise is the growth in the volume of activity in the health sector. Over the past few years, the volume of activity has been increasing at 7·2 per cent per year. Contributing to this trend has been an increase in the availability of resources. During the past ten years, at least 20,000 new hospitals beds were constructed in the public and private sectors and the number of health professionals rose from 600,000 to 1·2 million, The growth of the general population (0·6 per cent per year) and the change in the structure of the population towards a greater percentage of elderly people also accounts for the growth in the volume of activity. These demographic factors are however relatively slight and should not be considered too important.

Perhaps, the most important factor contributing to the growth in the volume of activity in France, has been an increase in insurance coverage, especially within the last five years. The interesting thing about this trend is that it has been the result of a conscious governmental decision. Despite the obvious consequences to the growth-rate of expenditure, the government has made efforts to step up coverage. By greater coverage, two things are meant: first, a greater number of French citizens covered by the health insurance scheme, and second, a greater number of services that are reimbursed by the insurance scheme. With the intent to assure equal health protection to all, the national health insurance plan has progressed in recent years to cover the majority of the French population, including migrant workers. Similarly, the tendency has been for there to have been an increase in the kinds of services to be reimbursed by the insurance scheme. Although in some cases service coverage has actually decreased, a large number of services have received a greater percentage of coverage. This increase in coverage has been a major factor in the increase in the volume of activity, primarily because it has motivated a greater demand for health care.

The other factors contributing to the rise in the growth rate of expenditure are related to the rise in prices. The average price increase per year during the past ten years has been close to 11 per cent. This high percentage is, of course, partly due to inflation, especially since inflation in the health sector is generally higher than in other economic sectors. Perhaps more important however, has been the arrival of modern technology. Facilities and equipment that are expensive to make and to use have resulted both directly and indirectly in price increases. Advanced technology has contributed to rising prices because it has failed to provide substitutions of care, and also because it has resulted in an increase in the number of highly qualified personnel. In recent years, nurses and other medical professionals have demanded higher wages, claiming that the level of their technical expertise merits higher pay. Supporting this claim is the tendency in most curricula to add more time for training doctors, nurses and dentists.

Conversely, government efforts to control the escalating rate of expenditure have stepped up considerably in the last five or six years, with the dual policy of supplementing revenue and cutting back spending. Although there were indications even in the late 1960s that health costs and expenditure would pose a problem, the government did not take the issue seriously until five or six years ago. Indeed, it was only in the VIIth five-year economic plan, (the last one to be drafted), that the health expenditure issue was even discussed. One method that the government has adopted to cope with rising expenditure is to increase the working force's financial contributions. This method is a viable solution in France because the health budget is entirely separate from the other social budgets. This means that when there is an increase in the demand for contributions to the health programme, contributors are aware that their increased contributions are going to the health budget, and not to public budgets that they might not want to support. Hence, the government has been successful in demanding greater contributions based on salaries. The government has also demanded that there should be a differential rate applicable to high income workers and to low income workers. Until recently, there was a relatively low ceiling in the health taxation system, which meant that high income workers were paying similar amounts as workers with lower incomes. Over the past few years, efforts have been made to raise this ceiling to make contributions more a function of earning levels.

The other principal method by which the government attempted to stem the tide of increasing costs in the health care system, is by restricting spending. Most of the measures that could achieve this objective are still experimental. Although the trend has shown increased coverage, as was mentioned above, insurance for some services has been cut back. The distinction between vital and non-vital medicine, for example, has formed the basis for the policy of allocating insurance reimbursements. The change in reimbursement for the cost of drugs over the past five years is a case in point. Five years ago, all medication was covered equally. Since then, laws have been passed which reduce the rate of reimbursement for drugs deemed 'comfort drugs' and increase the rate of reimbursement for drugs considered 'vital'.

In fact, although the government feared that such a cutback could be interpreted as a first attempt to decrease the coverage, there has been very little controversy over this measure, which was extended a year later to a number of non-essential medications.

The other major action taken was the setting up of a *'Tableau statistique d'activité des practiciens'*, which measured the volume of prescription dispensing to make physicians aware of how their dispensing of prescriptions compared to that of other physicians of similar status. It was originally proposed that there should be more direct control of the dispensing of prescriptions, but this was considered to be a transgression of the privacy rights of physicians.

Apart from these measures, it is striking to notice that there have been very few measures implemented over the past ten years, although the health system has been constantly strained by political tensions.

General framework

The French health care system is still evolving, as the regulatory efforts of the government gradually extend to the problem areas of the system. Each wave of governmental intervention and the accompanying legislation has been motivated by a different social condition or concern, with the general goal of offering better, more cost-effective care. Hence, the objectives of the French health care regulation are best presented chronologically, following the course of events since 1965.

The first major reform, the *Loi Debré,* was enacted in 1965 in order to improve the quality of the professional staffs of public hospitals. It called for the affiliation of major hospitals and medical schools and offered full-time positions at public hospitals to those physicians that would accept the triple function of teaching, practising, and researching. One of the aims of this law was to upgrade the quality of hospital care by attracting the best possible practitioners to the public sector.

In keeping with this plan, full-time physicians were offered relatively high salaries, the possibility of receiving private patients in public hospitals, and attractive retirement plans. Between 1965 and 1980, more than 15,000 full-time positions were created, altering dramatically the character of French public hospitals. Hence, this law played a significant role in the transformation of public hospitals from the poorly-equipped charity hospitals of the mid 1950s to the ultra-modern *'centre hospitalier'* of today.

The 1970 reform, the *Loi Hospitalière* was intended to be the institutional equivalent of the *Loi Debré*, reorganizing the administration and improving the facilities themselves.

It had a fourfold objective:

(a) to establish a means of assessing the needs of the population in order to organize more equitable and sufficient distribution of health services;

(b) to set up norms for the construction and rehabilitation of facilities and equipment;

(c) to make each hospital more responsible for its management by giving directors wider administrative powers;

(d) to achieve a balance between the private and public sectors in order to avoid wasteful competition between them.

More precisely, the instruments created by the 1970 law were the following:

The planning of facilities

The creation or the modification of any hospital bed (public or private) or of any costly equipment should be submitted for authorization by the Ministry of Health. This authorization would be delivered according to a certain number of criteria, including national norms and local environment data *(carte sanitaire)*. For example, 'indices' of bed equipment were provisionally set up at 1·7 to 2·3 beds for 1000 inhabitants for surgery and medicine, or from 0·4 to 0·6 beds for obstetrics and gynaecology. Within this range of concentration, each region would have established a regional mapping of the existing institutions and the planning of expected development in the area. At the regional level a 'Regional Committee for the health equipment' *(Committee Regionale de l'Equipement-Sanitaire)* composed of administrators of both public and private institutions, and of representatives of the medical associations, has to advise on the planned equipment. Then, a succession of administrative steps involves the central administration *(Direction des Hopitaux)* and a national committee for health equipment *(Commission Nationale de l'equipement sanitaire)* and finally, an approval from the Minister of Health.

The major objective of this part of the 'loi hospitaliere' has been to avoid any costly duplication of equipment and correct the uneven distribution of health facilities. Thus, it has had the reputation of a 'negative' regulation since it has much more often been used to refuse an authorization rather than to facilitate the development of health equipment. However, the objective of the *'carte sanitaire'* has not been achieved and does not cover long-term care facilities and rehabilitation centres. These institutions are regulated by means of budgetary measures, set up by the Social Security administrators.

Costly equipment such as telegamma therapy, linear accelecators, renal dialysis machines, nuclear medicine cameras, scanners, etc., are also regulated through the *'carte sanitaire'* mechanism. For each type of equipment a standard has been set up in order to limit the natural tendency to over-equip. For example, the diffusion of scanners has been largely limited in France, since the 'standard' was set at the level of one machine per million inhabitants. This level was reached in October 1980. At that time it was considered too low and it was changed immediately to one machine per 600,000 inhabitants to meet the physicians' recommendations. This change in the planned distribution of scanners, however, had no immediate effect, and in 1981, only three new machines were installed, despite the legal authorization of thirty. A cutback in the budget explains this delay.

The management of hospitals

The *'Loi Hospitalière'* defines the rules for the internal management of the hospitals, and establishes the respective responsibilities of the Director (an administrator in most of the public hospitals, a physician in most of the non-profit institutions, such as the oncology centres) and, of the Board of

Trustees *(Conseil d'Administration)* which is composed of representatives of local communities, local security administrators, and staff members. It also creates a special 'Medical Advisory Council' *(Commission médicale consultative* or CMC) which gives the Director advice on the budget of the hospital and the functioning of the medical services. In summary, this part of the law was intended to give much more initiative to the Director and the hospital staff. It is indisputable that it works quite well, and the staff often show a great deal of interest in the management of the hospital. However, the lasting complexity of the budget setting, to a great extent limits this involvement, to the sole power of criticism.

Hospital utilization regulations

The law provided that there would be a possibility of closing down hospital facilities if the hospital (or the private clinic) failed to meet the criteria that were used to give the initial authorization for opening. In the case of the public institutions, the agreement of the Board of Trustees would have been necessary. Thus, this provision of the law was never really applied, except in the case of severe incidents or accidents that could threaten the life of the patients. (Several hundreds of small maternity, and some abortion clinics were closed down through this regulation). In 1979, it became more and more apparent that the rate of growth of hospital expenditures was not compatible with the corresponding rate of growth of the Social Security financing. The newly appointed Minister of Health and Social Security announced on 25 July 1979 an 'emergency plan' to alleviate the deficit of the social security budget. In summary, this plan was intended to fix 'global objectives for growth' that would concern hospital care as well as ambulatory care; the objective was to set the rate of growth of expenditures very close to the rate of GNP, since that rate was a good reflection of the resources available.

In order to complete this plan, a series of amendments to the *'Loi Hospitalière'* were voted. For example, a law was passed on 31 December 1979 that gave the Minister a discretionary power to close down hospital beds considered as unnecessary (i.e. with an average occupancy rate below 40 per cent), without asking the approval of the Board of Trustees of the institution.

An estimated number of 7000 hospital beds were thus scheduled to be suppressed. This new provision of the law was not well received and triggered a fury of criticisms from both the majority party and the opposition, since the mayors of the cities were the Presidents of the Boards of Trustees. Thus, this measure was never really applied.

The search for an equilibrium between the public and the private sectors

This last provision of the 1970 law was interpreted by several economists as creating a 'legal chimera' by creating a 'hospital public service' in which the private sector could be included. According to the law, conventions and contracts could be passed to make the private clinics involved in taking care of emergency services or in the provision of specialized care.

In some instances, where the financial situation of the clinics was particularly unstable, the public sector has taken over the management of the private institution. But despite an initial high interest in this provision of the law (447 private institutions obtained a right to participate in the 'public service') the general mood has been uncertainty rather than satisfaction, and it would be hard to find anyone who believes that the respective role of the public and the private sectors are well defined in the French Health Care System.

The recent change in the political orientation of the country did not modify the stand-still competition between the two sectors. The communist Minister, Jack Ralite, made clear that he would not consider the private sector as 'competitive' but rather 'complementary'. When the question of distribution of new scanners was aired, he stated that priority was given to the public sector, since the needs of a machine could better be justified in large institutions. Thus the first thirty-one new authorizations granted in 1981 were all intended for public hospitals. But in March 1982, he made a reassuring gesture by giving four more authorizations to private clinics. Among those four, one concerns a large clinic in Le Havre, a municipality which is led by a communist mayor who obviously would have preferred the machine to be allocated to the public hospital of his town.

Although of minor importance, this decision shows that the new Socialist Government has no intention of questioning the existence of a private sector in the delivery of health services. In the *Charte de la Santé*, issued in May 1982, a paragraph states clearly that 'private institutions are an intimate part of the French system . . .'. The two associations of private hospitals reacted however to the publication of the *'Charte'*, not because of the paragraph but because it was considered as too short compared to the place devoted to the public sector. There has however been an important change in the structure of public hospitals. According to the 1958 law creating 'full-time staff positions' for physicians in public hospitals, there was a possibility of keeping a limited private practice within the public institutions.

During the past ten years a series of abuses and scandals were reported, some physicians deriving sizeable amounts of money from such private practice or omitting to declare it to the Inland Revenue.

There have been some attempts to 'regulate' these abuses in the past, but the question of maintaining such a privilege was often raised on the political scene. Francois Mitterand, during his campaign as a presidential candidate, committed himself to supress the 'private sector in the public hospitals'.

Bitter negotiations have taken place during the fall of 1981, which led to the creation of an association of physicians called *'Solidarité Medicale'*, (reminiscent of the Polish union against the communist government). In June 1982, however, the final decision was made to withdraw the privilege of caring for private patients in public hospitals. This decision will be fully implemented in January 1986.

To compensate for such a drawback, salaried physicians in public hospitals will receive a better social insurance coverage and a more generous retirement plan.

The control of hospitals

There is a regular control of hospitals in France. An initial accreditation is given by the Minister of Health following the advice of the National Committee for Health Equipment.

This authorization classifies the hospital into a category of institution that entitles it to provide care that will be reimbursed by the Social Security.

The utilization of services is supervised by a special body of inspectors called *'Practiciens-conseils de la Securité Sociale'*. These physicians number about 4000 and they belong to the Social Security Administration. They come from all sectors of medicine and, since they are well paid, these positions are highly sought after. The overall professional reputation of this body of inspectors however is often questioned by the hospital doctors whom they are supposed to control. Their task consists of giving their approval to the full reimbursement *(prise en charge)* of any costly procedure or prolonged stay in hospital. This system is cumbersome, sometimes causing delays since the authorization has to be given before the act is performed. A new mechanism of computerized *'a posteriori'* approval is currently being tested on the basis of a 'provisional length of stay' compatible with a probable diagnosis.

Apart from this system, which involves only the Social Security Administration, there is a control over the adequacy and the general conformity of the institutions with regard to standards of care. This control is imposed by the *'Medicins inspecteurs de la santé'*, a body of civil servants who belong to the Ministry of Health. These physicians are placed under the authority of the *Directeur Departemental des Affaires Sanitaires et Sociales* (DDASS). They number about 300 and are not as well paid as the *'Practiciens-conseil'*. Thus there is a dramatic scarcity of such inspectors, and many positions stay unfilled, especially in remote areas. Their task is to survey the current activities of the different institutions. They can work at random, or if an incident or an accident occurs. In fact they have very little time to organize any systematic control. At a national level, the *'Inspection General des Affaires Sociales'* (IGAS) represents a body of high-ranking inspectors. The majority of them are not physicians but administrators. They can give an expert opinion on request or when an important issues are addressed. Every year, IGAS publishes a 'special report' which is supposed to be the state of the art in a given area. For example, the 1980 report dealt with 'professionals in health', the 1979 report dealt with the 'institutions of health', and the 1978 report with 'health prevention services'.

On the administrative side, a periodic audit of hospitals, selected at random, is carried out by the *'Cour des Comptes'*, an independent body of finance experts who have a jurisdictional power of the whole French administration. In 1980, the report by the *'Cour des Comptes'* on hospital administration severely criticized the management of several hospitals, drawing attention to various abuses and neglects. This report led to measures of austerity called *'Plan Barrot'*, which lasted from August 1979 to May 1981 with the objective of forcing hospitals to tighten up their management and to reduce the growth-rate of their expenditures.

The growth of hospital expenditures and the productivity of health services

There were in 1980, about 3570 hospitals in France (1060 public institutions, 1750 proprietary for profit private institutions, and 760 non-profit voluntary private institutions). In terms of capacity the public sector is prominent (a little more than 400,000 hospital beds in the public sector compared to 175,000 hospital beds in the private sector). This is because the size of the institutions is very different from one sector to another, since 88 per cent of the private clinics have less than 100 beds, as compared with 80 per cent of the public hospitals which have more than 200 beds. (Eight per cent of the general hospitals in France have a capacity of over 1000 beds.) The relative importance of a strong private sector is thus an original characteristic of the French system. In the past ten years there has been a fierce competition between the three sectors (proprietary, non-profit, and public) each sector trying to prove that its management was providing better care for less money.

As a matter of fact, the evolution in the three sectors has been very different during the 1970–80 period; the capacity of the public hospitals increased only by 5000 beds (+0·4 per cent per annum) whereas the private sector constructed 15,000 new beds, but closed down about 250 small institutions (maternity mostly). The expenditures in the two sectors show also two different trends, with a rate of growth of 12 per cent annual increase in the private sector, as compared with 21 per cent in the public sector (1).

The volume of work performed in each sector however is quite different: the private clinics, with 28 per cent of the total bed capacity are responsible for about 39 per cent of the number of acute hospital days, especially in surgery, while the private sector has about 53 per cent of the total surgical activity with 47 per cent of the bed capacity.

These facts have obviously led to some value judgement as regards the productivity of the two sectors. That kind of discussion does however underestimate the influence of the case mix, which is very different from one sector to another. Several studies have shown that the private proprietary hospitals perform more 'medium range' operations whereas the public hospitals have a commitment to accept minor operations (that are not well reimbursed) and to perform heavy and costly procedures (open heart surgery, intensive care, . . .).

There is also an obvious differentiation among social and profession categories with regard to the selection of public versus private institutions, with a marked preference of high resource families using private services. There is an additional factor which makes comparisons between public and private sectors very hazardous. That is the pricing mechanism, which is fundamentally different. *In the public hospitals* the 'hospital day price' is a comprehensive tariff that is calculated on the basis of an anticipated activity, adjusted for an economic hypothesis about the change in the prices of goods and services. It is different from one institution to another. The doctors are usually salaried, and their incomes are totally independent from their activity. With a few exceptions, they display a total indifference concerning the price of the different services by the hospitals.

In the private clinics the 'hospital day price' is the same in all the institutions in a given regional area. It takes into account only the ancillary services of the clinic. The doctors are paid separately on a fee-for-service basis. Thus, the rules of the economic game are very much different, and any crude comparison is only speculative.

Despite this last remark, it would not be fair to ignore the rate of growth of the public hospital expenditures, which is indisputably higher than that in the private sector. Moreover, it does not prevent the rise of general dissatisfaction among the health professionals who suffer from excessive workload, which expresses itself in high absenteeism (an average 12 per cent) and occasional strikes and demonstrations.

It was not until 1975 that the government began to show serious concern about the problem of escalating expenditure. The general theory, until that point, was 'more is better', the only limitation being the availability of resources. Even so, most of the requests of equipment between 1960 and 1975 were met. During this period, the X-ray equipment and biological instruments industries flourished, and the hospitals were transformed entirely into modern and prestigious constructions.

In 1975, the oil-crisis drew the attention to the deficit in the health care budget. At that time, Social Security was placed under the jurisdiction of the Minister of Health. Prior to this change, the operation of health services had been separate from the source of resources, with little or no co-ordination between them. The continuous discrepency between the growth-rate of health care expenditure (and the corresponding rate of the insurance premium) and the reduced growth-rate of the national economy was considered by the government as a probable source of potential problems.

The Minister of Health and Social Security's first response was to advocate voluntary efforts to stem the growth of expenditure, and to state that a limit would be determined on the proportion of 'mandatory participation' demanded of the citizen. The actions that followed were of a more serious nature. Perhaps the most important action taken was the placing of a limit on the number of students entering medical schools.

Ambulatory care and the supply of doctors

The vast majority of ambulatory care in France is provided by private practitioners, generalists, and specialists. There is no limitation access to any of these physicians, nor is there any limit to the prescription of care to the patient. Total freedom to choose one's physician, total freedom of prescription by the physician, and total freedom to set up practice, are three among the four 'basic principles' upon which French liberal medicine is based. The fourth principle, freedom to negotiate fees, was abandoned in 1960 (Decree of May, 1960) when the de Gaulle Government proposed to the medical profession a system of individual annual contracts (Convention) with a fee schedule negotiated annually on a national basis.

In 1982, this system still prevails, with 92 per cent practitioner participation. Within this group of 'Medecins conventionné', 28 per cent of the specialists and 5 per cent of the generalists enjoy the privilege of being allowed to exceed the fee schedule because they are considered 'prestigious' by a college of peers. There still remains a small number of practitioners (2 per cent) who do not accept the 'Convention'. Their patients are thus reimbursed at a very low rate *(tarif d'autorité)* which is intended to be a deterrent.

In 1979 the Barrot Government proposed an intermediate system which would extend the privilege of exceeding the fee schedule to anyone who asked for it, at the expense of a fiscal and social disadvantage. This provision was intended to satisfy some physicians who were penalized by the uniform fee system of payment because they have to take more time in their practice (psychiatrists, acupuncturists, ...). There is a little doubt that the new system was also intended to open up the possibility of shifting the burden of the rising cost of physician's fees to the consumer, although it was never presented that way. Only 6 per cent of physicians choose this 'free-fee-sector' where the patient is reimbursed at a fixed rate which is the same as for 'conventionné' physicians. The leading physicians' association, the Confederation des Syndicats Medicaux Francais (CSMF) fought bitterly against this system, finding allies in the most leftist trade unions. Ultimately, during a demonstration in May 1980, police action illustrated the bitterness of the relationships between the Giscard d'Estaing Government and the medical professions. Thus, it could have been expected that this 'dual sector' would have been abandoned by the Socialist Government on the grounds that it paved the way to 'medicine for the rich and another medicine for the poor'. Surprisingly, there has been no attempt to question this system, either by the present government or by the physicians' associations.

As of January 1982 there were about 120,000 practising physicians in France. About one-third of them have an exclusively liberal practice. Another third have a mixed practice, comprising a salaried part-time position and a liberal practice. The final group is made up of purely salaried doctors, either in hospitals or in other types of institutions. Among the latter, a special mention should be made of the *'dispensaires'* or 'municipality health centres'. There are 915 such centres (540 medical centres, and 375 dental care centres), which are operated by local associations, trades unions, the Red Cross, the mutual aid societies, or municipalities. The originality in the management of these health centres lies in the fact that doctors are salaried, but the centre must be reimbursed by the social security on a fee-for-service basis, at a lower rate than for private practice (between 7 and 20 per cent reduction) in order to have fair competition with the private sector. Classically, private practitioners have always been hostile to any expansion of these centres. The preamble of the 1976 Convention states clearly that the Social Security Administration will not create its own health centres, a point that led to several months of negotiation. Today, the discussion over the future of health centres has been reopened, since the Socialist Government has declared that it favours the development of 'integrated health centres', leaving the initiative of their creation however to the local level.

Regulating the manpower supply

As has been noted two-thirds of the registered physicians in France practise private medicine. This supply of physicians is generated by the medical faculties of universities and by teaching hospitals, which are under the oversight of both the Ministry of Education and the Ministry of Health. The objectives of the regulation of this supply have principally been to render the supply adequate and not excessive to the population's need.

Even before 1960, there was concern over the number of doctors serving the French population. At that time, young doctors were setting up fees at 'bargain prices' to attract clients creating wasteful competition to established doctors. This competition was severely criticized, in particular by the *'Associations des médicins'* and it was suggested that there might be a surplus of physicians. This was the first time that the notion of there being a surplus of doctors was discussed. It was not until twelve or thirteen years afterwards that the question was brought up again. In the meantime, efforts were even made to increase the supply of physicians.

After the implementation of the *'politique conventionelle'*, which guaranteed patients high reimbursement percentages, the demand for health services grew faster than the supply. Despite the fact that the capacity of medical schools increased from 4000 new doctors per year to 6000 year in 1968, and although an act passed in 1971 embodied a selection procedure for admission procedure for admission to medical training, the general feeling at this time was that there was a shortage of physicians. New medical faculties of universities were thus opened, and the number of doctors per year rose between 1975 and 1980 to over 10,000.

At the same time as the number of new doctors per year was increasing, a concern was expressed by many that such an increase would eventually lead to a surplus. At first, this concern was considered 'conservative', and did not have much impact. In 1975, however, the Minister of Health proposed a rigorous policy for entrance into the second-year of medical school. Despite bitter opposition from medical students, this policy was implemented, and each succeeding year the number of students entering the second-year was reduced by 5 per cent. The objective was to stabilize the growth rate of the medical population to aim for an upper limit of 170,000 (one per 400 inhabitants) by 1980. The implementation of this policy was not well received, especially since the accompanying reduction in the capacity of medical schools was having an adverse effect on the budget of these institutions. The leftist opposition was particularly adamant against the selection policy claiming that the policy was tailored to the forming of an 'elite', when there was a need for more doctors prepared to accept work in underserved areas.

This points up the government's goals for the better distribution of the supply of physicians. Primarily because the government has always respected the four 'fundamental' principles of the French health care system, the distribution of reduced manpower has not been well regulated. There are more doctors practising in the South than in the North. There is a higher concentration in urban areas than in rural areas. Although many solutions to correct this uneven distribution have been suggested during the past ten years, the only effort that has been made, was the creation of an information centre intended to inspire doctors to choose an underserved area to set up practice. This information centre provides information about underserved areas and information about what a physician could expect in setting up a practice in a given area.

At first, an experimental centre was set up in Aquitaine. Then, because students were satisfied with the service (although not so much because this service was having a positive effect on the ill distribution of physicians), the government decided to make the information service nationwide. Apart from this effort, measures have not been taken to even out the distribution of physicians. The continued respect for the private practitioners' right to set up in practice when and where he wishes has been the main factor in the uneven distribution of physicians.

The new Socialist Government has not yet taken measures to correct this distribution problem. Neither has the new government shown any intention of increasing the quota for admission to medical training, although before being elected to office, the socialists and communists were against the 'quota' policy. In 1981, Jack Ralite, the Minister of Health, decided to leave the quota at 6400 per year and to make a thorough study of the population's needs for doctors services. In June 1982, the Director of Health decided that he will follow the line of his predecessors, and set the quota for medical schools at the level of 5800 per year in 1983.

Recent political changes in France

Since May 1981, the French Republic has been governed by a coalition of socialists and communists, after a general election that brought to an end twenty-three years of a 'Gaullist' political majority.

The newly elected President, François Mitterand, is a socialist. His mandate at the Presidency is seven years. The new Chamber of Representatives is also led by a majority of socialists, and is elected for a five years mandate. Thus, the current government of France is constitutionally assured of enjoying power for at least five years, without fear of any foreseeable change.

During the first year of Socialist Government, the accent was essentially placed on a reorientation of economic policy, giving priority to the fight against unemployment. To achieve this objective, the government placed its major thrust in stimulating the general market by elevating the purchasing power of consumers. An illustration of this policy has been the distribution of money to low-income families and the creation of new 150,000 civil servants' jobs, thus expanding the public sector. This policy was in marked contrast with the former government orientation, which was committed to reducing the role of the administration and to imposing a measure of 'austerity' in economic life.

The expected outcome of the new policy was a general growth in consumption which would allow the private sector to invest and create jobs. However, after one year of various incentives aimed at convincing private investors that the future was promising, the government realized, in May 1982, that the inflation rate was becoming a major problem and decided to take drastic measures to fight it.

In June 1982, it was decided to devalue the franc and a three month's freeze of wages and prices was decreed. Despite the fact it meant going back on agreed policies, these measures were approved by the socialists and the communists. In general however, the general climate of confidence in the Socialist Government that has prevailed since May 1981 has not been markedly affected.

One reason for the continuing popularity lies in the fact that the Socialist Government can still blame the former government for the 'heritage' of the previous situation.

The French health care system and socialism

Under the pressure of change in the medical knowledge, the different medical professions were forced to waver between making progress more accessible (especially in the public sector) and protecting liberal medicine. A subtle balance between public and private initiative has been so far preserved in almost all types of service, and does not seem to be doomed by the new Socialist Government, although the health sector was placed under the responsibility of a communist Minister.

In June 1982, the government published a declaration on health called the *'Charte de la Santé'* which is supposed to state all the political orientations in this domain. In the ambulatory care sector, it guarantees independence and freedom to private practitioners. It announces also that new experiences like 'health community centres' will be encouraged. In the hospitalization sector a priority will be given to the 'general hospitals' (non-teaching hospitals). A reform in the hospital professions is scheduled on the basis of a unique statute for all salaried full-time staff physicians.

Finally, the *Charte de la Sante* insists on the necessity to control health expenditures, saying that 'the health system must be accountable to the nation. Any wasted money is a precious resource that is lost for the community, and also hinders efforts to heal someone somewhere . . .'.

In order to achieve the objective of control, the French government will develop instruments for evaluation, in the public as well as in the private sector, and will implement a budgetary policy for the hospitals.

In terms of concrete changes, there has been little transformation in the functioning of the system. As already mentioned the major decision that has been made is the withdrawal of the authorization that full-time doctors call to see private patients in the public hospitals.

But various projects are currently underway and will undoubtedly raise some controversies next year. The most important reforms that are currently in discussion (and will then be presented under the form of a law), deal with the following issues:

Emergency care (Loi sur les urgences medicales)

Post-doctoral training (Loi sur la reforme de l'Internat)

Mental health (Loi sur le secteur psychiatrique)

Research administration (Statut de l'INSERM)

A new style of management has also emerged, which is characterized by a major participation of consultants who come from the trade unions and other associations.

Is this new orientation well accepted? A large majority of the medical community was far from satisfied by the former government. The French health care system relies very much on a tacit compromise between State intervention and liberalism, and is thus very sensitive to any political instability.

It is indisputable that a large majority of the general public likes the current type of organization of the health system. But the professionals are highly sensitive about the constant decline in their purchasing power (-6 per cent per year in the past two years for the private practitioners). The recent freeze on wages and prices occurred only two days after a promise made by the Ministry of National Solidarity to raise the doctors' fees, and thus stirred up a new dissatisfaction.

In the salaried sector there is also a lasting disgruntlement due to a shortage of personnel in the hospitals. An effort to hire about 15,000 employees in the hospitals has been partly offset by new measures reducing the working time.

Thus, one can predict that agitation and conflicts will affect the health sector in the next years, since the government will have to face the bitter resentment generated by the unmet expectations it has opened up.

However, one has to acknowledge the fact that the French health care system has been considerably upgraded in the last twenty years, and the economic crisis comes thus at a time when the system has been modernized and well equipped. Will the French recognize it, and make efforts to exploit the 'productivity reserves' in the management of the system? This is at least their intention.

REFERENCES

1. Délégation Générale à la Recherche Scientifique et Technique.
2. Centre d'Etudes sur les Sciences et les Techniques Avencées (CESTA).
3. Ticket Moderateur d'Ordre Public (TMOP).

Management without objectives

The French health policy gamble

VICTOR G. RODWIN

VICTOR G. RODWIN

Victor Rodwin is currently a Research Fellow at the Institute of Health Policy Studies, University of California School of Medicine, San Francisco. Over the past several years he has served as advisor to the Director of the principal French National Health Insurance Fund (CNAMTS) and as a lecturer in the Health Arts and Sciences Program, University of California, Berkeley and in the Department of Organization and Management Studies, University of Paris IX (Dauphine). Dr Rodwin is the author of *The Health Planning Predicament: France, Québec, England and the United States*. Berkeley, University of California Press, forthcoming in 1983. He is also editor of a recent French book (with J. de Kervasdoué and J. Kimberly): *La Santé Rationnée: La Fin d'un Mirage*. Paris: Economica, 1981. The English edition is forthcoming under the title, *The End of an Illusion: The Future of Health Policy in Western Industrial Nations*, Berkeley: University of California Press.

ACKNOWLEDGEMENTS

I am grateful to D. Coudreau and to J. C. Stephan for their generous help in my studies of the French health system. I thank J. Devevey for assistance with the figures and B. Voytek for efficient secretarial services. Above all, I owe thanks to Vlasta and Marc Rodwin. The research has been supported by the Institute for Health Policy Studies, University of California, San Francisco, and by NIA Training Grant No. T32 AG00045.

Management without objectives
The French health policy gamble

ABSTRACT

The combined behaviour of providers and consumers under French NHI has led to a dynamic proprietary sector, the growth and modernization of public hospitals, and a flood of new doctors. Medicine in France has become not only big business but good business. However, the price of prosperity in the health sector has been an explosion of health care costs. Although this has created pressure for the State to strengthen controls over the health system, French policy-makers have made an unambiguous gamble in favour of the *status quo*— they have taken stop-gap measures in order to avert more jolting structural reforms.

After highlighting the virtues of the French health system and the evolution of health policy, this paper presents the long-cycle trends in average growth rates of medical care consumption, and analyzes the two principal management options to balance the structural deficit in health care financing: methods to increase revenues and methods to control expenditures. Finally, the paper considers three unresolved problems in managing the French health system and postulates that the combination of NHI and *la médecine libérale* will survive only so long as these issues are avoided.

INTRODUCTION

Images of health systems abroad are usually distorted perceptions of what one would like to imitate or avoid at home. In the United States, we harbour images of barefoot doctors in China, and socialized medicine with long queues in Britain. The French envisage a 'big brother' state delivering medical care in Britain and a significant portion of the population of the United States—those without health insurance—walking the streets without care (1). Whatever images the British have developed about the delivery of medical care outside the NHS, this paper should help in assessing their neighbour's health system across the Channel.

In contrast to Britain, following the Second World War, France was not a pathbreaker in the domain of social policy. Although the Laroque Report was instrumental in laying the foundations for a social security system based on the notion of national solidarity, unlike the Beveridge Report, it did not reassess the role of the State in assuming responsibility for the general welfare (2). Nor was its influence as broad as that of the Beveridge Report. Whereas the British State increased its control over the health system in one swoop through the nationalization of hospitals and the creation of the NHS in 1948, the French State increased its control more gradually while involving business groups—the *patronat*—and trade unions in the management of the social security system. As a result of exercising such prudence before tampering with the financing of medical care, the French health system is characterized by the co-existence of NHI and private medical practice under fee-for-service reimbursement—what the French call *la médecine libérale*.

Douglas Ashford has observed that Britain created its welfare state 'by intent' and France 'by default' (3). The paradoxical result is that Britain—the former welfare leader —spends less (per capita) on health care than all other Western European nations, including France—the former welfare laggard (4). What is more, the British elected a Conservative Government which pledged to reduce social expenditures while the French elected a Socialist President whose programme involves increasing social expenditures. In the course of catching up with the level of British health expenditures, France has developed a prosperous health sector and captured the imagination of certain British politicians in the Thatcher Government (5). Is this phenomenon another case of the grass seeming to be greener across the Channel like French-style economic planning during the sixties? Or is the organization of medical care, *à la française*, a system worthy of imitation?

It is presumptuous to answer this question dispassionately; it provokes a host of value judgments and ideological predispositions about the proper role of the State in the social organization of medical care (6). For this reason, in the present essay I proceed rather indirectly so as to enable the reader to arrive at an independent judgment. I begin by sketching the broad features of the French health care system and highlighting its virtues. Then I attempt to fill in this image by reviewing the evolution of French health policy. Finally, I analyse the problem of rising health care costs and discuss some unresolved issues of regulatory policy and management based on my experience in working with the Director of the principal NHI Fund.

AN OVERVIEW OF THE FRENCH HEALTH CARE SYSTEM

The French health system is a prototype of continental European health systems: its distinguishing characteristics are collective financing, through the mechanism of NHI, and the coexistence of a public and private sector for the provision of medical services (7).

National Health Insurance

French NHI is part of the country's comprehensive social security system originally legislated in 1928 and implemented in 1930 (8). At first, NHI was mandatory for specific occupational groups and administered by private insurance and mutual aid funds. Since 1945, however, the Social Security Ordinance committed the State to devising a unitary NHI programme with equal benefits for all (9). This process of extending health insurance coverage and making benefits uniform has taken over thirty years and is still not complete. Virtually the entire population (99 per cent) is now covered under four NHI funds. The majority (75 per cent) are covered by the *Caisse Nationale d'Assurance Maladie des Travailleurs Salariés (CNAMTS)*—the NHI Fund for Salaried Workers (10). However, agricultural workers (8 per cent), the self-employed (7 per cent), and a set of special interest groups (9 per cent), have their own health insurance funds.

The self-employed are eligible for fewer benefits and required to pay higher co-payments than salaried workers, and the special interest groups such as miners, merchant seamen, railway workers, veterans, and public employees maintain their right to more favourable benefits. In spite of this pluralism in the structure of French NHI, one can safely say that the French have succeeded in eliminating financial barriers to medical care.

From the point of view of reimbursement, all four NHI funds have similar hierarchical structures to facilitate service to their subscribers. The CNAMTS, for example, which finances roughly 70 per cent of aggregate health expenditures and 30 per cent of the capital for hospital investment is organized around 16 regional health insurance funds and 122 local 'primary' health insurance funds. In French administrative law, the CNAMTS is a private organization charged with a public service. But in reality it is quasi-public since it falls under close ministerial supervision; and it is parafiscal since it is financed not directly from state revenues but almost entirely by employer and employee pay-roll taxes.

From the point of view of consumers, upon visiting their physicians, they typically pay the service charge, in full, out of their pockets. Subsequently, they fill out a form and present it to their local health insurance fund, either by mail or in person. The fund will then reimburse the consumer roughly 75 per cent of the charge as set by a national fee schedule. Thus, 25 per cent of the fee is financed as a co-payment—which the French call a *ticket modérateur*. If physicians refer their patients to hospitals, they do not have to pay directly. Instead, the hospital bills their health insurance fund for roughly 80 per cent of the charges and bills the patient separately up to a maximum of 480 francs over a six-month period. The same applies to diagnostic hospital services provided on an outpatient basis and to costly drugs and laboratory tests. In the hospital, patients are eligible for further benefits. If they are kept more than three days and are unable to work, beginning on the fourth day the local health insurance fund pays cash benefits.

La médecine libérale

As far as the provision of medical services is concerned, in the ambulatory care sector, the French—particularly the medical profession—are deeply attached to a set of principles associated with *la médecine libérale:* selection of the physician by the patient and vice versa, clinical freedom for the doctor, professional confidentiality and, above all, fee-for-service payment. In the hospital sector, the French are committed not merely to the co-existence of public and private non-profit hospitals but also to proprietary hospitals *(cliniques)* which account for almost 20 per cent of the total number of beds.

La médecine libérale can be traced to an often idealized past when the health sector was a cottage industry. Office and home visits were the predominant modes of medical practice and physicians were neither concerned about primary prevention such as occupational health programmes, nor about the diffusion of medical technology, nor about regional teaching hospitals. Since the passage of the first health insurance law in 1928, French professional medical associations have sedulously cultivated an image of the personal, symbiotic doctor-patient relationship. The principles of *la médecine libérale* were first elaborated in a document called *la Charte Médicale*, in 1927. In 1955, they were codified by executive decree in the *'Code de Déontologie Médicale.'*

Despite the strength and centralization of French public administration, there are few countries where private fee-for-service practice has been more established than in France. Since the Second World War, however, as in other industrially advanced nations, French physicians have practised in a socio-economic context whose growth and changing patterns have transformed the health sector from a cottage industry to a major industrial complex. In the face of such change, the French state has wavered between protecting the prerogatives of *la médecine libérale* and adapting the health sector to the demands of a modern economy. On the one hand, policy-makers have acceded to pressures from the medical profession and the hospital industry; on the other, they have protected the right of access to medical care by extending health insurance coverage and introducing controls over physicians and hospitals.

The case for the *status quo*

In one of his rare speeches on health policy, former President Giscard d'Estaing assured the nation that 'France will remain the country which through the pluralism of its health system, will succeed in reconciling *la médecine libérale* and the socialization of its cost (NHI)' (11). Political change has not altered national policy on this matter. Neither President Mitterand nor Communist Minister of Health, Ralite, have questioned the combination of NHI and *la médecine libérale*. Although the Socialist Party Programme called for aggressive development of health centres, and although Ralite has proposed a law to abolish private pay-beds as well as private consultations within public hospitals, the fundamental ways in which medical care in France is currently financed and organized remain unchallenged.

In the long-run, as I have argued elsewhere, the marriage of NHI and *la médecine libérale* may not survive as a distinguishing characteristic of the French health system (12). Rather than planning for the health system's gradual adaptation, however, and managing its transformation in relation to long-range objectives for health care reform, French policy-makers have made an unambiguous gamble in favour of the *status quo*.

The case for the *status quo* in French medical care organization grows out of a recognition that there are virtues associated with combining NHI and the private provision of services. Above all, there is an apparent freedom from resource constraints and management objectives. This is not to suggest that France has overcome the problem of scarcity. It does suggest that critical actors in the health system behave *as if* there were no resource constraints.

From the point of view of institutional providers, since they are reimbursed on the basis of patient-day rates, they have had a carte blanche to expand. From the point of view of physicians and other health care professionals, since they are reimbursed predominantly on a fee-for-service basis, they have been given pecuniary incentives to increase consultations and medical procedures. From the perspective of consumers, there are no gatekeepers to the medical care system.

They are covered under NHI for a wide variety of treatment modalities. Pathways through the system may lead to general practitioners as easily as to specialists, to solo or group practice medical offices, to a public hospital outpatient department or to dispensaries managed by municipalities, trade-unions, or non-profit associations.

The combined behaviour of providers and consumers under French NHI has led to a dynamic proprietary sector, the growth and modernization of public hospitals and a flood of new doctors. Medicine has become not only big business but also good business. In 1975 the average income of French physicians was 51 per cent higher than that of executives and 114 per cent higher than that of engineers (13). Using 1974 data, an OECD study indicated that the ratio of an average doctor's income to that of an average production worker's was higher in France than in all other OECD countries—7·0 compared with 5·6 in the United States and a low of 2·7 in the United Kingdom (14).

The price of prosperity in the health sector has been an explosion of health care costs. Over the past decade, average annual health expenditure increases have fluctuated around 17 per cent (in current prices). Although this has created pressure for the State to strengthen controls over the health sector, as we shall see, French policy-makers have succeeded in taking short-term stop-gap measures in order to avert more jolting structural reforms.

A BRIEF HISTORY OF FRENCH HEALTH POLICY

Following the Second World War until the beginning of the 1970s, the French health system grew without any apparent constraints. This expansion phase coincided with a period of triumphant success in the medical and biological sciences. Politicians, citizens, and health professionals believed, as a general rule, that more was better: more pharmaceutical products, more hospitals, more personnel, more innovation, and more expenditures. There was a broad consensus on this approach to health policy; to such an extent, in fact, that there was no political debate about priorities in the health sector—a sure sign of tacit agreement between major interest groups.

In the early seventies, the economic crisis struck and the situation changed. Signs of this change came as early as 1965 when the *Patronat* released its report on the future of French Social Security (15). Two years later, President de Gaulle centralized the formerly more autonomous social security funds to tighten control over social expenditures. But it is only several years later that the exponential growth of health expenditures was widely perceived and that policymakers began pointing out that this growth was not accompanied by a significant increase in life expectancy.

By the mid-seventies, questions were raised about the quality of medical care, the functions of a hospital within a health system, the prevailing method of fee-for-service reimbursement, and the effects of the CNAMTS' reimbursement policies on the structure and evolution of the health sector.

At the present time, these questions remain central to issues of regulatory policy and day-to-day management. Before reviewing the problems which they raise in more detail, however, it is helpful to highlight several turning points which have characterized the evolution of French health policy from 1945–80.

Negotiations with the medical profession

Since the first health insurance law in 1928, there have been a series of explosive conflicts between the health insurance funds and physician trade-unions (16). The controversy has repeatedly focused on the issue of fee setting. Physician trade-unions refused to abide by negotiated fees and sign contracts with the local health insurance funds because they did not want the State to be in a position to monitor and potentially control their income. Thus, until 1960, the law which was supposed to establish a negotiated fee was not enforced. The physician trade-unions even refused the 'Gazier Plan' proposed in 1956 despite the fact that it would have adjusted their fees to a cost of living index.

In 1960, two years after de Gaulle's rise to power, the government imposed a system of individual contracts on physicians thus forcing them to accept nationally set fees if they wished to be reimbursed for their services. In giving physicians individual choice in deciding whether to abide by national fees, a severe blow was struck at the collective power of trade-unions. The government's strategic move produced irreconcilable disagreements between physicians and divided the formerly unique trade-union, the *Confederation des Syndicats Médicaux Français (CSMF)* thus leading to the creation of a second national physician trade-union, the *Federation des Médecins de France (FMF)* (17). The system of individual physician contracts functioned for a decade and in 1970, 80 per cent of physicians in private practice had signed individual contracts with the government, thus agreeing, in principle, to abide by the nationally set fees.

In 1971, largely in response to the rising costs of medical care and to ideas promoted by the VIth Plan's Commission on Health and Social Transfers (18), a national collective contract was finally accepted by the government, the CNAMTS, and the physician trade-unions (19). The contract was made for four years and applied to all physicians except those who individually took the initiative to opt out. National fees were negotiated annually on the basis of a relative value scale—the *nomenclature*—and a system of statistical profiles on the procedures performed by each physician was established to monitor the volume of medical care provision. Until 1975, for the most part, physicians abided by the fee schedule while increasing the volume of their procedures. However, during this period, the system of physician profiles was not operational and health care costs continued to grow. In 1976, a new national collective contract, almost identical to the preceding one, was signed but it functioned with difficulty especially during the annual fee negotiations.

Within two years the difficulties had grown into open conflict between the State and the largest physician trade-union, the CSMF, which represents roughly 45 per cent of all physicians in private practice. In July 1979, the government blocked the previously agreed-to increases in physician fees, urged self-discipline in controlling the volume of medical procedures, and threatened to link future increases in fees to effective control of volume such that aggregate health expenditures be contained within a global budget. The CSMF called three strikes between October 1979, and June 1980. The final strike resulted in violence between physicians and the police and so in June when it came time to renew the collective contract, the CSMF opted out.

A new collective contract was signed on 1 July between the State and the FMF, which represents only 13 per cent of physicians in private practice. The innovation in this latest round of negotiations is that the collective contract applies to all physicians and that those who do not wish to abide by the national fees can sign a special agreement, thereby joining a 'second sector' in which they are free to determine their own fees 'with tact and reasonableness' so long as they indicate the fee on the patient's reimbursement form (20). The patient remains reimbursed on the basis of a national fee unless the physician has altogether opted out of the system in which case the patient is hardly reimbursed at all.

This crisis of 1980, significant as it is, is but the most recent one in a history of conflict between physician trade-unions and the State.

The Hospital Reform

In 1958, the Hospital Reform Act was passed to modernize the French hospital system by linking regional specialty hospitals to university medical schools (21). The principal provisions of the reform were to initiate a shift in the reimbursement of hospital-based physicians from fee-for-service toward salary payment and to restore the reputation of French bio-medical sciences which had progressively lagged behind since the beginning of the century. In the French tradition of reform by Decree, the Hospital Reform took advantage of Article 92 of the Fifth Republic's Constitution, which allowed the Prime Minister to pass an Ordinance and thereby circumvent normal parliamentary control. Since the architect of the reform, Robert Debré, was not only a distinguished pediatrician but also the Prime Minister's brother, implementation of this reform was closely monitored by the government. Not surprisingly, it succeeded in completely overhauling the hospital in spite of vigorous resistance by physicians who were hostile to the principle of being paid like civil servants, by the state.

Although there were measures taken to facilitate the transition, the Hospital Reform made salaried payment in hospitals the rule and encouraged full-time salaried work. In addition, it encouraged chief physicians to engage in research and teaching as well as in clinical work. Perhaps the principal innovation following the Hospital Reform was the emergence of new scientific, as opposed to clinical, disciplines within the large teaching hospital. New professors were hired in such fields as biochemistry and biophysics and they began establishing research laboratories as well.

Despite these changes, the Hospital Reform preserved some of the financial interests of the highest ranking clinical professors—*les grands patrons*. They conserved the right to hospitalize their private paying patients in 'private' beds within their *service* at the public hospital. And they were allowed to use up to four per cent of their beds in this capacity (this privilege is about to be revoked). In addition, new investment funds accompanied the Hospital Reform and thereby increased the hospital-centred focus of the French health system. The development of new medical technology and specialization contributed to the rising costs of hospitals and eventually to the Social Security Reform.

The Social Security Reform

In 1967, the Ordinances of 21 August subsequently ratified by the Law of 31 July 1968, produced a major reform. The reasons for this were largely due to a 'structural deficit' in health insurance financing: health care costs were rising faster than the wage base on which the pay-roll taxes were levied. Having come out of a social democratic tradition, the original founders of the social security system in 1945 believed that the individual regional and local funds should be managed by elected representatives. However, this did not provide the government with the degree of control which it wanted over the funds. Consequently, the 1967 Ordinances divided the responsibility for managing the system between representatives of workers (trade-unions) and of employers (the *patronat*). Since the trade-union movement is split (CGT, CFDT, FO) and the *patronat* is solidary, power has actually rests with an alliance between the *patronat*, the State, and the more conservative trade-union, *Force Ouvrière* (FO).

The main theme of the 1967 Ordinances was to co-ordinate the formally separate administrative branches of the entire social security system: health insurance including maternity, invalidity, and industrial accidents; family allocations; and pensions. Each branch was given a certain autonomy to manage its funds and the responsibility of keeping its financial flows in balance. In addition, the local and regional funds were placed under the administrative authority of national funds which are responsible for maintaining overall budgetary balance. On the health side of the social security system, the CNAMTS became the central banker for the entire health system.

Despite the 1967 reform, the CNAMTS has failed to eliminate recurring and growing deficits and consequently the Ministry of Finance and the Prime Minister have repeatedly intervened to increase the level of pay-roll taxes and raise questions about more fundamental reforms, none of which have yet been implemented.

The Hospital Law and health planning 1970–80

The Hospital Law and its subsequent regulations represent a new stage in the evolution of French health policy—one of planning and increasing regulation. The idea of medical progress was not questioned but subsequent to passage of the law, all new hospital construction, as well as capital expenditures, were supposed to conform to a national as well as detailed regional plans which were elaborated on the basis of national standards. This procedure is known as the *carte sanitaire* (22). Whereas all previous regulatory measures emanating from the Ministry of Health aimed to encourage hospital modernization and better management, the 1970 reform was far broader in scope. It proposed no less than a series of measures to reorganize the French hospital system by creating a new 'public hospital service' to which all private hospitals could become associated.

The Hospital Law aimed especially to control the growth of the private sector. It established regulatory commissions charged with authorizing hospital expansion and capital expenditure programmes in the private sector. In addition, the Hospital Law encouraged co-operation between hospitals within a region and sought to establish a 'harmonious distribution' of facilities based on identification of health 'needs'. The Hospital Law required the elaboration of a national as well as regional health plans. France's 21 administrative regions were divided into 284 health service areas (*secteurs sanitaires*) and each area was required to conform to national standards.

Despite the passage of the Hospital Law, however, the number of hospital beds in the private sector increased until 1978 (23) and health care expenditures have continued to soar. Since the early seventies, rising health care costs provoked concern about the state's ability to finance NHI thus casting doubt on the 'limits of solidarity' (24). The Ministry of Finance could no longer ignore the growth of health expenditures for they lead to social security deficits, increased fiscal and parafiscal pressures (from income and pay-roll taxes) and affect disposable income and the production costs of industry. Increasing costs of production get passed on to consumers either through real wage losses or price increases and this runs against French economic goals of developing an industrial sector that can compete in international markets.

THE COST EXPLOSION AND METHODS TO MANAGE IT

Long-cycle trends

Between 1960–80, as a per cent of GDP (Gross Domestic Product), the total consumption of medical services in France almost doubled from 4·3 to 8·1 (25). That represents an average annual rate increase of 15 per cent in current prices, and 7·5 per cent, in 1970 constant prices. Figures 1 and 2 depict secular trends—in current and in constant 1970 prices—of the average annual rate of increase for the three

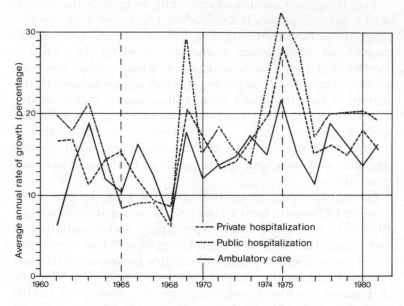

FIG. 1. Average growth-rates. Final medical care consumption in current prices.

Source: National Health Accounts (INSEE—CREDOC)

principal categories of medical care consumption: private hospitals, public hospitals, and ambulatory services in the private sector. Figure 3 depicts the average annual growth for aggregate medical consumption—public and private hospitals and ambulatory services combined—as well as for the expenditures of the CNAMTS (26).

In looking over the growth-rates of average annual health care costs, it is worthwhile noting the peaks and slumps in Figures 1–3 for they reflect the broader forces which appear to affect the growth of health care costs: hospital investment policies, macro-economic stabilization policy (particularly wage levels since 70 per cent of hospital costs are attributed to personnel), and political events.

The peak in 1960 probably corresponds to the initial stability of the Fifth Republic and to the individual contracts signed with physicians, which assured them of reimbursement in return for acceptance of nationally set fees. The

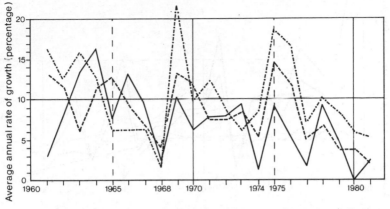

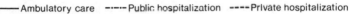

——Ambulatory care   ‒·‒·‒Public hospitalization   ‒‒‒‒Private hospitalization

FIG. 2. Average growth-rates. Final medical care consumption in 1970
constant prices.
Source: National Health Accounts. General Price Index (INSEE)

slump in 1964 is probably a reflection of Finance Minister
Giscard d'Estaing's deflationary stabilization programme of
1963. The slump of 1968 appears to reflect what the French
refer to as the 'Events of May' as well as the earlier Social
Security Reform of 1967 which tightened control over the
local and regional health insurance funds. And the peak in
1969 coincides with the wage increases negotiated at Grenelle
following the general strike.

Although health planning, particularly the *carte sanitaire*
procedure was in operation during the early seventies, its
effects on hospital investment and subsequent growth-rates
in health care consumption could not possibly be detected
before the late seventies for it takes six-to-eight years, on
average, to put a hospital into service from the date of the
initial authorization to proceed. Since the sixties and early
seventies correspond to France's expansion phase in the
health sector, and since wages of hospital workers increased
along with hospital expansion and modernization plans, it is
not surprising to note high growth-rates between 1974 and
1976. As for the slump of 1973, it probably reflects the energy
crisis and economic recession.

Of course, such explanations are speculative, at best (27).

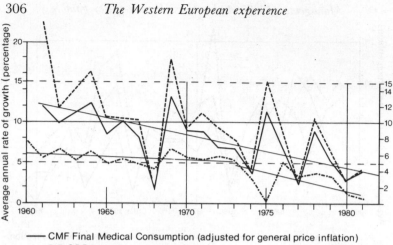

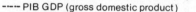

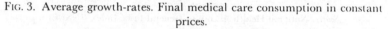

——— CMF Final Medical Consumption (adjusted for general price inflation)
---- PIB GDP (gross domestic product)
---- Health expenditures of the CNAMTS adjusted for general price inflation

FIG. 3. Average growth-rates. Final medical care consumption in constant
prices.

Source: National Health Accounts (CREDOC—INSEE)

This is not the place to analyse the determinants of rising
health care costs. The purpose of Figures 1–3 is merely to
visualize long-cycle trends and to suggest what Lévy *et al.*
have already argued in depth: that the growth of health care
costs, in France, reflects broad and complex processes of
societal transformation (28). An average annual rate of increase in health care consumption of 7·5 per cent (in constant
prices) over two decades is high. This point has been made
time and again in major reports on the problem of rising
health care costs in France. What is noted less often is the
secular decline in this growth-rate from 1960 to 1980 (see
Figure 3). Although, at first, this downward trend would
suggest that the problem of rising costs is improving, a look
at the secular decline of the GDP, in constant prices, over
this same period, indicates that since 1973 the growth-rate of
the GDP has declined faster. This explains why rising health
care costs continue to remain on the health policy agenda:
they are felt even more strongly.

Since 1977, the economic situation has exacerbated the
problem of rising costs, for growing unemployment as well as
slow economic growth have reduced the revenues of the NHI

Funds thereby increasing their deficit (29). What, then, can be done to balance the structural deficit in health care financing? In the crudest terms, the French State has two principal management options: to increase revenues and to control expenditures.

Methods to increase revenues

Increase pay-roll taxes

Pay-roll taxes for health insurance provided by CNAMTS are currently equal to 18·75 per cent of the taxable wage base. Employees pay 5·5 per cent on their full wage; employers pay 8 per cent on the full wage and 5·45 per cent on the wage below a ceiling of 7080 francs a month. Over the last eight years pay-roll taxes for employers as well as employees have been raised on six occasions as part of financial salvage operations to balance the social security budget.

Raise wage ceilings

In France, pay-roll taxes are assessed as a proportion of salaries beneath a ceiling. To raise or even to eliminate this ceiling would increase revenues while simultaneously reducing inequalities since those employers with employees earning wages above the current ceiling pay proportionately less than those with employees earning wages below the ceiling.

Extend the taxable base

Another method to raise health insurance revenues would be to tax capital in addition to labour or move toward a value added tax. The main argument for a move in this direction is that the present tax burden penalizes labour intensive industries and favours capital-intensive ones (30). Moreover, during periods of recession the present mechanisms encourage employers to reward overtime work rather than increasing the number of employees. On the other hand, one might reasonably ask whether it makes sense to tax new investments when these are all the more necessary to restructure the present economy.

'Fiscalize' the entire system

Whereas raising the wage ceilings and extending the pay-roll tax base represent methods by which to redistribute the tax burden of firms within the parafiscal system, financing social expenditures out of the government budget, as in Britain (through the fiscal system) is yet another option—one with very different economic and political implications.

Such a reform would eliminate the concept of contributory insurance schemes. Firms would be relieved of the tax burden they now bear but the State would be forced to increase taxes in order to finance the present level of social expenditures. Politically, this would shift power from a corporatist social security system managed by trade-unions, and the *patronat,* to the State. Consequently, French Social Security would fall under the public sector and be bound by its administrative procedures. Parliament would have to approve its annual budget, all health personnel including physicians would become civil servants and the degree of administrative centralization would most likely increase.

Increase private financing

Roughly 80 per cent of French health expenditures are collectively financed by the CNAMTS and the Ministry of Health. That leaves 20 per cent in the form of private financing by individual out-of-pocket payments. One way to finance the growth of health expenditures is simply to increase the share of private financing through co-payments or deductibles. This method would probably result in individuals relying more heavily on mutual aid funds and subscribing to private health insurance to protect themselves against their increased risk.

Methods to control expenditures

Price controls

Regulation of prices, in France, is a well-established tradition and the health sector is no exception to the imposition of administrative pricing. On the demand side, policy-makers can attempt to reduce utilization of services by adjusting the level of co-payments and deductibles. On the supply side, policy-makers can manipulate reimbursement rates for physi-cians in private practice as well as for private and public hospitals.

Demand-side policies are strictly limited in a society which has grown accustomed to NHI. Nevertheless, a number of minor measures can be taken whose effectiveness depends on the price elasticity of demand with respect to the service in question. In 1977, for example, the Council of Ministers reduced reimbursement rates for certain 'non-essential' drugs from 70 to 40 per cent of the controlled prices. In 1980, the government imposed a co-payment as well as a deductible for long-term hospitalization: co-payments above 80 francs a month for 6 months or above a total of 480 francs were thereafter assumed by the CNAMTS (31).

On the supply side, regulation of physician fees is one of the cornerstones of French health policy. As we have seen, negotiations with the medical profession have resulted in agreement by a large majority of physicians to accept nation-ally set fees. The problem, however, is that the *nomenclature* of professional procedures is more of an instrument for purposes of billing the NHI funds than an instrument for giving price signals to physicians so as to encourage them to behave in ways which are cost effective. Since the *nomenclature* is the result of negotiations between professional medical associa-tions, the CNAMTS and the government, it also reflects the relative power of medical specialty groups to negotiate ad-vantageous fees for the procedures controlled by their disci-plines (32). Thus, although negotiation of the *nomenclature* is a critical institutional mechanism for controlling reimburse-ment rates of physicians in private practice, it is not necessar-ily an effective instrument of price control.

Economists suggest that fee schedules be designed so that relative value points reflect relative costs (33). By this cri-terion, the *nomenclature* is a crude instrument. For example, the value of a particular surgical procedure is constant whether or not it is performed by a general practitioner, a certified surgeon, or a cardiologist, and regardless of the presence and degree of pre- or post-operative complications. In contrast, pricing rules for X-rays are more refined. They not only distinguish between reimbursement rates for radiologists versus gastroenterologists but also include amortization and operating charges based on the value of the technology and equipment required by the procedure. As for consultations and home visits, their rate of reimbursement is constant, regardless of whether the doctor spends five minutes or an hour, thus encouraging 'fast medicine' and multiplication of procedures.

There is an additional problem with the French *nomenclature*: the relative values are not annually adjusted for changes in technology—for example, economies of scale in the production of laboratory tests, or the introduction of microprocessors that reduce the unit cost of radiological equipment. Thus, there are built-in distortions which, on the whole, tend to encourage specialized diagnostic services and use of medical technology such as electrocardiograms and colonoscopes.

In addition to physician reimbursement rates, French policy-makers also control reimbursement rates to proprietary hospitals (*cliniques*) and to public hospitals. Both are reimbursed largely on the basis of costs incurred, the principal unit of reimbursement being the patient-day (*prix de journée*). In the public sector, the value of the patient-day for year $n + 1$ is calculated by dividing total operating costs, including teaching, research, and administrative costs, other ancillary costs plus the institution's deficit for year n, by the total number of patient-days. In the private sector, the patient-day is less of a catch-all category for, in contrast to the public hospital, operating room costs, expensive drugs, laboratory costs, blood transfusions, and prostheses are all billed separately on a fee-for-service basis.

From the point of view of price control over hospitals coordination is exceedingly difficult to achieve because the CNAMTS negotiates the rate of the patient-day for *cliniques*, whereas the Department Prefect, on instructions from the Ministry of Health as well as the Ministry of the Budget, sets the rate of the patient-day for public hospitals (34).

Volume controls

In an open-ended system characterized by fee-for-service payment under NHI the problem with price controls is that the volume of services tends to be adjusted to compensate for rigid price regulation. This is true for private practice in the ambulatory sector as well as for *cliniques* and public hospitals. Thus, policy-makers in France have attempted to control the volume of services provided.

In the ambulatory care sector, since the collective contract of 1976, the system of statistical profiles on the procedures performed by each physician was computerized. The rationale has been to control the quality of medical care and to sensitize physicians to the financial implications of their activities. The system is based on finding irregularities in medical practice and issuing sanctions to doctors who over-prescribe tests and drugs. This is exceedingly difficult, however, because criteria on proper workloads have not yet been agreed on. If the entire medical profession is influenced by reimbursement incentives to increase medical procedures, particularly specialty services and high-technology medicine, or if it is influenced by cultural norms to overprescribe drugs, the effect of the profiles will be negligible.

Since 1980, all French physicians receive periodic statements summarizing the consultations and procedures for which they have billed the CNAMTS through the intermediary of their patients. Enormous amounts of data have been collected on patterns of physician activity. Information is currently being collected by the CNAMTS on the socio-demographic characteristics of physician clientele populations. This is critical for it will one day enable the CNAMTS to go one step beyond pointing up disparities in the procedures performed by physicians; it will enable the CNAMTS to ignore disparities easily explained by such factors as age and sex and to investigate selectively the seemingly less justifiable disparities.

In the hospital sector there have been isolated attempts to control volume and regulate quality of care. However, there has been no systematic effort comparable to the physician profiles neither in the *cliniques* nor in the public hospitals. When volume controls have been imposed in the hospital sector, they have aimed largely at procedural issues to reinforce the price controls. For example, they have attempted to put limits on allowable rates of expenditure increase and to regulate administrative procedures such as hospital budget review (35). Although French hospitals are not financed on the basis of closed budgets, estimated budgets may be inferred indirectly once one knows the allowable patient-day rates and the estimated number of patient-days.

With respect to *cliniques*, more refined classification schemes have been devised within which to regulate expenditure increases of like groups of institutions. With respect to public hospitals, every year a Circular is issued by the Ministry of Health, after consultation with the Ministry of the Budget and the Ministry of Social Security (now called the Ministry of Solidarity) which sets the allowable rate of increase for all hospital budgets. In addition, entire categories of expenditure within hospitals have been strictly limited, and new positions for full-time staff have been denied by the Ministry of Health (36).

Capital controls

In contrast to price controls and volume controls which are short-run methods to contain expenditures, capital controls are designed to contain long-run health expenditures. They aim to limit hospital expansion and modernization plans, capital expenditures for new medical technologies, and the production of new 'human capital,' e.g., doctors. Although controls on hospital investment have been a part of national economic planning in France since 1946, controls on the supply of medical manpower are relatively new.

With respect to hospital facilities and capital expenditures, the *carte sanitaire* procedure originally aimed to promote redistribution of health resources. At the national level, areas of need were explicitly identified and standards were devised in terms of hospital bed/population ratios for specific medical services. At the regional level, resource inventories were carried out for each of the 284 new health sectors. The level of existing resources was compared to the national standards and public issues were made on the basis of the observed disparities. The result of this exercise was to identify 'substandard' regions and to legitimate new investments there. There was no corresponding decrease of hospital beds, however, in regions which were above standard.

Since 1976, the *carte sanitaire* procedure has served as an instrument for the planning of retrenchment. Over a period of ten years (from 1970–80) the rejection rate on hospital investment requests (in the private sector) increased from 55 per cent to over 80 per cent (37). As for the public sector, a series of new Circulars as well as a new law have increased the Ministry of Health's authority over the growth of public sector hospitals (38). In 1976, the government decided to stabilize the aggregate number of hospital beds in France. In 1979, the Law of 29 December granted the Minister of Health authority to close down hospital beds in the public sector. So far, no beds have yet been closed by Ministerial Decree. Under the previous regime, the *carte sanitaire* standards served as criteria for assessing where to cut. Under the present regime, however, policy-makers are talking of expanding hospital personnel not reducing beds.

Along with the December 1979 Law granting the Minister of Health power to close down hospital beds, as part of a long-term cost control policy, the French government passed legislation reducing the number of physicians trained, by cutting enrollments in the medical schools. In effect, since 1971 the Ministers of Health and of Education were granted the authority to control indirectly the supply of physicians by controlling entry into the medical school 'pipeline'. The criteria for controlling entry were supposed to reflect the university's capacity for training physicians. However, in 1979, when it was declared that the number of medical students accepted into their second year of training would drop over a few years from 9000 to 5000, there was no longer any doubt about the fact that France had imposed a *numerus clausus*. One may speculate about the reasons—no doubt partly to control long-run health care costs but also to conserve the prestige of the medical profession, or at least its income.

Structural change

Price controls, volume controls, and capital controls share one thing in common: they assume that the way in which the health system is presently organized will stay the same. If we relax that assumption, however, there may be other methods to control health care expenditures all of which are worth at least a brief mention.

Above all, changes in the financial and organizational arrangements for health services hold the promise of containing health care costs. The experience of health maintenance organizations (HMO's), for example, in the United States suggest that effective management may reduce hospitalization by as much as 30 per cent (39). In contrast to the French or British health systems, HMO's and other prepaid group practice organizations assume a contractual responsibility to provide or insure the delivery of a range of health services in return for a fixed payment from enrolled members. HMO's put physicians at risk for the expenditures they generate. Generally, the physicians work on a salaried basis with a possibility of earning an annual bonus depending on the organization's success in assuring low rates of hospital admission and short lengths of stay. Such an incentive structure discourages inappropriate or excessive use of ancillary services and of inpatient facilities while at the same time maintaining incentives for quality: an HMO whose reputation is questioned may suffer from disenrollment and find it more difficult to attract new members.

The experience of encouraging health centres (CLSC's) in Québec and imposing prospectively set annual budget limits on hospitals—so-called global budgets—is another approach to controlling health expenditures. Its significance lies in showing that there are possibilities for substitution of community-based ambulatory care for costly institutional services. Within the hospital sector, global budgets force policymakers to ascertain the relative efficiency of hospitals so as to distinguish between those with excessive and those with insufficient budgets. Although global budgets are no panacea for the problems of resource allocation in the health sector, at the very least they force explicit consideration of how to allocate limited resources among competing claims within the hospital sector.

Finally, still another experience in devising new financial arrangements for hospitals is now in progress in the state of New Jersey (USA). The New Jersey Health Department, in collaboration with all third-party payers and the state hospital association, have agreed to link reimbursement directly to standardized costs identified by analysis of case mix so-called diagnostic related groups (40). The innovative aspect of this experiment is the application of a primitive administrative technology capable of establishing a common language between doctors and administrators. The technology enables physicians to examine patterns of resource consumption for similar patients in their own practices over time, and also permits one physician to be compared with another, and one institution with another. Thus, a potentially powerful mechanism now exists for increasing the visibility of physician practice in a fashion which permits non-physicians to observe deviations readily and to evaluate them.

The combination of NHI and *la médecine libérale*, in France, has been so cherished that there has been no temptation to transform financial and organizational arrangements for the delivery of health care. Currently, however, there have been some signs of change. Inspiration from the experience of Québec has prompted policy-makers to experiment with global budgets in individual hospitals. Also, the new Director General of public hospitals at the Ministry of Health recently arranged for a French delegation to review the New Jersey experiment. In addition, members of the Cabinet at the Ministry of Solidarity are talking cautiously about experimenting with 'new forms of medical practice' such as health centres that attempt to combine social and medical services like the CLSCs in Québec.

Perhaps the most interesting structural change now under consideration concerns the future role of preventive medicine in the French health system. In March of 1982, Minister of Health, Ralite, received the report of an urgent task force he had appointed to make recommendations about what to do in the field of prevention (41). Thus, far, his first measure has been to designate four regions which will receive a starting budget with which to initiate a range of prevention programmes. Assuming that these programmes remain a political priority and that they are effective, it follows that one could reduce significantly the burden of disability and disease associated with alcoholism, smoking addiction, and poor working conditions. Of course, this may be a great illusion for all of these achievements will not prevent us from dying some day of a disease requiring costly medical technology and prolonged hospitalization. Nevertheless, the idea is enticing.

THE PRESENT PREDICAMENT:
SOME UNRESOLVED PROBLEMS

Faced with the problem of financing the explosion of health care costs, French policymakers have relied, above all, on revenue increasing methods—in particular on raising payroll taxes and raising the wage ceilings to which they are applied. As for the methods to control expenditures, outlined above, French policy-makers have relied largely on short-run methods such as price controls and volume controls. They have also reinforced the *carte sanitaire* procedure to regulate investment and limit enrollments of medical students so as to regulate the future supply of doctors. There have been no long-term strategies, however, to alter the financial and organizational arrangements for health care services in France.

To devise long-term strategies, it is necessary to specify explicit objectives and to reach agreement about the desirability of meeting them. Such is the conventional wisdom embodied in decision-making techniques such as 'management by objectives', PPBS, and zero-based budgeting. These administrative technologies were helpful during the expansion phase of the health sector when there was widespread agreement on the pursuit of such objectives as hospital construction and modernization. During the present containment phase, however, the old administrative tools no longer seem relevant (42).

In modern France—even the new France of socialist inspiration—no one appears to know what the future 'modern' health sector should look like. As for the present health care system, political debate has focussed more on the management of the entire social security system than on the social organization of medicine, the objectives of the health system, and alternative methods of achieving them. In this context, it is hardly surprising to note the absence of long-term strategies to alter the financial and organizational arrangements for health services in France. Even if one were to focus on the broader management of the entire social security system, it would be challenging, indeed, to identify a set of explicit agreed-upon objectives for reform. It is no small paradox that the French welfare state, in pursuing universal entitlements and national solidarity, has created rising expectations and virulent disagreement between major interest groups.

At the present time, the Socialist Government has proposed dismantling the 1967 Social Security Reforms and returning the management of the system to the trade-unions or elected representatives of the insured. In response, the *patronat* has threatened to have no part in the system. Such ideological conflict is frequent and unfortunate, for it detracts attention from the more fundamental problems of health sector management: substantive health policy issues; institutional issues; and political issues.

Substantive health policy issues

Four critical problems—all widely recognized by French policy-makers—have periodically been addressed, then quietly dismissed and remain, to this day, unresolved.

First, there is the problem of the appropriate role for hospitals within the health system. France was one of the first European countries to classify and eventually reorganize its hospitals in relation to the concept of regionalization (43). The 1958 Hospital Reform Law envisage the regional teaching hospital as the pivotal institution around which the health system functioned. In contrast, a 1969 task force made a case for regionalization of health services so as to enable substitution of ambulatory community-based care for hospital care, whenever possible (44). Most recently, the Gallois Report criticized the lack of co-ordination between hospital services and *la médecine libérale* and urged the government to strengthen the organization of health services outside the hospital sector (45).

In spite of the attention devoted to this problem, the administrative and organizational separation between hospital services and *la médecine libérale* remain a major obstacle to continuity of care in the French health system. In addition, poor co-ordination often leads to excessive reliance on hospital care for services which would be best provided outside an institution, for example, long-term care for the elderly. Under the present government, it appears that the communist Minister of Health favours a hospital centred health system whereas the socialist Ministry of Solidarity favours reinforcing the community-based ambulatory care sector. Unfortunately, there is no explicit guiding policy on this matter.

Second, is the problem of deciding what responsibilities to give to preventive medicine and public health. Programmes in occupational health and safety, environmental control, and health education need to be supported by epidemiological research and evaluation. This has traditionally been a weak area in the French health care system.

Third, is the problem of negotiations with the medical profession as well as other health professionals such as dentists, physical therapists, and midwives, over their fees. The CNAMTS and the government have often acted as if these negotiations were the essence of health policy. There is a confusion here between what is and what ought to be. Usually the negotiations have, in fact, constituted the essence of health policy. But that reflects more about the poverty of health policy than about the importance of the negotiations. Ideally, health policy goals such as redistributing physician manpower should serve as criteria in the negotiations over fees. In practice, however, the agreements with the medical profession are a reflection of corporatist politics with the resulting fees largely determined neither by relative costs, nor by health policy criteria but rather by skill in bargaining and brute power (46).

Fourth, is the problem of devising appropriate information systems for purposes of long-run planning and day-to-day management. To do this, it is essential to specify explicit health policy goals. It is also essential to dismantle certain routine data collection efforts which are no longer useful for purposes of monitoring and evaluation, in order to make room and develop capability for devising badly needed information systems.

In contrast to Britain, the French have highly disaggregated information on the activities and prescribing behaviour of French physicians in private practice. With respect to hospitals, however, the CNAMTS is unable, at this time, to calculate its total reimbursement payments, over a given period, to a particular hospital. The CNAMTS knows what it pays to *all* general hospitals *(centres hospitaliers)* in France for reimbursement of patient-day fees but it cannot yet distinguish, for example, between patient-days in surgery and patient-days in intensive care.

Institutional issues

When viewing the health sysem from the outside, it is odd to note that the CNAMTS finances health care expenditures without exercising management controls on what is provided; the central government, through the Ministry of Health, exercises titular control over all public hospitals even though it finances only a small fraction of total health expenditures; and physicians determine the mix and quantity of resources used even though they share no financial responsibility, neither in hospitals nor in private practice. From the point of view of institutional analysis, the most critical problem in French health policy is the lack of effective linkages between health care payers (the CNAMTS), the providers, and the State Administration as regulator (47).

Since the CNAMTS controls the purse strings, it sets implicit policies and these policies do not necessarily coincide with the goals of health policy; in fact, they often work at cross-purposes. For example, provider reimbursement incentives encourage the multiplication of medical procedures and of patient-days spent in hospitals whereas policy-makers at the CNAMTS and in the Ministry of the Budget are concerned with controlling rising health care costs (48).

In 1976, a group of students from France's elite National School of Public Administration (ENA) published an analysis of the relation between the CNAMTS and the public hospital. In their analysis they suggested that 'the contradictions between the exigencies of good management and the rules of hospital remuneration should be eliminated' (49).

They explained that 'the relations between health insurance and the public hospital are more influenced by factors resulting from their historic evolution than by a rational distribution of skills and responsibilities.' Finally, they questioned the legitimacy of an administrative system in which two health planning institutions—the Ministry of Health and the CNAMTS—can follow divergent policies. Since 1976, this situation has remained the same.

Political issues

At some point in the future, it will be interesting to see if a number of fundamental policy issues will be identified and explicitly confronted, in France, or if they will be avoided and, if so, how? These issues revolve around the following questions: What kinds of political and institutional mechanisms will be established to decide what proportion of the GNP to devote to health? By what criteria should health and social expenditures be allocated? How can revenues and expenditures be kept in balance? Who should finance these expenditures and how (e.g., income taxes or pay-roll taxes)? How can France move from the present system of administrative centralization and rigid controls to one more open to local initiatives and more adaptable to the evolution of new medical technology, new management methods, and emergent risk factors? What mechanisms will be devised to monitor the quality of medical care and to evaluate its impact on health status? Finally, how will health care be rationed and will the procedures for health care rationing be explicit or implicit? (50).

A CONCLUDING COMMENT

The unresolved problems of French health policy are captivating for the intellectual but not for the policy-maker. For the policy-maker, these problems are more likely to resemble the labour that greeted Hercules in the Augean Stables. Health policy-makers in France tend to keep their heads high and protect the marriage of NHI and *la médecine libérale* from the menacing storm of rising health care costs.

Like captains of a ship in a stormy sea, French policy-makers strive to keep the present system afloat. The key ingredient to hold the ship on course is short-term policy—sensitive negotiation with physicians, representatives of the private and public hospital sector, the *patronat*, and trade-unions; careful avoidance of sensitive policy issues; and delicate day-to-day management *without* long-range objectives.

If this health policy gamble is won, the social organization of medical care in France will be preserved, structural reform forestalled, and the case for the *status quo* vindicated. If the gamble is lost, it means that the storm of rising health care costs is strong. The ship keels over, and as the pressures to face trade-offs explicitly grow, management without objectives will no longer be appropriate. French policy-makers will be forced to contemplate the unresolved problems outlined in the preceding section. Should this occur, the French image of the British NHS may require reappraisal and French policy-makers may find themselves looking back across the Channel!

NOTES AND REFERENCES

1. A student of mine at the University of Paris IX—Dauphine, Dr Henri Philippe, did a content analysis of the French medical press which revealed a systematic bias against the British NHS. See e.g., the *Quotidien du Médecin*, whose reporter in London, Annie Daguerre, sends back at least two reports a week on the problems of 'nationalized medicine'.

2. W. BEVERIDGE, *Report on Social Insurance and Allied Services*. (London: HMSO, 1942); P. LAROQUE, *Réflexions sur le Problème Social*. (Paris: Editions Sociales, 1953).

3. D. ASHFORD, 'The British and French Social Security Systems: Welfare States by Intent and by Default.' Paper prepared for delivery at the 1981 Annual Meeting of the American Political Science Association. The New York Hilton, September 3–6, 1981.

4. The most recent figures from the OECD Directorate of Social Affairs for Manpower and Education indicate that in 1980, as a per cent of GDP, health expenditures for the United Kingdom were equal to 5·7 in contrast to 8·1 for France.

5. I am referring, for example, to the former Minister of State for Health, Gerard Vaughan's interest in NHI systems abroad.

6. For further elaboration on this point, see my *The Health Planning Predicament: France, Québec, England and the U.S.* (Berkeley: University of California Press, forthcoming in 1983, Chapter II). See also A. CULYER, A. MAYNARD, and A. WILLIAMS, 'Alternative systems of Health and Care Provision: An Essay on Motes and Beams' in, M. OLSON (ed.) *A New Approach to the Economics of Health Care.* (Washington, D.C.: American Enterprise Institute).

7. The principal sourcebook on the administrative setup of the French health system is by D. CECCALDI, *Les Institutions Sanitaires et Sociales.* Paris: Edition Foucher, 7th ed., vols. 1 & 2, 1979. Other helpful sources, in English, are: BARONESS PIKE of Melton Mowbray, *The French Health Care System.* Prepared by Economic Models Limited of London for the American Medical Association, Chicago, 1979; M. TRAHAN, *Health Insurance in France, Australia and Canada.* (Ottawa: Department of National Health and Welfare, 1981). Also see P. CORNILLOT and P. BONAMOUR, 'France' in I. DOUGLAS-WILSON and G. MCLACHLAN, (eds.) *Health Service Prospects: An International Survey.* (London: Nuffield Provincial Hospital Trust 1973).

8. R. F. BRIDGMAN, 'Medical Care Under Social Security in France,' *International Journal of Health Services,* **4,** 1971.

9. J. J. DUPEYROUX, *Droit de. la Sécurité Sociale.* (Paris: Dalloz, 1979, 8th ed). For a more critical appraisal of the French Social Security System, what J. P. DUMONT has called an 'unfinished cathedral,' see his *La Sécurité Sociale Toujours en Chantier.* (Paris: Les Editions Ouvrières, 1982). Also see S. COHEN and C. GOLDFINGER, 'From Real Crisis to Permacrisis in French Social Security.' in L. LINDBERG, R. ALFORD, C. CROUCH, and C. OFFE, (eds.) *Stress and Contradiction in Modern Capitalism.* (Lexington, Mass.: D. C. Heath, 1975).

10. The literal translation of CNAM is the National Sickness Insurance Fund. However, since the more customary American term for sickness insurance is health insurance, I have taken the liberty of referring to French NHI.

11. VALÉRY GISCARD D'ESTAING, Speech presented to the Academy of Medicine on the occasion of the bicentennial of the birth of Laennec. Paris, February 17, 1981. Parentheses are my own.

12. V. RODWIN, 'The Marriage of NHI and *La Médecine Libérale'*, *Milbank Memorial Fund Q.* **59**(1), 1981.

13. CH. GLARMET-LENOIR, *Les Revenus avant Impôt et les Tarifs des Médecins Conventionnés en 1977. Evaluation 1962–1977.* (Paris: CREDOC).

14. OECD. *Public Expenditure on Health. Studies in Resource Allocation, No. 4,* (Paris, 1976).

15. *La Sécurité Sociale et son Avenir.* Paris: *Patronat Français,* Supplement to vol. 253, June, 1965.

16. H. HATZFELD, *Le Grand Tournant de la Médecine Libérale.* (Paris: Les Editions Ouvrières, 1963).

17. J. C. STEPHAN, *Economie et Pouvoir Médical.* (Paris: Economica, 1979).

18. *Santé et Prestations Sociales.* Sixth National Economic Plan. (Paris: Documentation Française, 1971).

19. L. THORSEN, 'How can the U. S. Government Control Physicians' Fees under National Health Insurance? A Lesson from the French System.' *International Journal of Health Services*, 4(1), 1974.

20. *Convention Nationale Destinée à Organiser les Rapports Entre le Corps Médical et les Caisses d'Assurance Maladie.* (Paris: CNAMTS, May 1980).

21. H. JAMOUS, *Sociologie de la Décision—La Reforme des Etudes Médicales et des Structures Hospitalières.* (Paris: Editions du CNRS, 1969).

22. G. MOREAU, 'La planification dans le domaine de la santé: les hommes et les équipements,' *Revue Française des Affaires Sociales*, Numéro Spécial, no. 4, October-December, 1980. For a thorough review of the application of the *carte sanitaire* to policies on medical technology, see R. FUHRER, 'Policy for Medical Technology in France', Chapter 6 in *The Implications of Cost Effectiveness Analysis of Medical Technology, Background Paper #4: The Management of Health Care Technology in Ten Countries.* (Washington D.C.: Office of Technology Assessment, 1980).

23. J. DE KERVASDOUÉ, 'La Politique de l'Etat en matière d'hospitalisation privée. 1962–1978. Analyse des conséquences de mesures contradictoires.' *Annales Economique de Clermont-Ferrand,* 1980, Vol. 16.

24. See e.g. the report of the Finance Committee to the Sixth National Economic Plan: *Economie Générale et Financement.* (Paris: Documentation Française, 1971).

25. These figures are based on the most recently available OECD data. Directorate of Social Affairs for Manpower and Education.

26. Figures 1–3 are based on estimates from the French National Health Accounts compiled by CREDOC from INSEE data. Final medical consumption (CMF) represents the greater part of aggregate health expenditures including categorical programmes such as maternal and child health, school and university programmes, the health service for the military, biomedical research, administrative costs, and capital formation.

In Figures 2 and 3, current medical care consumption is deflated by the 1970 INSEE general price inflation index.

In Figure 3, the growth of the CNAMTS' expenditures is always higher than those of the CMF because they are more sensitive to the growth in hospital expenditures and because health insurance coverage has increased over the past two decades.

27. See e.g. discussions of this issue by the *Commission des Comptes de la Santé*, Ministry of Health and a discussion paper presented to the World Health Organization by B. MAJNONI D'INTIGNANO, 'Cost Containment Policies: France'. Paris: *Assistance Publique,* March, 1981.

28. E. LEVY, M. BUNGENER, G. DUMENIL, and F. FAGNANI, *La Croissance des Dépenses de santé.* (Paris: Economica, 1982).

29. A recent projection by the National Institute of Statistics and Economic Studies (INSEE) indicates that even assuming relatively high growth rates (3 per cent), in 1986 the deficit for all social expenditures (health insurance, pensions, and family allowances, combined) will exceed 66 billion Francs and perhaps even reach 120 billion, M. FEROIDE, E. RAOUL, and H. S. DYNIAK, 'Securité Sociale et évolution macro-économique', *Economie et Statistique,* April, 1982.

30. C. ROLLET, 'Pourquoi modifier l'assiette des cotisations sociales,' *Droit Social*, September/October 1978.

31. Decree No 1 80–8, January 8, 1980. *Journal Officiel*, 8–1, p. 65.

32. G. DE POUVOURVILLE, 'La nomenclature des actes professionels, un outil pour une politique de santé?' *Revue Française des Affaires Sociales*, 1981.

33. REINHARDT, U. 'Alternative Methods of Reimbursing Non-institutional Providers of Health Services,' in *Controls on Health Care, Papers of the Conference on Regulation in the Health Industry*, January 9, 1974. (Washington, D.C.: National Academy of Sciences, 1975).

34. The mechanics of hospital reimbursement in France is extremely complex. For more detail, see P. COUDURIER, *Les Prix de Journée*. (Nancy: Berger Lerrault, 1971); M. GADREAU, *La Tarification Hospitalière*. (Paris: Editions Médicales et Universitaires, 1975); B. MAJNONI D'INTIGNANO, 'Tarification, gestion et financement des hôspitaux. De nouvelles perspectifs?', *Hôspitaux de Paris*, Winter, 1981. For a discussion in English of these issues, see W. GLASER, *Paying the Hospital in France*. (New York: Center for the Social Sciences. Columbia University, 1980).

35. These regulatory mechanisms are discussed in more detail by R. LAUNOIS and D. LETOUZE, 'Analyse economique des mesures prises en France afin de maîtriser la croissance des dépenses sanitaires,' in *Droit et Economie Médicale*. (Paris: Economica, 1981).

36. Ibid.

37. G. MOREAU, *op. cit.*, no. 22.

38. The two Circulars date from 1 August, 1977 (BOSP 77–34 no. 13315, and from 3 March, 1978 (Circular No. 536, BOSP, 78–14, no. 14658). Law no. 79–1140.

39. This issue is more complicated than this passing reference would suggest. For a thorough review of the evidence, see H. LUFT, *Health Maintenance Organizations: Dimensions of Performance*. (New York: John Wiley & Sons, 1981).

40. R. FETTER, Y. SHIN, J. FREEMAN, R. AVERILL, and J. THOMPSON, *Case Mix Definition by Diagnosis Related Groups*. Supplement to *Medical Care*, **18**(2), February, 1980.

41. *Propositions Pour une Politique de Prévention*. Rapport rédigé sur sa demande, à l'intention de Monsieur le Ministre de la Santé, March, 1980 (mimeo).

42. V. RODWIN. Health Planning in International Perspective. Chapter 13, Section II, 'France: Health Planning Under NHI,' in BLUM, H., *Planning for Health: Development and Application of Social Change Theory*. (New York: Human Sciences Press, Second Edition, 1981).

43. R. F. BRIDGMAN, 'Hospital Regionalization in Europe: Achievements and Obstacles,' in C. ALTENSTETTER, (ed.) *Changing National-Subnational Relations in Health*. (Washington D.C.: Fogarty International Center, 1976).

44. Groupe de travail sur la prospective de la santé, *Réflections sur l'Avenir du Système de Santé*. (Paris: Documentation Française, 1969).

45. GALLOIS-TAIB, *De l'Organisation du Système de Soins*. (Paris: Documentation Française, 1981).

46. On the corporatist context of physician politics and for parallels and contrasts to the French situation, see DEBORAH STONE'S incisive analysis of health care in the Federal Republic of Germany, *The Limits of Professional Power.* (Chicago: University of Chicago Press, 1980).

47. V. RODWIN, 'On the Separation of Health Planning and Provider Reimbursement: The US and France', *Inquiry,* **18,** Summer, 1981.

48. B. MAJNONI D'INTIGNANO, 'Les instruments de maîtrise des dépenses de santé sont-ils performants?' in *La Santé des Français.* (Paris: PUF, 1980).

49. 'L'assurance maladie et l'hopital public,' in *Revue Française des Affaires Sociales,* special issue, July/September 1976, p. 206.

50. These questions are explored in J. DE KERVASDOUE, J. KIMBERLY, and V. RODWIN, (eds.), *La Santé Rationnée: La Fin d'un Mirage.* (Paris: Ecomonica, 1981).

PART
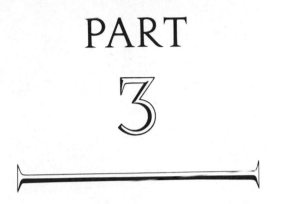
3

*The
English speaking
countries*

The English speaking countries

The United States of America
Canada, and Australia

The European experiences show quite clearly that the Netherlands, Belgium, the Federal Republic of Germany, and France are having similar debates about the public/private mix not too dissimilar from those in Britain. Although the goals of the several policies adopted in each country may differ at any point in time, and constantly change in emphasis through time, the nature of the policy debate cycle, with the constituent elements of equity, access, cost, freedom, regulation, etc. is very similar. It cannot be stressed enough that this is not surprising given the similarities of the powerful interest groups which operate in all health care markets and the inherently complex nature of these markets.

It has been evident in recent years that for all the similarities of the goals of medical care the several experiences of the American, Canadian, and Australian policy-makers show some apparent diversity in goal (objective) setting and the development of policies to achieve these goals.

All the authors were invited to comment on the current scene. McNerney explores the diversity of the US health care market with its complex cross-currents in policy design, development, and evaluation which has tended to follow American traditions. In particular he discusses current moves to contain costs by competition, consumer choice, and other policies which reflect the concern with ever-rising costs. Evans analyses the Canadian experience especially with the use of global budgets, since it has been claimed that these have 'capped' expenditure and altered the nature of the policy debate there. He also discusses the intellectual basis of privatization in a unique way which can be related to the present British dilemma. Deeble gives an up-to-date account of the recent

329

history of Australian health affairs and the changes in system, the insurance part of which was nationalized by the Whitlam and denationalized by the Fraser Government and discusses whether such changes are likely to affect the evolution of regulatory action, the need for which does not seem to have disappeared as the public/private mix alters apparently towards a larger 'private' sector. The realities of regulation by government, pressurizing carriers and providers are starkly presented.

All of these essays have powerful lessons for the British policy-maker concerned with the effect of alterations of mix, and there is no substitution for reading them closely. Indeed it is hoped it will be possible for the reader to distil from these accounts not only the nature of the goals policy-makers and societies are seeking to achieve but the limitations which seem to follow changes, in the effort to shake-off regulation. All too often the nature of these goals and what their achievement entails, is lost in the rhetoric of the political debate. But if values are quantified in real terms and the intent of politicians identified, there is a surprising degree of concurrence between the aims of different politicians in different countries. There is concern everywhere about 'value for money' i.e. the efficient use of scarce economic resources, which implies that costs are minimized and benefits maximized. There is also concern about 'distributional justice' or 'equity': all politicians seek to direct resources to the poor, the aged, and the chronically ill so that they are given access to 'adequate' health care (a concept often ill-defined but nonetheless dominant).

These two goals, efficiency and equity, require careful elaboration and the creation of effective policies for their achievement. This identical challenge is facing policy-makers in the United States, Canada, and Australia as well as in Europe. It is evident that differences about the proportions of the public/private mix and in particular, heated debates about changes in this mix, may obscure these goals all too often; but they exist nonetheless and require resolution everywhere.

The control of health care costs in the United States in the context of health insurance policies

WALTER J. McNERNEY

WALTER J. McNERNEY

Walter J. McNerney has had a long and distinguished career in many of the aspects of health care. Before becoming Professor of Health Policy in the Kellog School of Management, Northwestern University in 1982 he was President of Blue Cross Association of the United States from 1961–78, when he became President of both Blue Cross and Blue Shield Associations until he relinquished these appointments in December 1981.

Professor McNerney's experience has been very wide, covering financing and delivery of health care, as well as management in various capacities. The Blue Cross and Blue Shield organizations themselves cover most of the important aspects of health care within the US. Between them they enrol approximately 84 million persons in the private market for health insurance, where organizations actively compete with many new financing and delivery systems, insurance companies, and health insurance arrangements. Both organizations also serve approximately 35 million persons under government contracts, including 27·5 million under Medicare. The 'Blues' also cover 5 million additional persons under the Federal Employee Program.

Prior to 1961 he was Professor and Director of the Bureau of Hospital Administration, the School of Business Administration in the University of Michigan, and directed the celebrated Michigan study, the Report of which was published in two volumes as *Hospital and Medical Economics* (HRET: Chicago, 1962).

Professor McNerney has been a member and occasional Chairman of a number of important Committees in the US concerned with health education and health policy in both the public and private sectors. He is the author of several important policy essays over the last twenty years. He has been the recipient of numerous awards in the US for outstanding achievement and, as an alumnus of Yale, was the recipient of the Yale medal for outstanding service to that University in 1979. He is a charter member of the Institute of Medicine of the National Academy of Sciences, Washington D.C. He is also immediate Past President of the Federation of Voluntary Health Service Funds.

The control of health care costs in the United States in the context of health insurance policies

ABSTRACT

In the US cost containment is the major driving force behind legislative and private sector health strategies. Faced with intolerable deficits, the Congress appears determined to end its open-ended commitments to low income groups and the aged. Similarly, employers are increasingly determined to control health care costs as a major component of the fringe benefit structure.

To contain costs the Reagan Administration feels that competitive forces should be encouraged through a variety of means, e.g. increasing the numbers of financing and delivery systems available to individuals and employees, and involving persons more directly in health transactions through cost-sharing, both at the time of purchasing health insurance and at the time of illness. It is claimed that greater competition and more consumer involvement will make it possible to provide more care with less expenditure, without compromising the quality of care.

Others claim that normal market forces cannot cope with complex human services and heavy regulation is needed. Some support the concept of competing delivery systems, but minimal cost-sharing, under the thesis that the individual is not able or willing to influence doctors or hospitals upon which he or she deeply depends.

Cost-sharing, one of the major market strategies, is now under close examination. Unfortunately, the fact base is slender. Where data are available to show changes in use patterns related to cost-sharing in various forms, corresponding data on effectiveness or quality of care are lacking. As a result, cost-sharing takes on a highly subjective character, to some representing enlightened conservatism—a way to energize the market, to others a serious underestimation of how deeply the public feels about security and predictability. To others, it represents a practical way to draw the boundaries of expenditure, letting the user decide when he's had enough. Some however feel this is an avoidance of responsibility. Inevitably, boundaries should be drawn by the community as a whole. The cynical note that cost-sharing permits the government and the employer to shift financial burdens to the individual. Critics note that cost-shifting adversely affects the poor disproportionately.

It appears however that cost-sharing will have increased but selective use in the future, i.e. applied to non critical services and to premiums, as one disciplinary tool among many, and that more attention will be paid to competing delivery systems.

For Britain, the key concept may be 'selective use', that is application of cost-sharing to small repetitive services to sharpen cost awareness at the margins of productive health services. Periodically, the NHS needs an inventory and evaluation. Cost-sharing should be weighed, but not as a central concept or as a powerful remedy. Allied market strategies bear evaluation as well as requiring demonstration.

THE CURRENT PERSPECTIVE: MARKETS, COMPETITION, CONSUMER CHOICE

Cost containment in both government and the private sector

Currently, the most actively debated health care issue for government and the private sector is cost containment, that is how to limit expenditures, moderate demand, or increase productivity through either incentives or regulation. Between 1960 and 1980, total personal health care expenditures per capita increased approximately 630 per cent in the USA without discounting for inflation. Over the last five years, the increase was approximately 77 per cent (1). In 1960, health care expenditures comprised 5·3 per cent of the GNP, in 1980, 9·4 per cent. With a flat economy, troublesome federal deficits, high unemployment, and widespread concern among business leaders about rising costs of fringe benefits as a percentage of pay-roll, it should be expected that health care costs will be high on the national agenda for the next five to ten years. The government is a doubly interested party, primarily in respect of its own financing programmes designed to implement its own policies, but also in an equally important aspect of public policy for the effect of rising health costs on the economy in general.

Cost containment has not always been of prime concern. In the 1920s and 1930s, modest government programmes and fledgling prepayment programmes, such as Blue Cross Plans, struggled to protect individuals against the unpredictable costs of health care and to help keep beleaguered hospitals open. In the 1930s, 1940s, and 1950s, the primary concern was the improvement of access to care. During this period health prepayment and insurance grew substantially and the government made significant commitments to hospital construction, education, and research. Effective demand accelerated. Interest was expressed in the need to organize delivery systems, but it was subordinate to concerns about the aged and low income groups.

In the late 1960s, we experienced a transition from this concern over the generation of effective demand, to a greater concern over excessive demand and costs. Major legislation, passed in 1965, to provide government benefits to persons over the age of sixty-five and to low income persons under the Medicare and Medicaid Acts (2), triggered the transition. With widespread private prepayment and insurance schemes, these programmes, pressing against marginally productive providers of care, started an acceleration in costs that is now of national concern. It is also perceived to be part of the government's overall problem in stabilizing the economy. In the late 1960s, a series of legislative interventions was started to moderate cost increases that ultimately included a national planning programme with regulatory provisions to control hospital bed growth, regulations to control utilization in hospitals and allied facilities and special financial *plus* regulatory support for alternative delivery systems, e.g. Health Maintenance Organizations that were purported to be more efficient. The main features of these Organizations are that they are delivery systems that provide comprehensive and co-ordinated institutional and professional services for a fixed *per capita* amount. These systems use significantly less acute hospital care for their subscribers than the more traditional alternatives. As a result, overall costs are usually less for comparable services.

The quest for cost containment reached its regulatory zenith in the Senator Kennedy proposals of the early and mid 1970s (3). The essence of the original proposal was to raise most of the money required for health services through taxation and to spend it through a hierarchy of Federal, regional, and state units with regulatory authority regarding allocation and control over overall amount devoted to categories such as hospitals, drugs, nursing homes, etc. Even with a Democrat controlled Congress, the proposals failed to muster a majority. They were too extreme for a society that views with suspicion top-down planning in general.

The deregulation of the health economy

Currently, the Reagan Administration is on a significantly different tack, i.e., to deregulate the health economy and rely to a greater extent on market forces. This is characterized by such notions as *consumer choice and competition* among delivery and financing systems, to provide suitable incentives and controls. As a significant part of public policy a 'safety net' would be provided for *disadvantaged persons*, e.g. the poor, handicapped, and aged, but it is asserted that others would be better served by less government and greater personal involvement in the transactions with doctors and hospitals that ultimately determine costs. With this policy the Administration has implied that better care should cost less. It is important to the perspective to note that the health field does not stand alone as a target for change. Similar strategies have been offered for housing, food stamps, and other programmes. Decisions have not yet been taken by the Congress on several key points, but the debate now centres on *market forces* reflecting traditional American values that have recently been rediscovered.

The rapid shifts from the effect of regulation to incentive, from the prominence of the collective (in Government) leadership to the pre-eminence of the individual; from the concept of equity, to the lash of competition, and the idea of devolution from national to local trust, reflects marked changes in public attitudes favouring decentralized control, and reflecting clear disillusionment with several of the federal programmes promulgated in the 1960s and 1970s. Further, in the 1970s, the labor movement started to lose membership and influence and thus sparks as well as a potentially combustible mass were lost.

A slow change?

Although rapid, the shifts will not be extreme. Congress is still pragmatic; there are few persons of influence stationed at the ideological extremes of the debate, and the general public distrust of simplistic remedies persists. Thus, some new ideas will be adopted and others will not. We will not return to Kennedy formulations in the near future, nor will we set off in entirely new directions. It is likely that we will evolve on the path of a sine curve whose vertexes are limited by the changing but still centripetal forces of the pluralist society which is a feature of America. In this context, the healthiest point of view seems to be to be open to new ideas, not to effect national reforms without testing them in real-life situations but to discontinue programmes that are unproductive or counterproductive while preserving the programmes that are going well. In essence, 'if it works, don't fix it', where things are not working, make manageable changes, and move on.

These general assertions require greater elaboration to bring out certain universal truths which apply to health systems generally and which may best be considered under *'Public and private initiatives'* and *'Cost-sharing'*, a notion which is currently in vogue. There must also be some speculation about *'The way ahead'*. There is also a *'Postscript'* which tentatively explores the relativity of our experience to certain recent developments in the UK.

PUBLIC AND PRIVATE INITIATIVES

The Federal Government

In pursuit of a reasonably balanced budget (4) by 1984, an election year, the Federal Government wants to opt out of an open-ended commitment to the elderly and poor and, perforce, plans to *cap* its commitment in these sectors, leaving the rest to the States and the private sector. This strategy, only in preliminary legislative form, is justified by the rationale that competition and deregulation, popular concepts in the business community, will improve efficiency in health services to the point that all persons will be served but at better cost/benefit.

The aim of this strategy seems clear from its immediate effect which would be to shift costs *to consumers*, through cost-sharing and tighter eligibility rules, *to carriers* who would end up paying for at least part of uncovered costs and *to providers*, particularly those with teaching programmes and/or serving low income populations.

Recent estimates of large Federal deficits, together with concerns over sharing health care costs fired by inflation, have simply served to heighten the interest of the Administration in pro-competition legislation. Initially, the legislative proposals which seem to be favoured have featured such concepts as: yearly election by individual employees of benefit options from among a variety of financing and delivery systems (*versus* employer selection of one bargained by management and labor); a pegged employer contribution *versus* employer payment of the whole, or a major part of the premiums; changes in the tax laws to limit the tax deductibility or tax credits for employer contributions and/or employee contributions, and a move to a voucher system for Medicare, and, possibly, Medicaid, recipients. The voucher system would be designed to enable persons to purchase coverage in the open market among *approved* plans. Above all however it would afford the Federal Government an opportunity over time to limit its contributions through controlling the value of the voucher. Clearly these concepts are meant to shift responsibilities away from government by putting the individual person or patient in greater control, through exercise of options, larger deductibles and co-payments and through tax changes to make the individual more aware of relative costs.

State government actions

Among the States, there are similar concerns about unlimited commitments and rising costs. Most States are not able or willing to pick up much of the Federal slack because of limited resources (5), competing social needs, e.g. schools and transportation, and a lack of administrative experience or expertise. In general, States are more inclined to put pressure on the private sector, through tighter regulation of insurance carriers (e.g. mandating the offer of selected benefits), limits on payments to hospitals for State or Federal/State welfare recipients, more restricted benefits and tighter eligibility standards for those on public assistance.

Thus, a lack-lustre private economy faces the prospect of seeking to pick-up most of the slack either through individual payments, greater productivity, or through insurance schemes. The ability to do this will depend ultimately on the strength of the economy generally. Health care financing is linked inexorably to the effectiveness of the Presidents's overall economic proposals. If these proposals do not work, undoubtedly other health care strategies will have to be devised.

Private market reactions

Among private business concerns, there is a deep and growing concern over costs. A feeling persists, as with government, that excessive demand is a major problem and that private carriers, among others, are not working hard enough to effect economies in the system.

The US Chamber of Commerce reports (6) that employee fringe benefit values now equal 37·1 per cent (including legally mandated programmes of Social Security, Workman's Compensation, and Unemployment Compensation) of salary in many companies and are growing faster than salary increases. If the trend continues for five years, benefits will be prohibitively expensive. Already several large companies, are significantly above the average.

As a result, across a wide front, employers have become much more demanding and discriminating as purchasers of health insurance. For example, in selecting a carrier, they pay much more attention to such elements as; the size of the carrier's administrative costs and reserves, the timeliness and accuracy of claims processing, responsiveness to employer and employee enquiries, field service through marketing personnel, cost containment efforts to drive down claims costs, detailed utilization and cost reports (carrier and employer), flexibility of benefits tailored to company needs (instead of the carrier forcing its products on the employer), and flexible financial arrangements (e.g. when premiums are paid or prepaid).

In most industries representatives of management make the benefit determinations. Labor influence has waned in all but a few industries. Within management, financial officers, as opposed to human relations officers, are more active in decision-making and laying greater stress than ever on cash flow, and on account specific information relating to costs. It is significant that where carriers are non-responsive, management is turning increasingly to self-insurance and using the carrier, if at all, for administrative purposes, for example, payment of claims. Under self-insurance, some companies are indeed negotiating special rates with hospitals and doctors, and contracting with medical foundations or hospitals for utilization review services. To the extent self-insurance involves companies with the better risks, the total insurance pool is reduced and weakened and the consistently healthy further separated from the ill.

The company Chief Executive Officer is now becoming involved. For years his concern has been focussed on the size of the fringe benefit package overall, not with any of the particulars. On 3 November 1981, the Businessman's Roundtable (7), a prestigious group representing the country's largest companies, established health care as a top priority on its action agenda for the next three years. There is action at local level too. Thus recently in Des Moines, Iowa (8), a group of businessmen banded together to address health costs aggressively. They were dissatisfied because they 'sought to cut a deal with doctors and failed' and, were determined to limit both hospital utilization rate increases and cost increases, the latter to 10 per cent or less.

This is by no means a unique case. Uncertain about the future of government planning, businessmen across the country in over 60 major cities, have started or joined community coalitions, and the number is increasing rapidly. In 1976, the Federal Government made a strong commitment to area-wide planning of health programmes and facilities under Public Law 93–641. An initiative was established involving national goals, supporting state health plans and regulatory authority controlling hospital bed construction, and other major capital expenditures. Provision was made for Federal as well as State and local government fundings but specifically excluded most private funding. The Reagan Administration has proposed that this Law be terminated in 1983 as part of the overall deregulation thrust and be replaced by local voluntary planning, on the basis of local initiative and largely private funding. This action, of course, is consistent with the free market notion that priority, distributive, and directional challenges will be met largely by the market, that is as the result of a myriad of economic votes cast at the grass roots level, as opposed to deliberations made in concert at the community or national level. With competition legislation in trouble, PL 93–641 could well be modified rather than terminated. The prospect of an unregulated capital structure and widespread cost reimbursement without new market intermediations is too painful to accept.

Some coalitions, e.g. New Britain, Connecticut, cover all social, welfare, and health services. They seek to establish regional priorities, reduce overlap among services, and tighten co-ordination among programmes. Others are focussed on the concept of health itself. Major strategies of these include development of a fact base, utilization review (e.g. in Cleveland, Ohio, a 17-person board of employers, carriers, hospitals, and doctors are undertaking a 100 per cent review of admissions and length of stay through contracts with a professional standards review organization, incentive reimbursement, and health promotion). The pattern varies considerably with the community. Intentions are commendable but, to date, there are few outcomes to report. Some have broad programmes, others highly selective. Some are comprised only of businessmen; others (gaining popularity) include provider representatives and doctors as well.

A number of companies are initiating educational programmes for their executives who serve on Hospital or planning boards, to acquaint them with the firm's concern over costs and discuss options for changes in the delivery system. Illinois Bell, for example, conducted a survey of the health programmes in Illinois and concluded, among other matters, that few hospital administrators challenge medical staffs sufficiently or take into account community needs. On the basis of the survey, they started a successful training programme.

Organized labor, on a self-admitted four-year's holiday from comprehensive National Health Insurance, is now looking at coalitions with interest, less interested in cost-sharing as a concept, but more aggressively interested in area-wide planning, the fostering of alternate delivery systems, and the promotion of environmental medicine.

In essence, employers, deeply concerned about cost-shifting by government, and a bit queasy about the Federal Government abandonment of both planning and utilization reviews (the PSRO programme), feel the need to limit their expenditures for health benefits, as fringe benefits in general and health costs in particular, grow beyond other expenses.

Thus, the compression of government on health care costs and delivery mechanisms is being intensified by private action. The effect is one of mutual reinforcement.

Provider and professional responses

Frustrated by a tighter money supply, government regulation, inflationary forces, rapid technological change, malpractice suits, the rising demands of the aged, high labor costs, and increased specialization, providers and professionals are reacting. In the last year or two, we have seen the beginning of a quiet revolution in programme and structure that seems to favour formal and informal co-operation among hospitals and allied institutions and the development of a myriad of smaller, free-standing institutions. In many areas the stand-alone acute general hospital appears in jeopardy. Some of the more conservative initiatives among hospitals include *shared service arrangements, group purchasing, management engineering, energy conservation, preventive maintenance, in-house construction* and *increased emphasis on outpatient care.*

Bolder initiatives include *vertical and horizontal* integration (31 per cent of hospital beds are now in multi-hospital systems operated under a variety of holding companies), in response to the need to achieve economy of scale, to improve use of scarce management skills, to minimize the impact of regulations and to improve access to capital. These systems, both those that are highly centrally managed and those where management is decentralized, are aggressive and specifically attentive to financial viability. They will probably become the dominant form of health delivery in the 1980s. Although the trend is unmistakeable, bottom line figures in support of economy of scale are largely anecdotal. There are supporting data from selective ventures like joint laundries, but overall economy of scale is currently, largely an article of faith.

In any event, as hospitals, and hospital systems, are forced to compete for their portion of a decelerating GNP, it is conceivable that the less efficient and effective institutions will be forced out of the market. Those that remain will be tougher in negotiations with government and private financial mechanisms.

The traditional, *non-profit institutions are also being challenged by a growing number of investor-owned institutions* astute at finding market niches, network management, and management of government or non-profit institutions on contract. Along with new and innovative alternative delivery systems, such as Health Maintenance Organizations, these new institutions will confront carriers with more aggressive demands, and fewer and larger units, each with more sophisticated management.

Characteristic of a deregulated market, while there is a great deal of aggregated effort, there is also a significant amount of functional separation of services going on as mentioned above. A variety of narrowly focussed services have developed separate from or loosely connected with hospitals, e.g. ambulatory surgery centres, 'store-front' emergency centres, and birth advice centres, financed to a limited extent by insurance and to a greater extent (to date) by direct out-of-pocket payments. The delivery system is thus literally going in two directions at once. Among aggregates in larger management structures, the physician is required more and more to have a subordinate position, while some of the free-standing services afford physicians entrepreneurial opportunities, often competitive with the hospital or hospital systems. In passing, it should be noted that airlines, brokerage houses, banks, and other industries that were deregulated, have experienced a similar process.

Just as HMOs (and in the UK recently, the BUPA) have combined the financing and delivery of care, one can expect that some of the networking hospitals will begin to sell their services directly in the market, as opposed to the procedure of going through carriers. This, in turn, may lead to more per capita arrangements under which physicians' fees and other arrangements will be determined within competing systems as opposed to across systems through carriers.

A halt to growth and societal shifts

For the last fifteen years, a major characteristic of the health sector has been its 'growth', which has reflected the overall economic well-being of the country which crested in the late 1960s and early 1970s. The public and private health policies of the 1980s will probably reflect far less growth, and less optimism, as the growth of real personal income slows and the more intense competion of a mature market (9) is realized.

Evidence of greater fragmentation of the health economy is manifest, involving, as mentioned, a variety of financing and delivery patterns, and account specific demands *versus* community demands. This has been accompanied by a dispersion in power in medicine among the American Medical Association, State, and Local societies, Specialist societies, etc., as well as among hospitals (see the American Hospital Association, Catholic Hospital Association, Association of American Medical Colleges, Federation of American Hospitals, strong State Associations, etc.) There has also been a marked growth in special interest groups, e.g. an association of hospices. Overall, there is less interest in National Health Insurance with top-down directions and regulations and more interest shown in the possibilities of local variety and choice.

All of these developments have been associated with significant societal shifts elaborated by a new breed of 'futurists': viz: *a shift from an industrial to an information society, a decline in unionism* (now less than 20 per cent of the work force), *growth in entrepreneurialism* (6 times the number of new firms in 1980 as was the case in 1960), *a change in political structure* (two party to issue politics), *a lower tolerance for taxes and government programmes, change in family make-up* (more emphasis on individuals, fewer children, more one-parent families) *marked shifts in population and plan locations, geometric growth in technology* (continually unsettling old ways of doing things), *fewer hierarchies and more net working, leaderships with more limited mandates* and *from a mandated top-down society* to one in which local decisions are paramount.

Much has happened in a short period of time. The market for health services has matured and become more competitive. The overall economy has experienced decelerated growth serving to intensify competition in established territories: and, a lot of fundamental underlying changes are occurring in our political, institutional, and family frameworks, shaping all of our institutions, including health institutions. Furthermore, the speed of change is accelerating. It is a testing time for all, challenging, but also unsettling and intimidating. Not all institutions are coping. There is a great deal of anxiety evident among various health groups. For example, in the hospital field there is tension between the American Hospital Association and the new Federation of American Hospitals, representing the investor-owned hospitals. Medical centres are deeply concerned about how to provide tertiary care, education, and research, at a reasonable and affordable price. Indeed, the health field reflects some of the uneasiness felt in industry. The stock market reflects the fact that although business firms are publicly supportive of government initiatives, they are deeply concerned about how they are working. The concept of cost-sharing has also emerged as one of several market forces catalyzing responsibilities and accountability. As a long-standing issue it deserves elaboration.

COST-SHARING

Definition and implementation

Of long standing interest to many parties, public and private, cost-sharing is now at the centre of the stage as a part of the Reagan Administration's determination to rely on market forces as much as possible in order to discipline the health field, and to depend less on regulatory forces such as areawide planning and mandatory utilization review to rationalize the system. Cost-sharing in this context refers to payments by both employers and the individual or the government and the individual when benefits are purchased (at a flat rate or per cent of premium) or at the time of illness, in the form of co-payments, deductibles, or payments for services not covered by insurance or prepayment. Cost-sharing appears to be a natural ally of consumer choice. The theory is that employees and other individuals under public and private programmes are able to select from a variety of benefit options on a periodic basis. In effect, it *involves the individual* more directly in transactions including physicians and other health services *at the time of illness* just as *consumer choice involves the individual* at the point of *selecting a carrier.*

The thrust of the Reagan Administration is not without reason. Clearly, Federal costs overall, perceived to be more profligate than private expenditures, have to be controlled, if inflation is to be moderated: and health care costs are a significant part of the Federal budget. Regulatory concepts legislated over the last fifteen years in the health field have not worked as well as expected (were expectations reasonable?), e.g. Certification of Need under the Planning Act.

Most agree that there is still excessive fat in the health system. And, there is truth in the allegations promulgated by *Enthoven and others* (10) that the health field lacks free entry, the consumer is too well insulated from most transactions, and providers appear to be automatically rewarded for both efficient and inefficient care. In any event, they certainly share too little in the risk.

It is also true that the Administration's thrust is not without challenge. *Eli Ginsburg and others* (11) have pointed out that market concepts have limited applicability to such fields as health and education and that no amount of social engineering will totally overcome the difficulties. Followers of this persuasion point out that competition is inevitably compromized by professional requirements. Entry to the market must be limited, not everyone can practice medicine or nursing. There is not a standard commodity where the concept of price can rule. Consumers lack sufficient information to make consistently sound choices and, in fact, if ill enough, have no choice but to get care. There will always be ambivalence about 'need' versus 'demand' as the primary animating force of the market: and, unlike most markets, there is a generally obverse relationship between need and ability to pay.

Thus, because cost-sharing is now centre-stage, it does not mean that consensus has been achieved about it. But, new and old arguments are being aired and given greater attention against the backdrop of a broadly enunciated market oriented programme involving health and a wide group of public services.

Cost-sharing under premium payments

For the past thirty years at least, there has been a steady trend in health insurance toward greater employer (versus employee) payment in absolute or percentage terms, particularly among large accounts where many employees now pay 100 per cent of the premium. The overall percentage of employer payment is approximately 70 per cent. This trend reflects labor's interest in security, the power of tax incentives (employer and employee premium payments are tax deduct-

ible), the threat of comprehensive National Health Insurance
and a general underlying concern for security and predictability across the population as a whole that is not well
appreciated by many in public or private life. In regard to
this last point, it is interesting to note that a majority of
employees under the Federal Employee Benefit Programme,
that involves consumer choice and a *pegged* employer contribution, have selected over the years more expensive coverage
even though significantly greater premium cost-sharing is
involved (12). In the last year or two there has been some
movement away from comprehensive benefits as the price of
health services has become unacceptable. Security and predictability have their outer limits as the extent varies by
individual or family. In this respect a recent *New York Times*
survey (13) of 1530 adults revealed that 45 per cent would be
willing to pay a higher deductible if it would reduce the cost
of health care, on the other hand 33 per cent thought it best
to have all of a person's medical bills covered by insurance
even if it increases total medical costs. More declared Democrats felt this way than Republicans.

This trend shows unmistakable signs of moderation and
might even be reversing. With fewer numbers, organized
labor is losing its influence in determining fringe benefits
under collective bargaining and in shaping legislation. Management is in a far stronger position, because it now pays
more of the bill, and can capitalize on labor's weaknesses. As
mentioned, there is growing concern among many employers
that fringe benefit costs, a major percentage of pay-roll for all
employers (a special survey of 186 companies revealed that
the average was 24 per cent in 1959 and 41·4 per cent in
1980, and growing faster than salary increases) (14), are
getting out of hand, particularly in the light of increasing
international competition from labor efficient or low cost
countries. Even the Federal Government, acting as an employer under the Federal Employee Programme, is seeking to
reduce its contribution to premiums (15).

To increase employee sensitivity to premium costs, the
Reagan Administration is eyeing new and different tax incentives in addition to cost-sharing provisions. The current
incentives encourage purchase of insurance or prepayment

by offering tax deductions to employers and employees. This practice goes back to the 1940s when wages were often frozen during the war and the cost of benefits when paid by the employer were designated as proper and unfrozen costs of doing business. The Administration would, however, like to stem demand for insurance and prepayment by limiting the amount that is deductible for the employer or the employee or both. Because workers, unionized or not, would resist a wholesale change, compromizes are being aired, such as a national or regional limit on the current exclusion from the income subject to Federal Income Tax. These are intended to cause employees to reconsider marginal health benefits in the future, and of exemption of currently negotiated contracts until the limits and current values intersect.

Cost-sharing at the time of illness

Many of the same dynamics as apply to the payment of premiums hold in this context. Employers would like to see employees more responsible for disciplinary services at the time of illness, in support of market-type versus regulatory intervention and, of course, to reduce the costs of fringe benefits. Labor and several in the Democratic party still oppose cost-sharing at the time of illness, to any significant extent, under the thesis that an ill individual in need of service is relatively defenceless against persons and organizations on whom he or she must depend on for help. In any event it is felt that hospitals and doctors are better disciplined by highly organized delivery systems (e.g. HMO's), occupational health programmes developed to improve working conditions, environmental interventions, e.g. clean air, proper disposal of pollutants, establishing limits on physician manpower (more manpower generates more use) and the promulgation of more aggressive health promotion programmes. In effect, labor and others want *the community* rather than the individual to make the hard decisions. The opposing philosophies of employers and employees will be put to the test shortly when the next round of labor regulations get fully underway. Recently, the Ford Motor Company settled with the United Auto Workers and, contrary to prediction, increased cost-sharing was not included in the Agreements (16). On the other hand, under the Federal Employee Programme where the Federal Government acts as an employer and several competing carriers are involved at risk, under the Blue Cross/Blue Shield high cost option programme, for the first time, a $25 a day, co-payment for inpatient care was included (17), along with a cutback in the scope of benefits, including mental health benefits. Although the pressure from employers for more cost-sharing is growing, it is a bit early to predict how much change there will be. Interestingly, the AHA and AMA are supporting cost-sharing (18), even though their constituents could become exposed to bad debts, because they deem excessive demand as a major part of the cost evaluation problem and do not think hospitals and doctors should be doing most of the rationing of care.

In fact, the application of cost-sharing will differ with the account. For example, some accounts may elect to stay with comprehensive hospital benefits, feeling that $25 saved up front may be more than added in services or length of stay; some add 'wrap-around' major medical coverage involving deductible co-payments for doctor and other services. Faith in UCR (Usual, Customary and Reasonable) payments to doctors is diminishing and doctors, most of whom are doing well financially, can charge bad debts against income and thus minimize the impact of cost-sharing under major medical coverage. Other accounts may turn to HMOs and allied delivery systems that minimize cost-sharing and rely on the effectiveness of internal incentives to produce efficiency within an overall per capita rate. For many such systems, not all health services are included, and patients still have out-of-pocket expenses, even though of a lesser amount.

Hopes, fears, and weaknesses of policies

The preliminary pronouncements of the current Administration portray *the advantage* of cost-sharing as a way to:

1. stimulate rational, cost-effective purchasing decisions by consumers (overall use and cost will decline);

2. cause the consumer to be more resistant to price increases than governments or carriers seem to be and to shop

more aggressively for comparisons than he or she would under 'free care';

3. achieve broader benefits with the same premium, and

4. reduce the cost of insurance (admittedly, largely a transfer).

The *reservations* about cost-sharing have been born of years of experiences which are not unknown to decision-makers everywhere. Thus:

1. persons can and do purchase supplemental benefits which vitiate the effect of cost-sharing. If cost-sharing really is a significant policy one could count on supplemental benefits being a bargaining issue and further count on the fact that the Federal Government will not outlaw them;

2. with given cost-sharing provisions, low income persons pay higher out-of-pocket amounts as a percentage of income than high-income persons;

3. cost-sharing increases carrier administrative expenses (more so if income classifications are taken into account) and increases the frustrations of subscribers who try to figure out who pays for what;

4. many consumers lack either the information or the know-how to make 'rational' purchase decisions and demonstrably some decisions among low income groups can result in under-care; and

5. varying applications of cost-sharing can shift care towards the least restricted benefits, and, depending on the structure, increase rather than decrease overall costs.

In pointing out the *potential weakness* of individuals playing control roles, it has to be recognized that the *alternative of carriers or governments* exercising controls introduces certain frailties. The contrast is not absolute; too often these institutions fail to use the financial leverage they have *vis-à-vis* providers or they retreat philosophically behind the 'skirts' of the user individual. With all of the rhetoric, there has been little aggressive pressure put on hospitals and doctors. The control strategies in general have been permissive.

One of the leading thinkers behind the competition legislation, Alain Enthoven (19), makes a clear distinction between *incentives, reform,* and *economic* competition. He envisages consumer choice as a method of creating market conditions 'favourable to the growth of cost-effective, comprehensive care organizations that serve their members well', e.g. HMOs, organizations that employ rational economic incentives, that 'cut cost substantially without cutting the quality of care.' He stresses that 'economically self-sufficient consumers' are made 'cost conscious at the time of annual choice of a health care financing and delivery plan'. He sees the cost-sharing school as making every consumer cost-conscious at the time of each medical purchase, and the basic concept, lamentably, as one of leaving 'intact the existing dominant system of insured fee-for-service solo practice.' Enthoven favours too, incentive reform and feels that cost-sharing not only has a number of practical difficulties, such as those cited above, but that 'the cost-increasing incentives of fee-for-service for the physicians are supposed to be offset by the physicians concern for the patient's pocketbook'. Clearly, the two concepts are not mutually exclusive, but at least one new of the leaders in 'new thinking', regards incentive reform leading to new delivery systems as the key to capitalizing on market forces. (He does not pretend that if HMOs become more expensive than fee-for-service medicare they will face the same prospect of growth); and he eschews in general the use of cost-sharing. Incidentally, Enthoven also spells out in detail the number of conditions needed to make a supplier incentives reform, work well. The list is fairly extensive, *supporting the notion that it does, in fact, take significant regulation to harness market forces.*

The fact base is slender

Given such a pattern of somewhat loaded and speculative considerations, it becomes more important than usual to sift through the facts we have, particularly because the cost-sharing issues are now becoming national, i.e. they extend considerably beyond the exercises of an individual employer account to the sphere of legislative debate.

In essence, what we ought to seek to know is the effect of cost-sharing on access, preventive and other care, quality of care, claims and administrative costs.

In fact, relatively little is known about cost-sharing and its direct effects. The underlying reason is that cause and effect are separated by a large number of hard-to-control, independent variables as has been pointed out by the Blue Cross and Blue Shield Associations (20). There are many problems in determining changes in the use of a particular service by a single population group resulting solely from changes in the price to the user of that service, viz:

Many factors beside price change the use of a particular service, e.g. number and type of providers, number and types of beds and doctors, and types of reimbursement or financing methods.

When two or more populations are involved for comparison purposes, such groups may differ on important demographic (age, sex, race), economic (income) and other factors (e.g. benefits included—or the configuration of diagnoses involved).

Retrospective studies seldom involve random samples. Most people, given a choice, pick benefits that suit their needs. Thus, it is hard to separate need from the insurance effect in measuring use.

For all studies, the number of variables makes studies long and expensive. Prospective studies, as those being conducted by the Rand Corporation have proved, can be extraordinarily expensive.

It is difficult and expensive to measure qualitative differences among services and thus to address such questions as 'how did reductions in costs come about' and 'what were the health status consequences'?

Results of cost-sharing

Despite the difficulties, there have been many studies on cost-sharing over the years (21). Among them the duplication is great and the yield of usable information for governments and the private sector is low. It would be unproductive to include here more than passing reference to somewhat mixed outcomes for each type of cost-sharing (e.g. deductible, co-insurance) and for each setting (e.g. hospital, ambulatory service). Roughly these are:

Deductibles can reduce the length of stay in hospitals.

If large enough, co-insurance will tend to inhibit hospital admissions.

Reasonable co-payments seem to have little effect on the use of the hospital but significant effects outside the hospital.

The effect varies with the amount of cost-sharing, in most instances.

Of particular interest is the recent Report of the Rand Corporation on the health insurance experiment (22). It is important, however, to recognize that the report issued in December 1981 is only an interim report. Only approximately 40 per cent of the person years under study have been recorded. No data are yet available out of the South Carolina site. We will have to wait approximately another year before all populations have a three-year documented exposure.

It is difficult to project what new facts will unfold a year or two from now. References in the preliminary report to health status suggest a lot of work was still to be done. Appreciable resources have been spent on ascertaining the effects on health status of differences in health insurance plane. To provide data for such analyses, Rand adopted a comprehensive strategy for measuring health status and changes in it over time. Health status was assessed according to six distinct concepts, based on a preliminary report, including physiological health, physical health, mental health, social contacts, health habits, and general health perceptions. Dental health was also evaluated. Sources of health data included medical screening examinations and various self-administered questionnaires. Rand feels that they have made numerous and significant advances in methods for assessing health status, but one hears that individual self rating (good, fair, poor) is involved and that such surrogates are being used as disability days, symptoms (to be rated retrospectively by medical experts), inpatient diagnoses, etc. as opposed to direct assessment. With National Institutes of Mental Health Rand negotiated an additional contract to look at the effect of cost-sharing on the particular use of mental health services.

Some of *the major findings* of the interim report attracting attention are:

Confirmation that co-insurance can reduce total health expenditure and 'free care' can cause expenditures to increase 50 per cent.

Most of the variation in expenditure appears to be in quantity of services versus price of services and the variation in the fraction of users across plans accounts for one-third to one-half the difference in use among plans (depending on the site and year).

Co-insurance measurably affects expenditures on ambulatory services.

The skewing of use in groups is confirmed by the finding that the expenses of one per cent of the persons accounted for 28 per cent of total expenditures.

Expenses *per* hospital patient showed no consistent relation with payment. Thus, cost-sharing after admission is of limited value (it is important to keep in mind that losses are limited to $1000 in the design for all plans).

Cost-sharing unrelated to income differentially affects lower-income families and results in lower use.

The alleged *weaknesses* in this very expensive study (approx. $70m over 12 years including benefit payments) can be summarized as follows:

In the absence of sound health status measures, or measures of effective use, the preliminary results are hard to interpret, as Rashi Fein asks in his comments in the *New England Journal of Medicine*, 17 December 1981. Is more or less good or bad for the individual or for the community? What are the trade-offs? Health status data forthcoming may shed light on these points.

The absence of data for the over 65 group severely limits the applicability of the results to major users.

The general protocol needs to be examined when a fuller report is available. What are the implications of 15 per cent initially and 20 per cent of the sample subsequently backing out of the trial?

We must keep in mind that the benefit design overall (specifically the stop-loss provision) affects the co-insurance impacts.

None of us should be in a mood to put down the Rand Study. The issues targeted are important, both in the US and probably abroad too. We should wait for further, more refined reports, particularly as they bear on the subject of health status.

The need for better criteria and further research

The study does however prompt us to realize that other approaches are needed, e.g.:

with the assistance of physician panels, develop criteria of medical effectiveness for high frequency diagnoses or complaints

select a probability sample of hospitals and offices in a few areas.

sample patient records within the above and apply the effectiveness criteria.

for cases that fall outside the criteria, to interview the doctor and patient, regarding clinical, family, financial, working, living, geographical, and other information.

and thus, to be able to measure economic and social factors associated with use (including how the bill is paid), against criteria of proper or effective use.

This particular line of approach sketched above, first employed at the University of Michigan (23), provided useful insights as to the relationship between cost-sharing and over and under use and appropriateness of use of health services.

The Rand and other findings (see note 21) begin to prompt questions and uncover some perplexing dilemmas. For example:

If the cost-sharing is high enough to reduce use, will it produce less care than is needed, according to medical consensus?

If cost-sharing is too expensive, will the benefits sell in the market; if it is too low, will the protection become too expensive?

The finer the tuning of cost-sharing to specific benefits (based on research) the harder one's eligibility is to comprehend and the more expensive it is to administer (by the carrier).

In the United States, such perplexities rarely promote causes led by zealots. We tend to sift through our experiences and apply the lessons pragmatically at random.

THE WAY AHEAD

The shape of the debate

The health field will be the subject of great debate in the 1980s for the many reasons cited. But, health is highly valued in the American culture and the current system of health services is generally rated well. Young persons still rate the profession of medicine above most careers. And, as health services have expanded, they have elicited higher expectations and greater financial investment. As a result, it is likely that changes will be made over time on an incremental scale, short of a rupture to the economy as a whole.

The President's proposals regarding the need for greater consumer choice and involvement among vigorously competing health plans are currently being assessed by the Congress. Enough practical problems have arisen so that it is safe to predict that none of the 'pro-competitive' bills will pass in its present form. Business and labor leaders, carriers, teaching hospitals, and others have raised enough questions to suggest that legislative changes in the next two years will be limited. What appeared at first to be a promising set of proposals now appears to have some serious flaws which may be of interest to other countries contemplating change. As pointed out, the exercise of option by an employee can lead to selection problems favouring the young and well, and to impairment of the insurance pool. Some carriers may not compete by motivating providers to become effective, but instead, avoid confrontations with doctors and hospitals through cost-sharing (e.g. deductibles and co-insurance) and selective underwriting practices (e.g. taking mainly good risks). Management and labor might lose interest in pressuring the system when individuals make the key choices. Similar concerns are being expressed about the use of a voucher system for the aged and low-income beneficiaries, whose problems are compounded by the unique problems such persons often have evaluating alternatives.

These flaws are not entirely speculative. For example under the Federal Employee Benefit Plan, involving over 10 million employees and dependents residing in all 50 states, the problems of selection have been significant (24). In essence, with yearly enrollment opportunites, the well have tended to select lower premium cost plans from among several options and the sick have tended to select higher premium cost plans, all aided by a fixed employer contribution. The aggregation of the sick has driven high reference premium costs significantly higher and, in fact, for too many, beyond reach. Thus, the needy are placed in jeopardy. In effect, the insurance pool has been excessively fragmented. Risk-sharing has been unduly compromised in the name of incentives. In this same programme, it is equally apparent that not all carriers do wish to get involved in improving the effectiveness of the delivery system. Given such a large and lucrative market, some organizations started carrier functions to capitalize on selective opportunities whose ultimate aims were to solidify membership for other purposes.

As the debate unfolds, the possibility clearly arises that it would indeed take, ironically, more regulation to make competition work than we have now. Certainly, people cannot be allowed to make bad choices in any major piece of legislation. If employer contributions are to be capped, the question arises how this is done equitably in a country with widely varying cost levels for the same service, and widely varying age and sex compositions among working groups in the same area.

At the same time, a seemingly insoluble dilemma has arisen. It is generally agreed that competitive forces take 5–15 years to have a significant impact while the Federal Government needs to save money now. Further, in the short run, moves to save *significant* amounts could cause access problems and if such moves are not made, budget objectives will not be reached.

Possible policy directions

As a result of these various factors, again, we are unlikely to see a very comprehensive piece of health legislation in 1982. The most likely *proposals* will probably include:

Limits on tax deductions or credits for employers and/or employees.

Voluntary choice programmes at the work-site with tax incentives for employers to expand options, at least modestly.

Strong encouragement for demonstrations of innovative financing and delivery systems.

Possibly, a *voluntary* voucher system under Medicare.

Selective use of cost-sharing (not methodically related to income) for various individuals and groups above the poverty line.

Stop-loss catastrophic protection involving full payment of services beyond a given level of out-of-pocket payments (to help prevent indigence among individuals and families because of health expenses).

Use of prospective payment to providers under Medicare (instead of cost-reimbursement) joining providers in the risk.

Selective use of regulation (cut-backs in some current regulations deemed ineffective or counterproductive, but probably the addition of others).

It is not beyond the realm of reason to contemplate government caps on expenditure and costs, despite all protestations to the contrary, if health care costs continue to escalate during 1982 as they did in 1981 and the Federal deficit projections through 1984 remain pessimistic.

The prospect before us

The most likely scenario involves a public/private partnership, greater decentralization within government, and the *concept of a minimum standard* (benefits, quality of care) for all above which individual options will be exercised rather than equality for all, based on the underlying assumption that the exercise of options will increase efficiency and productivity and thus enlarge the resource pie to be cut for the benefit of all.

As has been pointed out, inherent in the picture is *cost-shifting from Federal Government to States* and from *government to the private sector* justified (by the current Administration) by the necessity, in the face of inflation, unemployment, trade deficits, and a slack economy, to energize the economy through a reduction in Federal Government expenditures (24). *States* are weighing the trade-offs between added authority and added expense. There has been neither universal or enthusiastic acceptance of any given programme as yet. Seventy or eighty voluntary coalitions have been formed at the local level to address cost-containment challenges. It is early to tell how these will come out. However, is heartening to see such representatives sitting down together to deal with community health problems in manageable bites, even though there is widespread uncertainty about whether voluntary solutions will work and what interventions specifically will be effective. It remains to be seen whether the persons who have assailed government interventions can now, given the opportunity, measure up to the requisite private initiatives, while balancing the welfare of the community against that of the individual.

With the prospects of less government funds in the offing and tougher negotiations with employers and carriers, *providers of care* have begun to restructure their institutions. In fact, the changes have been remarkably bold in some instances, and certainly rapid in institutional terms.

Caught between sharing greater risks (through cost-sharing and fewer government beneficiaries) and a growing number of such incentive reimbursement schemes as per capita payments or prospective payment (where the efficient hospitals get to keep savings while others must absorb excess), as well as the prospect of tighter money for capital and innovative investments, *hospitals and allied institutions* are seeking new ways to orchestrate capital and management, achieve economy of scale, and minimize the impact of regulation through ingenious corporate structures. Undoubtedly, the delivery system will change significantly in the 1980s.

How *the individual* will respond to cost-shifting by government and some carriers is not yet clear. Given the weakness of the fact base, cost-sharing issues are best seen as in a state of flux with governments, carriers, employers, providers, and individuals trying to protect their own interests and with government clearly ambivalent about its dual obligation to minimize expenditure *and,* at the same time, protect low income groups. In such an unstable environment, the *overall economic and political forces* will exercise great weight. In this context, such questions arise as, will decentralization of government and a reduction in government expenditure last? Do individuals and local communities want more responsibility? Will low income and concerned aged persons rebel as voters? Is reliance on market forces in health realistic in general?

It is interesting to look at the notions which seem to be circulating within the Reagan Administration. Some within it feel strongly about the details set out above, and other related questions. One hears thoughts expressed such as: 'if individuals try hard enough, they will succeed'; 'the consumer is sovereign'; and 'the government is not necessarily responsible ultimately for public services'.

Thus, in a sense, how cost-sharing concepts are interpreted becomes a sign of the times. In the Kennedy era they were anathema. Today, they are used, in part, as code words to signify faith, or at least qualified faith, in the market.

Yet *consumer choice* concepts are now having a hard time, a year after their introduction. *Cost-sharing* is now under the microscope. It is likely that the outcome in the next few years will reflect a balance or compromise among perceived 'facts', the overall popularity of risk versus security and the tensions involved in balancing our international market struggles against a protected society.

It is difficult to predict what will happen between 1982 and 1984, two election years. It is likely that the leaning to the market side will continue but that finer distinctions will be drawn between incentive reform and cost-sharing, with the latter relegated to a more significant but selective role driven by costs and hedged by supplementary courage and the former given greater and increasing emphasis. Community and group oriented intervention will prevail over individual incursions, but both groups will be involved.

Americans are increasingly aware that other countries face many of the same cost rise and cost containment issues and that there are no easy answers available for import. As opposed to the 1960s and early 1970s, our attention is now inward, convinced that our health system must fit our society overall. We are becoming increasingly aware that the middle course between incentive and regulation and between centralization (Federal) and decentralization (States), probably, in this context, makes the most sense. In the next two or three years, we will probably see more use of incentives *and* more regulation, but with more regulation used to support incentives, and greater State and local participation in health services with less reference to sweeping, nationwide solutions. Since 1965, impressive gains have been made in morbidity and mortality. The gap between high and low income groups has been considerably narrowed. Access for lower income groups has clearly been improved, as measured by such surrogates as physician visits and hospital admissions (25). The challenge is to sustain this progress at levels we can or choose to afford.

POSTSCRIPT

In summary

In the US, it is commonly agreed that the health field will not experience the same overall growth in the 1980s as it did in the 1960s and 1970s. In part, this is due to the fact that alternative goods and services are beginning to assume higher relative value at the margins. But, it is also related to two other critical events, (1) the country turned conservative four or five years ago and became less inclined to spend government funds, and more inclined to seek local solutions (*before* President Reagan was elected) and (2) the health field has matured, and characteristic of matured markets in the US, we see more competition, more discerning buyers (individuals and groups), greater segmentation, greater threats to the inefficient carriers and providers, and slower growth (nevertheless better growth than in many fields and reasonably recession-proof). Competition, promoted by sophisticated purchasers looking for productive alternatives has energized the providers and professionals. We are experiencing a literal revolution in new delivery structures. The corollary process of deregulation inherent in the public mood, as it has in banking, brokerage houses, and other industries, has encouraged the development of large aggregations of providers generally under some form of holding company arrangement *and* a proliferation of smaller services separate from the hospital, for example, ambulatory and surgery, that are dedicated to small market niches.

Thus, the current Administration is reflecting a public sentiment, as well as giving the sentiment leadership. Whether the legislative thrusts involving consumer-choice, cost-sharing, deregulation, and decentralization, some of which are being implemented, will succeed is still uncertain. States are eyeing new responsibilities and trade-offs uncertainly and the private sector has clearly mixed feelings, torn between the privilege of greater freedom on the one hand and the greater financial responsibility, resulting from cost-shifting (already estimated to be $6b) on the other.

Whether and how market forces apply in the health field forms the centre of the public debate. To date, major issues have not been resolved. As a result, new legislation is narrowly focussed.

The debate has made it abundantly clear that we need better information regarding the effectiveness of, cost-sharing and area-wide planning, and we need better articulated public policy. Whatever one's predeliction is towards incentives versus regulation, the public debate should clarify such long-standing issues as social justice versus efficiency, one standard of care versus the concept of minimum standard, how to deal with health in an ageing society (e.g. separate out maintenance and dying services?), whether parameters to public versus private expenditures should be established before services are rendered, and what, more precisely, are the essential elements of a public/private sector partnership? These issues are too important to be left to the market alone, particularly given its uncertain application and the certainty of its long time span in taking effect.

In the last analysis, the debate will be coloured by the tone of our general economy which, at the moment, is stagnant with the depth of the recession hard to fathom.

Lessons for the UK?

This essay has mainly been concerned with the most actively debated issue in the US. It is not a review of the varied, complex field of health, but the influence of cost which clearly is a dominant factor in health care policies. What are the lessons for Britain? Differences between the US and Britain, in tradition, social purpose, and population base among other matters, are significant. One must sift the US experience carefully, to identify common bases.

One point in common is that both countries, as all 'developed' countries, are experiencing cost problems and for many of the same reasons, i.e. inflation, expanding technology, and growing consumer expectation.

Reactions have however differed sharply regarding how to establish priorities, assure adequate care for all persons, and contain costs. Britain has chosen to place the health system in a formal structure and exercise tighter controls over policy planners and expenditure decisions, while laying heavy emphasis on equity and equality of service.

The British Health Service has, since 1947, made outstanding contributions. But, thirty-five years of experience and changing environment, have also raised some questions. A few are being aired, for example:

Should private initiatives in health services be encouraged as a matter of public policy?

If so, under what means? Is there a prospect of the use of tax or other incentives?

If tax incentives are offered to employers and employees, will they become more interested in cost-containment, as they have in the States?

If the private sector were more broadly involved, to what degree should market forces be relied on, to what degree should regulatory standards (affecting both financing and delivery of care) be exercised to protect the public interest?

If the government and private sectors are to envisage a co-operative relationship, should the bounds be tight or loose? All degrees are seen in the States, for example, the private sector is quite independent when carriers underwrite risks; the same carriers act as agents of the Federal Government under the Medicare programme.

At a time when devolution seems to be the keynote, what are the relative advantages of unitary control over linkages among different units superimposed on a solid base?

Will selection take place in Britain as it has in the US if options are offered; and if so to what advantage the government or the private sector? What steps can be taken to minimize the problem?

Do new delivery systems being based in the US, for example, HMOs, have any potential in Britain, possibly on a dem-onstration basis, to test regional or area structures?

Can geographical distribution and productivity problems which involve the practice of medicine be attacked partly through judicious use of incentives?

Major changes are probably out of the question at the moment, but certain operating, capital, and morale problems deserve attention. Possibly the balance of political power is now too close to support even minor changes. But, if our maturation experiences are of any consequence, it might be well for Britain to explore a few avenues. It is not beyond reason to expect Britain, like the US, to see health services as having a reciprocal relation with the economic health of the country and the health of the economy as being vital to the health of the people. In this context, Mr Reagan is now weighing cuts in defence and social programmes (including health) against interest rates, inflation, and unemployment.

If there is reason to believe that some change is necessary in Britain, involving the private sector, it might be well to start a series of modest explorations into some alternative linkages between government and private institutions be-yond those that already exist. It seems inevitable that the private sector will continue to thrive in one way or another as was indicated in the 'Special Report' in *The Times* of 17 June 1982, which touched on issues not unfamiliar to those with experience of insurance systems in the US, and concerned with health policies generally (26). Why not agree on some mutual objectives and working relationships? At least an agenda could be agreed upon.

If this were to come about, both the private sector and the government would need to educate their representatives regarding the issues. This in itself would be helpful to the country, but it would be an essential antecedent to productive negotiations. Probably some new skills would be needed as well. With the size of the stakes they could be well afforded. Given the rapid changes we are all experiencing in health services, it is also essential to think five to ten years ahead. It is apparent that some developments are already underway in Britain, for example, involving private hospitals, that could affect long-term government strategies. These developments should be part of at least a plan, not treated as an outside event.

Finally, although it may seem gratuitously obvious to say it, conversations must start with an honest recognition of differences and an avoidance of winning, at someone else's expense, within a spirit of negotiation, if progress is to be made.

The current surge of change is so strong, technically, if not socially, that nothing less is required.

NOTES AND REFERENCES

1. DEPARTMENT OF HEALTH AND HUMAN SERVICES, HCFA, *Health Care Financing Review*, September 1981, p. 37 (article: ROBERT M. SEBSON and DANIEL R. UALDO, 'National Health Expenditure, 1980').

2. *Medicare,* Title XVII of the Social Security Act was passed in 1965 and implemented on 1 July 1966 to protect the elderly from the high cost of health care. In July 1973, coverage was extended to permanently disabled workers and their dependents and to persons with end-stage renal disease. *Medicaid* was implemented in 1966 by Title XIX of the Social Security Act as a joint Federal-State programme to provide medical assistance to the aged, blind, and disabled persons, or members of families with dependent children. If a State chooses, Federal matching funds are

made available for medical benefit for persons in the above categories who have income too high for costs assistance but not adequate to pay their medical bills.

3. First Kennedy Bill: Senate 4297, 27 August 1970. Second: Senate 3, 25 January 1971.

4. There is a great deal of dispute about what constitutes a reasonably balanced budget for 1983, but many would settle for a $50–100b deficit as opposed to the $100–200b deficit now projected with further gains in 1984. Probably, this will require delegated tax cuts, some tax increases, a reduction in defence spending and cut-backs in social programmes.

5. In seven of the last ten years, state deficits have risen faster than the Federal deficit.

6. US CHAMBERS SURVEY RESEARCH CENTRE, US CHAMBER OF COM-MERCE, *Employee Benefit Report, 1980*. (Washington, D.C.).

7. Established in 1972, the Business Roundtable is an association of business executives who examine public issues that affect the economy and develop positions which seek to reflect sound economic and social principles. Working in task forces on specific issues, the participants direct research, prepare position papers, recommend policy and speak out on issues. Health is such an issue. For a good summary of health issues, see: The Business Roundtable, *An Appropriate Role for Corporations in Health Care Cost Management*. (Washington, D.C., February, 1982).

8. JOHN K. IGLEHART, *NEJM, Health Policy Report*, 14 January 1982, p. 124.

9. A 'mature market' is one in which there are a multitude of products available to the vast majority of the community. In the health field specifically, most health services are widely dispensed and most persons have access to care through public and private financing programmes. Several years ago, competitors among several different delivery and financing systems started beaming on the same market. Winning market share is now often at someone else's expense. As buyers become more sophisticated and demanding the result is an increase and segmentation of the market. Overall market growth is slower and there is, perforce, a stake out of weak competitors.

10. ALAIN C. ENTHOVEN, PhD., 'Consumer-Choice Health Plan', *NEJM*, Part 1, 23 March 1978, Part 2, 30 March 1978, pp. 650–8 and pp. 709–19.

11. ELI GINSBERG, PhD., 'The Limits of Competition in the Provision of Health Services'. An interim Report to the Health Services Foundation, Blue Cross, and Blue Shield Associations, 12 June 1981 and 'The Competitive Solution: Two Views', *NEJM*, 6 November 1980, pp. 1112–15.

12. (1) US GOVERNMENT, CIVIL SERVICE COMMISSION, *Annual Report of Financial and Statistical Data, Civil Service Retirement, Federal Employee Group Life and Federal Employee Health Benefits and Retired Federal Employees Health Benefits, 1961–76;* (2) US GOVERNMENT, OFFICE OF PERSONNEL AND MAN-AGEMENT, *Federal Fringe Benefit Facts, 1977–80* (Note: in recent years a trend toward the selection of more economical coverage is developing).

13. *New York Times*, 'The Price of Health: examining the medical system', 5 part series, 28 March–4 April 1982.

14. US CHAMBER SURVEY RESEARCH CENTRE, US CHAMBER OF COM-MERCE, *Employee Benefit Report, 1980.* (Washington D.C.).

15. DONALD J. DEVINE, Director, OPM, 'Preliminary Analysis, Federal Employees Benefit Programme', 11 September 1981.

16. *Chicago Sun-Times,* 'Ford, UAW Reach Pact Helpful to Both Sides', 14 February 1982, p. 7 ('All major health benefits stay, including progressive surgical, medical and dental plans. Those with 10 years of service will get up to 24 months of group health coverage, if laid off, as opposed to the current limit of 12 months.').

17. US GOVERNMENT, OPM, *Government Wide Service Benefit Plan Brochure,* NOBRI 41–25, January 1982, p. 3 (Under high-option BC/BS coverage, a $25 co-payment has been added to the basic coverage in 1982 for a maximum of 10 days of general, acute, inpatient care; under the low-option basic plan, the amount is $30; deductibles (currently $200) and co-payments (currently 20 per cent) have been in place for supplemental coverage for several years).

18. (1) JOHN ALEXANDER MCMAHON, *Statement of the AHA on Consumer Choice Approaches to Financing Health Care,* to the Subcommittee on Health, House Ways & Means Committee, 30 September 1981, p. 4. (2) AMA, *Proceedings of the House of Delegates,* 18–22 June 1978, pp. 32–33, and 3–6 December 1978, pp. 103–104, and 203.

19. Unpublished remarks, testimony before the National Council on Health Planning and Development, Department of Health and Human Services, 18 March 1982.

20. BLUE CROSS AND BLUE SHIELD ASSOCIATIONS, *Executive Summary, A Critical Literature Review on Cost-Sharing* (ref. David H. Klein, SVP), Chicago 1981, and *Report on Front-End Deductibles,* 4 Sept 1981, Chicago (ref. William E. Regan, EVP).

21. ——, *Literature Review on Cost-Sharing,* Chicago, 1981 (ref. David H. Klein, SVP).

22. JOSEPH P. NEWHOUSE, PhD., *et al.,* 'Some Interim Results from a Controlled Trial of Cost-Sharing in Health Insurance', *NEJM,* December 1981, pp. 1501–07.

23. MCNERNEY, *et al.,* 'Hospital and Medical Economies, Character and Effectiveness of Hospital Use'. (Hospital Research and Educational Trust: Chicago, 1962, pp. 361–592).

24. BLUE CROSS AND BLUE SHIELD ASSOCIATIONS, *Testimony,* Committee on Post Office and Civil Service, Subcommittee on Compensation and Employees Benefits, US House of Representatives, 17 November 1981.

25. DAVID ROGERS, MD, 'Overview, the Elderly and the Independent', Duke Conference, 15 March 1982 (unpublished).

26. *The Times,* 17 June 1982, 'Private Health. A Special Report'.

Health care in Canada
Patterns of funding and regulation

R. G. EVANS

R. G. EVANS

Bob Evans is Professor, Department of Economics, University of British Columbia. He has been at UBC since 1969 and was Visiting National Health Scientist, University of Toronto, Department of Health Administration, 1977–78.

His primary interests are in research and teaching in the economics of health care, and more generally in the public regulation of economic activity, particularly of 'professional' occupations, and the sources of and responses to problems of market failure. His research has covered hospital behaviour and costs, analysis of particular programmes in hospitals (day care surgery, care by parent), physician price and output behaviour, dental and pharmaceutical insurance and delivery systems, patterns and economic effects of occupational regulation, determinants of regional variations in surgical utilization. He is the author of many essays and has written or edited several books on these subjects and is on the Editorial Board of the *Journal of Health Politics, Policy and Law, Health Services Research* and formerly on *Canadian Public Policy*. He is currently writing a textbook on the economics of health care.

He has been a consultant at various times to governments of Canadian provinces, Canada, and USA on matters of health research and policy.

Health care in Canada
Patterns of funding and regulation

ABSTRACT

Since 1970, the ratio of health care expenditures to GNP in Canada has been roughly stable, in the neighbourhood of 7 per cent, in contrast to most other developed countries. The contrast is particularly striking with respect to the US, which has a very similar health care delivery system, the critical difference being that by 1970 Canada had fully implemented its universal public insurance systems, covering virtually all hospital and medical expenses. In the previous two decades, when both countries financed care through a mixture of public and private insurance and direct payment, their cost escalation was virtually identical.

This paper examines the processes of cost containment in Canada, noting its pressure on medical fee schedules and incomes rather than manpower use, and on hospital physical capacity and budgets rather than on patterns of hospital practice. Constraint has not led to problems of queuing and costly forms of non-price rationing, rather it has influenced providers's decisions as to what care to provide. And the key lever has been direct reimbursement control, not regulation *per se*. Unlike the US, where extensive regulation of health care is generally regarded as a failure, Canadian provincial governments have restrained expansion by monopolizing the payments system. They have not, however, made much effort to improve efficiency of resource use either by regulation or by reimbursement.

The result is a programme which is enormously popular with the public, and has been very successful in terms of access promotion and equitable distribution of care and of expenditure burdens. It is under heavy attack, however, by physicians and hospitals for its failure to expand their share of national income. Successful cost restraint is reinterpreted as 'underfunding', for which the cure recommended by providers is more private funding. In particular the steady pressure by physician associations for the right to bill patients directly

371

indicates a belief, on the evidence well-founded, that in contrast to some of the more naive economic analyses such direct
charges will serve to raise physician incomes and medical care
costs.

'Underfunding', in the sense of failure to fund efficacious
care, has not been substantiated. Indeed there is evidence of
significant remaining inefficient and ineffective care, suggesting that the underfunding/privatization argument is primarily aimed at increasing physician incomes and expanding
their access to publicly provided capital equipment. In fact,
further reductions in care use and costs could be achieved in a
number of identifiable areas, with no risk to patients' health.
But the failure of governments to manage health care delivery
as successfully as they have contained its costs has made
defense against such attacks unnecessarily difficult, and the
basic structure of the public plan may be at risk. The paper
concludes with an outline of the alternative strategies for
Canadian health policy in the 1980s, and their likely effects.

WHY LOOK AT CANADA AT ALL?

The funding system in comparison with the US

Because Canada is the black swan; one refutes the proposition that 'all swans are white'. Developed societies are not
subject to some iron law of escalation of health costs. (1)
Although many countries have during the 1970s experienced
steady increases in the share of national income devoted to
health care, Canada has not (2). Table 1 reports Canadian
health care expenditure in total, per capita, and as a percentage of GNP over three decades, and contrasts the very
different US experience. While the Canadian percentage has
fluctuated between 7 per cent and 7·5 per cent since 1970,
the US has risen to nearly 10 per cent. Moreover, as Table 1
and Figure 1 show, the divergence between US and Canadian experience dates from 1971, when Canada's national
medical insurance programme became complete nationwide.
Earlier, when Canada's funding system was broadly similar
to that of the US, so was the cost experience. And the two
delivery systems have remained broadly similar, with medical services provided primarily by private practitioners reimbursed fee for service, and acute care hospitals owned by

Table 1. *Health care expenditures in Canada and the United States, 1950–80.*

	Canada Personal health care expenditures			United States All Health Care Expenditures		
	Total $MC	*Per capita* $C	*% of* GNP	*Total* $MUS	*Per Capita* $US	*% of* GNP
1950	535·4	39·03	2·9	12662	81·86	4·5
1953	734·9	49·50	2·9	15745	96·84	4·3
1956	988·2	61·45	3·2	19246	112·32	4·6
1959	1362·5	77·93	3·9	24878	137·94	5·3
All health care expenditures						
1962	2533·2	136·32	5·9	31404	165·88	5·6
1965	3362·1	171·15	6·1	43003	217·42	6·2
1968	4814·2	232·56	6·6	58864	288·17	6·8
1971	7122·3	330·21	7·5	82764	393·09	7·8
1974	10247·5	458·21	6·9	115610	535·99	8·2
1977	15395·2	660·99	7·4	169994	768·77	9·0
1979	18836·4	795·14	7·2	212200	943·0	9·0
1980	Not yet available			247200	1070·0	9·4

Notes.

1. Prior to 1960, Canadian statistics reported only personal health care expenditures—expenditures on hospitals, physicians, dentists, and prescribed drugs—and excluded other professional and institutional services, non-prescribed drugs and appliances, and expenditures on public health, prepayment and administration, research, and capital formation.

2. The Federal Department of National Health and Welfare assembles Canadian data and releases them in publications and interim unpublished materials. They are always subject to revision in both estimate and concept; data here are the most recent available to the author ATP and deviate slightly from earlier published figures.

Source. (3, 4, 5, 6, 7, 8).

voluntary societies, municipalities, or universities, and run by boards of trustees. In both countries, medical staff organizations representing private practitioners with admitting privileges at, but not employed by, the hospital exert significant influence over hospital management.

There are numerous differences in detail between Canada and the US in the organization and delivery of hospital and medical care, but they are nowhere near as significant as the differences in funding. Moreover, the contrast between Canadian cost experience pre- and post-1971 as well as between Canada and the US makes clear that it is the funding system

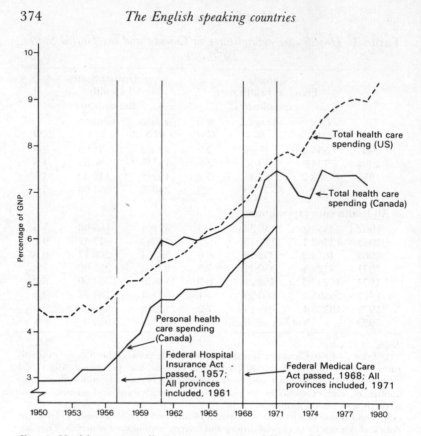

FIG. 1. Health care spending as a percentage of National Income, Canada and U.S., 1950–80.

which is critical. The universal public insurance programmes in each province which reimburse all hospital and medical costs through direct budgetary allocation and fee schedule negotiation, respectively, make expenditure control, not easy, but possible. The fragmentation of funding sources between private out-of-pocket payment, private for-profit and not-for-profit insurance, and public programmes, which characterizes the US now and Canada prior to the public plans, does not.

Comprehensive coverage

Moreover this control has been achieved with comprehensive coverage both of people and of services. The whole population is covered for, effectively, *all* needed services. The former system of private insurance excluded a significant proportion of the population, particularly those in most need, and could not assure coverage of very large costs. US experience bears this out. Fifteen years after the US launched its Medicare and Medicaid programmes to supplement private insurance 10 per cent of the population still had no insurance coverage at all. Over half the uninsured are low income people (9). Fragmented coverage is both more costly and less complete, as people 'fall through the cracks' (10).

Universal public insurance has also contributed to a more equitable distribution of service availability across the population. A number of studies have documented a shift in utilization by income class, the pre-insurance positive correlation of income with use being now reversed (11—16). Although information on the relation between utilization and need is rather inadequate, such as there is suggests improvement post-insurance.

Another consideration was the administrative cost of running a payments system. In Canada, overhead or insurance administration costs are about 3 per cent of health spending. Prior to the public plan, they ranged from 10 per cent up to over 50 per cent of private premiums; present US experience indicates private insurance costs of about 15 per cent of covered expenditures. To private insurers, these load factors are sales revenue and the source of profits. But to the patient, consumer, or taxpayer, they are simply the excess burden of an inefficient insurance mechanism, to which must be added the indirect compliance costs of patients and providers dealing with a multiplicity of different insurers and contract provisions.

It is not surprising, then, that two recent reviews of the Canadian health insurance system, each conducting public hearings, have found overwhelming popular support for present arrangements—with one (and perhaps two) major exceptions (17,18). The medical profession is very disturbed

precisely *because* the system has successfully controlled expenditures—which are also their incomes or the revenues of
hospitals where they practice. And provincial governments
find that costs, while a relatively stable share of income, are
still very large. Moreover the process of control forces governments and providers to bear the costs of negotiation and
conflict with each other. As these conflicts become increasingly severe providers are trying to pass the burden back to
patients. If provincial governments acquiesce, Canadian experience in the 1980's will be much less favourable.

The longer-term viability of the Canadian funding system,
with its built-in conflicts of interest between providers and
the public plan and its ambiguous incentives for government,
is thus in some question. At the beginning of the 1980s,
physicians' organizations across Canada have mounted a
strong campaign to replace Medicare with something closer
to a US style system of independent physician fee setting and
direct charges to patients over and above the negotiated fee
schedule.

A monopoly regulated insurance system

Regardless of how the future unfolds, however, comparison
of Canadian and US experience over the past decade points
an important lesson. The Canadian system is a monopoly
insurance system, not a public *service*, a monopoly maintained
by legislative exclusion of private insurers. There has been
little intervention in the delivery system itself. Provincial
governments do not practice medicine, nor direct the behaviour of hospitals, except insofar as they determine what
activities (in general, not specific cases) will or will not be
reimbursed. The issues of fee-for-service versus salaried practice, of state-owned hospitals versus independent boards of
trustees, of public versus private provision of health care
generally, have been resolved by leaving the pre-public insurance delivery system more or less in place.

That system has always been heavily regulated,—to talk
about a 'free market' in medical care prior to the public
insurance programmes is nonsense. Private associations with
statutory authority, in Canada as in the US, regulate the

entry to, and the professional and economic conduct of members of, occupational groups, and serve some shifting blend of their own and the wider public interest. Hospital behaviour is likewise heavily regulated, being influenced by public statute, by collectively established accrediting bodies, and by their own medical staffs. This regulation predates public insurance, and was not significantly modified by it.

But the public monopolization of the payment process has also served as a powerful, if indirect, form of regulation. Just as the power to tax is the power to destroy, so the power to fund is that to create, shape, and limit. The superposition without reconciliation of this public, indirect regulatory system on an essentially unmodified private direct self-regulatory structure is in a nutshell the source of the growing conflict over health care in Canada.

SOME MYTHS ABOUT RATIONING: IN CANADA AND ELSEWHERE

Free choice versus rationing, spurious alternatives

The vastly different experiences of Canada and the US have, when not completely ignored in the latter, frequently been dismissed as a result of 'rationing'. The image is created of direct state intervention, preventing patients from receiving services they desire and are willing to pay for.

The image is of course false, and on two levels. It is an inaccurate description of how health care is allocated in Canada. And at a more abstract level it misinterprets or distorts the concept of rationing itself.

Every elementary economics text opens with a discussion of scarcity, and the consequent necessity, imposed in every society by the niggardliness of nature and/or the greed of men, to ration. All societies develop institutions and processes which ration available resources among competing uses, and the resulting products among people. Private ownership, markets, and a price system form one such set of social institutions, which has significant advantages in rationing certain kinds of commodities. But not all. 'One man, one vote' is a statement that access to political representation is not well distributed by markets. 'To no man will we sell, deny, or delay justice' makes the same point. Of course money *does* buy political and legal representation, judicial advantage if not justice. And both political and judicial systems use up scarce resources of human time, energy, capital, and raw materials. But market allocation of their benefits is generally viewed as leading to individual and social outcomes inferior to those available through alternative rationing institutions (19).

Whether or not one accepts this view, which is merely a generalization inferred from the behaviour of most human societies, the point remains that rationing is inevitable for all resources in all societies. The issue is simply that of how, through what institutional framework? And what criteria should be used to choose among alternative institutions? Market systems ration by ability, and willingness, to pay— wealth and information. To characterize one system as 'rationing', and another as 'free choice', is simply rhetoric, politically advantageous perhaps, but economically meaningless.

Modes of rationing, the health care utilization process

A variant of the 'free choice versus rationing' rhetoric recognizes the common problem of rationing scarce resources. But it defines the criteria for choice and specifies the processes involved in non-price-rationing (NPR), on *a priori* grounds, such that price rationing (PR) is inevitably superior. One may assume, for example, that NPR always functions through some variant of queuing, and that non-monetary access costs in NPR systems increase to a market-clearing level. These time and effort burdens are pure waste—in a PR system the same time could be used for productive work or leisure and society as a whole would be better off. (The distribution of welfare will differ, but in a competitive market system with full information, any desired redistribution can be gained by wealth transfer without the burden of queuing.)

But mechanical application of the queuing model to

health care neglects the critical role of providers of care in influencing patients' desired, as well as actual, care use. Patients initiate care episodes by contacting physicians, physicians advise and direct further utilization. This advice and direction depends *inter alia* upon resources available for further care—hospital space, or diagnostic and therapeutic capacity. NPR operates on the patient's desired use through the provider's recommendations, and it does not require a confrontation between patient wants and constrained resources or facilities. A shortage of primary care physicians could show up in queuing, but in fact appointment times are very short in most parts of Canada; for urgent problems virtually non-existent, and there is concern about an overall physician surplus.

Hospitals *are* showing signs of increasing strain from NPR, but this strain is partly a result of the *physician* surplus impinging on a constrained bed supply, not a growth in patient needs, and partly a deliberate policy to induce physicians to economize on bed use. In a fee-for-service system physicians' earnings depend on access to 'free' social capital, and this access is increasingly constrained.

One may, of course, bypass the question of how NPR systems work in practice, and postulate, as an ethical norm, that consumer/patients ought to receive whatever they are willing to pay for and/or that direct intervention in the interchange between consumer and provider is offensive *per se*. Questions of how much wealth or information is available to back up willingness to pay are sidestepped by assuming some implausible or wholly unspecified processes which ensure that these are optimally or satisfactorily distributed among all transactors—leaving the ethical norm resting on a further set of hypothetical propositions. The superiority of PR then rests on its conformity with *a priori* ethical principles defined over allocation processes, whatever results these achieve must be the best available, and actual outcome data are irrelevant (20).

The price system, thus conceived, is like Pangloss's Divine Providence which, assumed beneficent and omnipotent, ensures that whatever happens, this is the best of all possible worlds. If one accepts the faith, then PR is always to be preferred to NPR, and further discussion is pointless. Pangloss can be ridiculed, but not refuted. If on the other hand one is seriously interested in policy alternatives, and the evaluation of different institutions and processes for resource allocation, then one must focus on health system outcomes. These can be objectively measured, though not easily or perfectly, such that reasonable men may examine various forms of evidence as to how different rationing systems work. No particular system of rationing should be accorded a privileged position *a priori*.

The relationship between utilization and health status

Of course rational men may disagree over the relevant dimensions of 'working'—what outcomes matter and how much. Canadian policy is built on the presumption that there exists some objectively identifiable relation between health care use and health status, at the individual and collective level. People have 'needs',—as opposed to preferences, demands, or willingness-to-pay,—for health care which would be judged, by an external, technically competent observer, to improve their health status. Further, the recognition of a need, unlike a more general want or demand, implies some degree of obligation on others in a community, to assist in meeting it.

Direct and self-regulation of providers, and universal public insurance, are both based on the belief that uninformed and unsubsidized consumer choices in an unregulated market will lead to patterns of utilization which do not correspond to needs. The operational definition of needs is exceptionally difficult, both because there is no universal agreement as to the 'best practice' response to any given health situation, and because, as we move out from 'hot' abdomens, through silent gallstones, to anxiety, the boundary between health and well-being in general is very difficult to recognize. Judgements of need made by practitioners and facilities planners are at the margin difficult, often arbitrary, and sometimes inconsistent, but the effort to respond to needs remains the principal policy guide.

Figure 2 provides a simplistic framework for this approach.

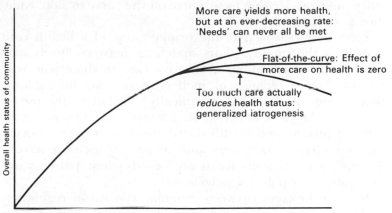

More care yields more health, but at an ever-decreasing rate: 'Needs' can never all be met

Flat-of-the-curve: Effect of more care on health is zero

Too much care actually *reduces* health status: generalized iatrogenesis

Overall health status of community

Total volume of resources (real inputs, not $) devoted to health care

FIG. 2. Alternative specifications of the relationship between health status and health care resources.

The health status of a community, aggregated in some unspecified way, depends on the resources (human time and skills, equipment, etc.) devoted to health care. Of course many other factors—diet, living conditions, occupations,—matter too, perhaps much more, but the *raison d'être* of a health system is its expected influence on health.

Diminishing returns, however, set in; if the most efficacious interventions are supplied first, then the payoff to additional resources, in terms of needs met, falls as effort increases. The pay-off may become zero—flat-of-the-curve medicine—or even negative—more care may be hazardous to health. We know this last happens in the case of many specific interventions. The figure makes the point about indefinite rise at declining ratios.

Such a curve represents an abstraction. Real world health systems will lie below, not on it, either because production is technically inefficient—sheer waste—or because interventions are not provided in decreasing order of payoff. If full technical efficiency could be achieved, and in addition all resources used where their efficacy is greatest, then a society's health system would lie on the curve. But if the curve slopes upward indefinitely—as it may—there will remain an inherently political decision as to where on the curve to stop, what 'needs' to leave unmet.

From this perspective, the primary test of a health care system is the quality of its matching between needs and utilization, its provision of effective care to those who will benefit, and avoidance of ineffective or harmful services. Secondarily, it should be technically efficient in the use of resources. At yet another level, a system will generate patterns of income and wealth distribution, as between providers and users or taxpayers, and as among users/taxpayers, depending on how its funds are raised—these patterns too are matters for political judgement.

But the linkages between different systems of regulation and funding and their outcomes, in these dimensions, are researchable questions. Such research is far from value-free; important judgements are made about which forms of evidence are relevant or convincing, and these are influenced by the researchers' values and preferences. But even if positive and normative can never be rigorously separated, the classification of issues into researchable questions and political choices can still help to narrow, focus, and sometimes even resolve, areas of disagreement. Pangloss cannot however do so.

GLOBAL EXPENDITURE CONTROL: HOW IT IS DONE AND WHY IT HAS WORKED

The process

The process of health expenditure control in Canada can be subdivided into short-run and long-run, and differs for physicians' services and hospital care (21). Outside these two sectors, dental care expenditures are effectively uncontrolled (and rapidly increasing) and there is a wide diversity of provincial pharmaceutical programmes. The principal federal initiative has been limitation of patent protection— issuing licenses to import generic equivalents of patented drugs—which has tended to hold down ingredient costs (22).

The negotiation of periodic binding fee schedules has been the key factor restraining expenditures on physicians' services. As shown in Table 2, physicians' fees escalated more rapidly than prices generally prior to 1969, but fell substantially behind thereafter. This constraint is easing substantially in the 1980s; it is the principal target of physician associations attempting to win the right to charge patients above the negotiated fee schedule at their own discretion.

As important as level of fees, is schedule structure. Canadian fee schedules provide little differentiation among types of office visits, penalizing practitioners who perform long and detailed examinations, but also restricting 'fee schedule creep', i.e. by physicians reclassifying a visit or a procedure into a higher paying class. Very large swings in 'volume', or procedure reclassification, were documented in the US when the ESP programme froze fees. Quebec likewise experienced 4 per cent per year 'creep' in physician incomes from 1971 to 1975, on a constant fee schedule which provided three different visit classes; 'major complete' examinations rose dramatically. Canadian fee schedules now provide limited scope for this.

Secondly, fees are paid only for services of practitioners, not their employees. The practitioner may hire assistants, but he must perform the act. The possibilities for procedural multiplication by task delegation are sharply limited. If the physician wishes to respond to fee constraints by recalling patients more frequently and recommending more services, he must also work more hours. There is scope for faster servicing, the 'revolving door', but this is limited both ethically and physically.

(One might fear that this limitation would discourage the substitution of auxiliaries for physicians, so raising costs. But such substitution is severely inhibited in all fee-for-service practices, for more complex reasons. Dentistry in Canada and medicine and dentistry in the US display the same underutilization of auxiliaries despite absence of fee schedule restraints.) (26).

Finally diagnostic services, which provide the greatest possibility for expanding billings without extra effort, are to a large extent centralized in hospitals or, in some provinces,

Table 2. *Physician fees, the consumer price index, and physicians and hospital beds per capita, Canada, 1957–81.*

	Index of Physicians' fees[1]	Population per active civilian physician[2]	Consumer price index	Beds per (000) Capita[3] public general hospitals	P.G. and allied special hospitals
1957	64·1	1282	70·8	4·7	5·4
1958	67·6	1264	72·6	4·7	5·6
1959	69·6	1242	73·4	4·8	5·7
1960	70·5	1234	74·3	4·8	5·7
1961	71·6	1226	75·0	4·9	5·5
1962	73·8	808	1217	75·9	5·0	5·8
1963	75·1	795		77·1	5·0	5·9
1964	76·7	785		78·6	5·1	6·0
1965	79.0	779		80·5	5·1	6·0
1966	80·4	763		83·5	5·3	6·1
1967	87·0	749		86·4	5·3	6·2
1968	91·6	744		90·0	5·4	6·3
1969	96·6	714		94·1	5·4	6·3
1970	98·1	689		97·2	5·5	6·4
1971	100·0	659		100·0	5·4	6·4
1972	101·4	636		104·8	5·5	6·5
1973	102·3	619		112·3	5·5	6·4
1974	107·4	605		125·0	5·5	6·6
1975	114·2	585		138·5	5·4	6·7
1976	121·8	577		148·9	5·2	6·6
1977	132·0	565		160·8	5·2	6·8
1978	140·2	558		175·2	5·2	6·7
1979	150·6	551		191·2	5·1	6·7
1980	164·8	542		210·6	5·1	6·7
1981	184·2	535		236·9		
Feb 1982	194·5			252·7		

Percentage increase per annum

1957–69	3·5	−1·5	2·4	1·2	1·3
1969–76	3·4	−3·1	6·8	−0·5	0·7
1976–81 (or 80)	8·6	−1·5	9·7	−0·5	0·4

Notes.

1. Prior to universal insurance, physicians' fees actually collected rose substantially faster than list fees, as collections ratios were rising and billing patterns shifting. Data on physicians' gross receipts suggests that their apparent 1·1 per cent annual gain in 'real' fees may actually have been in the neighbourhood of 4 to 5 per cent *per year* in the 57–69 period. After public insurance, billings 'creep' has been limited to about 1 to 2 per cent per annum.

2. 'Active Civilian Physicians' includes interns, residents, and salaried physicians providing medical care. Prior to 1962, series covers only Active Fee-Practice

approved private laboratories. Thus the opportunity for the average US physician to supplement his earnings with a private lab or radiology facility are largely foreclosed in Canada. The fee schedules restrict the practitioner to an 'income-leisure tradeoff'. Incomes can only rise faster than fees if working time increases.

Service volumes keyed to physician supply

In the longer run, however, servicing volumes rise proportionately with the supply of physicians. More manpower implies more utilization and more expenditure for a given fee schedule. Accordingly efforts have been made to limit supply. Immigration of physicians, which had exceeded domestic production in the late 60s and early 1970s—1347 in 1969—was cut sharply in February 1975. By 1979, immigration was only 298. But the output of domestic medical schools, designed to meet a late 60s population boom which never came, will keep the MD/population ratio rising for the foreseeable future (27). And despite a general federal and provincial policy of restraint, 'maverick' medical schools have occasionally been able to hoodwink or otherwise extort from provincial governments further expansion. This continuing increase in physician supply represents a serious failure of manpower policy and a significant threat to expenditure control now and in the future.

The hospital cost-control process is both simpler and more complex. It is simpler, because provincial governments can determine hospital budgets. At the beginning of the 1970s, most provinces shifted from line-item to global budgeting, enabling them to impose annual percentage increases. But in constraining global budgets, provincial governments have had difficulty capping the long-run rise of relative incomes

Physicians, who receive 50 per cent of or more of their incomes from fees. Growth rates are linked in 1962.

3. Public general hospitals provide primarily acute-care services; allied special include chronic, convalescent, rehabilitation, paediatric, and maternity hospitals. Both hospital series data are fiscal years (April/March) from 1977 on, all others are calendar. Hospital data for 1981/2 are not yet available.

Source: (23, 24, 25, 27).

for hospital workers (24,28). Consequently cost-constraint implies reduced hospital employment, which at some point may threaten quantity or quality of services. The issue is as yet unresolved.

The 'how' and 'why' of expenditure restraint

The longer-run control of hospital system capacity, beds and major equipment, and the limitation of duplication and underutilization, have been critical aspects of expenditure restraint. Canadian hospitals, unlike their US counterparts, are reimbursed for operating but not capital costs. They must seek separate grants for expansion. Thus while US hospitals can fund expansion from their own resources or from capital market borrowing, and have been able to evade efforts by public bodies to regulate their growth, Canadian hospitals' access to capital is a public investment decision taken (supposedly) in the light of the province's needs for a 'balanced and integrated' hospital system. The process is not perfect, and is often rather *ad hoc,* but on balance it has been substantially more successful in constraining hospital investment than the US free-for-all.

As important as the 'how' of expenditure restraint, of course, is the 'why'. Other publicly funded systems (e.g. Sweden) have shown rates of cost escalation in the 1970s which look more like the US. The answer appears to be two fold,—sole source funding, at an appropriate level of government. One public agency, the provincial Ministry of Health, is responsible for all costs. Providers cannot play one reimburser against another, or charge patients for amounts insurers refuse to pay. The 'cost-pass-through' of the decentralized, fragmented private system, in which the costs of expenditure increase fall eventually on the consumer of the product made by the firm which paid the premium which funded the insurer which paid the claim by the physician who directed the care that Jack received, is not available. And the 'sole source' is at a level of government with sufficient expertise and political credibility to confront and constrain providers.

But it remains a difficult issue, because the conflict of

interest between health care providers to whom health care expenditures are income, pure and simple, and the general taxpayer, is so clear cut. There is always a temptation, a sort of governmental 'moral hazard', to shed the confrontation and to limit government expenditures by transferring costs to private individuals. Insofar as sole source funding is a critical feature of global cost control, such a shift would lead to an expansion of overall health expenditures but perhaps, at least for a time, a fall in governments' outlays. Over the longer-term, of course, governments' outlays might well be higher in a multiple funding source system. But government time horizons are short.

The 'underfunding' argument and direct charges

It is significant that medical associations in Canada, federal and provincial, appear to follow this analysis. They argue that health care is 'underfunded', and although their case has yet to win acceptance outside medicine (18), they regard the development of 'private' funding sources through extra-billing or otherwise as the best means of increasing health expenditure. Essentially they argue that the public tax and expenditure system has led to a sub-optimal allocation of resources to health care, or an insufficient allocation of income to health care providers (specifically physicians)— they are not always clear as to the distinction. This short-fall should then be made up by a private 'tax' levied by physicians or hospitals on patients, whose proceeds would go to health expenditures/incomes.

Whether or not the Canadian health care system is in fact 'underfunded'—so far the principal evidence of underfunding offered has been the observed expenditure control—and if so whether privately levied taxes on patients are an appropriate response, the position taken by Canadian medical associations stands in sharp contrast to conventional economic analyses of 'privatization of funding' or 'patient participation', i.e. direct charges to patients. They are arguing that direct charges will meet their objective of *increasing* expenditure, and from their powerful efforts in this direction one must assume they are sincere. The usual economic argument is that direct charges will *reduce* expenditures (or at least utilization, the assumed pricing process is frequently naive or obscure). Clearly they cannot do both.

The economic argument contains serious gaps in both theory and evidence, and the analysis by Canadian physicians is probably correct (29). They are not energetically striving to cut their own economic throats. Most obviously, they note that physician incomes and prices, and medical costs, are higher in the US, where about a third of medical bills are paid out-of-pocket, than in Canada, where about 5 per cent are. The argument that increasing direct charges to patients will tend to lower health expenditures rests on a confusion between health care utilization and the initiation of a health care episode, as well as a failure to consider the provider's response to any such change.

Possible effects of direct charges

It is certainly plausible that, *ceteris paribus,* patients who face out-of-pocket charges for health care will be less likely to seek care in response to any given set of symptoms and more likely to question or to fail to comply with medical advice. Indeed it would be surprising if such a response did not occur. From the nature of health care, however, it would also be surprising if it were very strong. A number of attempts have been made, mostly in the US, to measure this response, all indicating utilization responding much less than proportionately to price change (30). Most recently, preliminary results from the Rand experiment, carefully insulated from provider responses, suggest ambulatory medical visit rates among the able-bodied non-elderly might fall about 30 per cent in a shift from complete to virtually non-existent insurance coverage, with total expense falling 20 to 30 per cent (31).

More important, the *ceteris* are not in fact *paribus* in the real world. If utilization drops, so do physician workloads and, in a fee-for-service system, incomes. Their response will be to recommend more care for each illness episode, and over the longer run to educate patients to be more sensitive to symptoms in initiating care. The 'demand for care' is shifted up at any given out-of-pocket price, a process currently being observed in the US as the physician/population ratio and medical prices are both increasing rapidly (32). This effect was deliberately excluded from the Rand experiments; it shows up in the US as increased (price-adjusted) service rates per visit or per hospital day, and in Canada as increased visits and procedures per capita.

If extra-billing becomes common in Canada, then utilization might well fall for a time. The fee increase would buffer physician incomes against workload loss, with no need to recall patients more frequently or service them more intensively. The result would be a combination of lower utilization *per capita* with higher physician incomes and medical expenditures. Some tendency has been observed in particular provinces for utilization *per physician* to rise less rapidly when fees are rising more rapidly, and conversely.

If direct charges were collected by provincial governments, and did not flow into physician incomes, the physician response would be such that utilization would fall very little, if at all. The critical variable in a fee-for-service system is the physician's income, which must fall (for a given physician stock) if expenditures are to be reduced. Threats to income will be resisted; if they take the form of reduced external 'demand' the response will be more internal generation of services. Fee increases, on the other hand, increase incomes without extra servicing, hence the enthusiasm for extra-billing.

Out-of-pocket payments by patients might have, however, a more general significance. Proposals for increasing the efficiency of health care through competitive market forces require patients to be responsible for some at least of the expenditures on their behalf. More efficient providers (lower cost and/or higher quality) can then expand their market share at the expense of less. But such market share competition requires (in addition to very strong informational assumptions) that purchasers select among providers on the basis of cost to themselves. If neither direct charges nor premiums vary across providers then competitive forces cannot work. The stagnation of capitation-based group practices in Canada is partially due to their inability to attract patients by passing on savings.

Whether the difficulty of reconciling competitive forms of delivery with universal first dollar coverage is a serious issue depends on how significant are the advantages anticipated from such alternatives. This is a speculative and contentious area; but two points are clear.

First, universal coverage with expenditure control in Canada is fact. The advantages alleged for pro-competitive policies are based on analogies with other industries whose applicability is itself speculative. There is no working experience, anywhere, with a fully privatized, unregulated health care system. Very serious questions of access and quality control in such a system are left unanswered. Proposals for a system of (regulated) private competitive prepaid group practices address these questions, but their experience, while by no means non-existent, does not yet provide answers.

Second, half a loaf is *not* better than none. We do have working experience with systems, dentistry for example in Canada and the US, where direct public regulation of delivery, or participation in insurance, is largely absent, but an extensive web of self-regulation on the supply side restricts the entry and conduct of providers. The result is that competitive forces do *not* function, at least not to promote efficiency and lower costs, in either country (26). A shift from public regulation, directly or through the public insurance monopoly, to pseudo-markets regulated by professionals or by collusive oligopoly or cartel, has no obvious attraction on theoretical or empirical grounds. 'Provider sovereignty' does not lead to either cost control or efficient production—quite the contrary.

BEYOND EXPENDITURES: 'UNDERFUNDING' VERSUS 'COST-CAPPING'

Expenditure for what? The income/expenditure identity

Discussion of health care often treats expenditures as ends in themselves. Where spending approaches 10 per cent of GNP, the US or Sweden, the system is criticized for its inability to control expenditure. Where the ratio is substantially lower, Canada or the UK, providers argue that care is underfunded. Yet the present level, whatever it may be, cannot be an argument for either more or less spending. The serious question is, what do we get for our money? Would more spending buy additional or higher quality health care, and if so, would we as a society value it more highly than the other things, public services, private consumption, investment, we would have to give up? Or would expenditure control free resources whose contribution to our well-being would be greater elsewhere? And how effectively are resources in health care being used at present?

Figure 3 provides a way of organizing this question. Health care 'costs' in any society are identically equal to expenditures on health care and to total incomes earned in providing health care. Total expenditures can be factored as shown into total quantities of different types of goods and services produced, and their average unit prices; and total incomes into numbers of income recipients and average incomes received. Most health care production is labour-intensive, most of the income earned is received in the form of wages or professional fees for labour services,—but it also includes profits, rent, interest, and dividends. Regardless of the form of income, or object of expenditure, one cannot influence expenditures without influencing incomes, and conversely.

More medical services, or wealthier physicians?

In the case of physicians' services, the 'underfunding' versus 'cost-capping' discussion takes a very simple form. Either it is a thinly veiled argument for more pay for physicians, or it is an allegation of a shortage of medical services. More spent on physicians' services must take the form of higher fees (and incomes) for a given workload, or it must purchase a greater service workload.

There are three possible responses to a shortage of medical care services: (i) encouraging physicians to work longer and harder, (ii) increasing the productivity of physician time by making more use of auxiliaries, (iii) training or importing

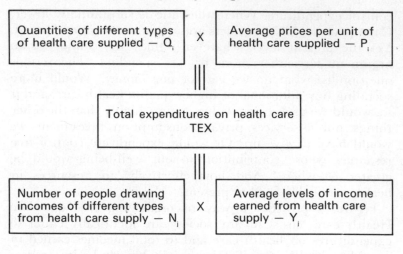

$$\Sigma_i P_i \cdot Q_i \equiv TEX \equiv \Sigma_j N_j \cdot Y_j$$

FIG. 3. The health care sector income/expenditure identity.

more physicians. But as noted above, Canadian policy has been to curtail immigration, and to try to limit medical school growth. None of the advocates of underfunding have suggested a change in these policies, or alleged a physician shortage. As for auxiliaries, all analysts agree that fee-for-service private practice leads to a severe under-use of physician substitutes and over-use of high-priced time (as indeed it does for dentists, lawyers, and accountants) (26,33,34,35). But none of the 'underfunding' advocates has suggested that their use be encouraged. Nor has there been any suggestion that physician working hours are too short. It seems fair to conclude, then, that insofar as it pertains to services of physicians, the underfunding debate is about incomes.

This is less clear among those who argue for expenditure control; here we find the bald view that physicians make too much money associated with concern over unnecessary servicing and severe under-use of auxiliaries. This suggests substantial *over* funding,—the same level of health could be produced with less care, and of care at lower cost using the alternative 'technology' of physician substitutes—if there were some way of disposing of the physician surplus.

It follows that, at least in Canada, the underfunding argument is *either* a plea for higher physician incomes, *or* a case for more spending in hospitals. The focus on extra-billing, having no connection with the latter, suggests the former rather strongly. And indeed this is not surprising, since universal public medical insurance in Canada has been associated with a surge in physician supply but a considerable fall in their real incomes relative to the rest of the population. In the fifteen years prior to Medicare, physician incomes rose from about 3·25 times the general average in the early 1950's to over 5·5 in 1971. In the 1970's much of that gain was lost. The process of both physician cost escalation prior to Medicare and cost control after it has thus been primarily a fee and income, not a real health care, phenomenon (36). It is of course quite plausible that at some fee and income levels, either too high or too low, there would be adverse effects on either the quantity or the quality of medical services provided. Extreme constraints on incomes might induce an 'internal emigration' by providers which would reduce the efficacy or quality of care. But there is no evidence that fluctuations within the observed range have had this effect. Nor does it appear that physicians who have used extra-billing (where permitted) to raise their fees have adopted significantly different practice styles as a result, though some appear to see fewer and less severely ill patients, (37). The more serious effect of fee restraints appears to be their erosion of physician acceptance of the public plan, and the political backlash thus generated, on which more below.

The hospital setting: underfunding or overprovision

In the hospital sector, the underfunding issue is more complex. Wages are about 70 per cent of operating expenditures, and increases in the relative earnings of hospital workers have been an important source of cost escalation. Like physicians, hospital workers moved ahead rapidly in the 1960s (24). During the 1970s, however, their relative income status continued to improve slowly (28). Provincial governments, fearful of the political consequences of a hospital strike, have found control of incomes in this sector more difficult.

Their response, control of global operating budgets and restrictions on new capacity, implies that when wage gains outrun these limits, the hospital sector must either reduce non-wage expenditure or cut staff. If there is 'managerial slack' in the system, then service volumes, levels of care activity, can be maintained by increasing productivity. In terms of Figure 3, average incomes rise, and numbers of income earners fall, but service volumes and unit prices of outputs are unchanged. But such a policy can persist only if productivity continues to rise.

In 'normal' industries, technological advance tends to hold down the unit costs of output. Health technology, however, is commonly identified as a source of cost increase. It expands the range of interventions available and so increases numbers of services provided by and numbers and levels of incomes drawn from the industry—in short, sales. Indeed a serious concern expressed by those who believe the system suffers from underfunding is that the Canadian hospital system, restricted to grow at the same rate as the rest of the economy, is unable to take full advantage of the dramatic expansion in technological prowess currently underway.

Yet technological prowess by itself is not an objective, any more than expenditures, at least not for society generally. The critical question is not, is Canada adopting new technologies less rapidly and less extensively than, say, the US, but are Canadian patients being denied access to efficacious, health improving interventions as a result? The answer is probably no.

New innovations in health care tend to be tested for safety rather than efficacy, although even safety testing varies considerably from drugs and devices, which are extensively tested, to surgical procedures, which are not. Efficacy is a secondary consideration; the profits of the manufacturers and marketers of new techniques depend on sales.

Moreover in a fee-for-service system physician earnings also depend on interventions; the billings which a physician can generate depend on his/her access to 'free' capital equipment in the hospital system. Increases in the physician/population ratio, combined with constraints on hospital space, personnel, and equipment, lead to a reduction in such 'free' capital available *per physician* if not per patient, and help to explain physicians' sense of shortages and capacity pressure. In Canada in the 1970's, acute-care beds per physician have fallen nearly 30 per cent, and this fall is continuing.

Nor is the problem a simple one of manufacturers selling equipment, or physicians recommending interventions, known to be inefficacious. A particular intervention will generally be useful for a particular problem. Once available, however, it tends to be used far beyond its range of efficacy. The CT scanner is a commonly cited example of an unquestionable diagnostic breakthrough—for some purposes—being used extensively in situations where its anticipated therapeutic pay-off is close to, or at, zero.

The literature yields numerous other examples of specific diagnostic procedures overutilized in settings in which it could be determined in advance that the pay-off would be nil. Electronic foetal monitoring, for example, may in total be doing more harm than good (38). Indeed the most costly misuse of diagnostic testing is not the expensive, prominent 'high technology' but common tests, endlessly repeated at great expense, for no information gain (39). Some efforts have been made to try to reduce the tendency of physicians to overprovide such tests, but powerful economic and professional incentives are at work (40).

Apart from testing, the medical literature contains numerous discussions and examples of unnecessary hospitalization; lengths of stay prolonged unnecessarily (41), surgery or diagnostic admission of dubious value (42), failure to use well-established ambulatory alternatives (43), and a depressing inability of the hospital system to learn from and apply demonstrated less costly approaches to care (44). Hence the view that in Canada the problem is not underfunding but a failure of hospitals to make effective use of the funds they have. And as the US example makes abundantly clear, adding more funding only accentuates the problem.

The diagnosis of 'overfunding' is shared by advocates of a shift to more reliance on competitive market forces. Those who are serious about private competition, de-regulation, as opposed to those who merely seek continued private regulation free of public oversight, hope to shrink the health sector, or at least constrain its growth, reducing utilization through 'deterrent' charges or health maintenance organizations and letting market competition bid down prices and incomes (20,45). 'Overuse' in this context, however, is unrelated to efficacy and is defined in terms of production cost greater than willingness/ability to pay (46).

If the marginal pay-off to investment of further resources in health care is now relatively small, then in terms of Figure 2, we may have reached a point at which the curve is almost, if not actually, flat. Or, given the substantial evidence of inefficient care, we may be too far below the curve to know what its shape is, and would be well advised to redeploy and use more effectively the resources currently available before adding more.

Aggregation is deceptive; there may well be areas of care where, and social groups for whom, more would yield health benefits. But there are other areas where the marginal payoff appears to be negative. The underfunding argument side-steps all questions of efficacy and baldly assumes that more is better, in defiance of the clinical evidence.

On the other hand, the clinical evidence is seriously incomplete. A good case can be made for a substantial increase in research as to the pay-off to different types of health care interventions. This has been actively pursued in the US by the Office of Technology Assessment, but to a much lesser extent in Canada. Even more critical, however, is the problem of how to manage the health care system to make use of such efficacy information as is available. Canada's success in expenditure control has been based only to a limited degree on such management; the control over hospital capacity has restrained some of the more prominent forms of 'technological hypertrophy' observed in the US.

What seems quite clear, however, is that although the centralized public funding system has had only limited managerial success so far, it has at least established some of the institutions through which such control could be exercised. A move to a more fragmented mix of public/private funding sources, on US lines, would make any form of public management impossible, while the health care system by itself seems incapable of dealing with issues of efficacy and efficiency in resource use. It just wants more. Whether a radical deregulation of health care supply would change this behaviour is questionable, since no one has ever tried, and despite the US rhetoric no one is trying now.

ENDS OR MEANS: WHAT IS THE PUBLIC/PRIVATE FUNDING DEBATE REALLY ABOUT?

Tax structure is not health policy

It is a curious feature of debates over health care funding that they are often not about health care at all. The central issues of health care policy, at least in the economic domain, are efficiency of resource use, efficacy of activities performed or foregone, and the provider income patterns generated as a result. But debates over social insurance or general revenue funding, insofar as they assume no change in how, or how much, providers are paid for their activities, what levels of capacity are to be provided, or how, if at all, usage of health care by individuals is linked to their contributions to it, do not in fact bear on the health care system as such.

In Canada, provinces have chosen different mixes of premium, income tax, and sales tax finance for their share of health expenditure. The Federal contributions in respect of health programmes come out of general revenue, principally income tax. But premiums, in those provinces which retain them, are effectively compulsory, and are unlinked to expected or actual use. The national income accountant treats them as a tax, regressive if not shifted, and arguments over their use follow left-wing/right-wing attitudes toward progressive or regressive taxation. Providers of health care, particularly medical associations, tend to advocate premium finance, but it is not clear whether they believe that provincial premium revenues, though not earmarked, will be easier to bargain for, or whether they reflect their upper-income members' preference for regressive taxation.

The UK discussion over social insurance versus general revenue finance, insofar as it is divorced from questions of how, and how much, health care providers are paid, seems equally a debate over progressive versus regressive taxation with no bearing on health care issues.

Why private funding?

The more interesting question is how particular funding mechanisms link to particular health care system outcomes. From this perspective we noted that in the US, privatization of both funding and delivery of health care, reducing the role of government as regulator and payer, is widely viewed as a way of constraining expenditure increases. In Canada and the UK, by contrast, it is seen as a way of expanding levels of health care spending. System-wide cost experience as well as more detailed analysis suggests that the UK/Canadian view is correct.

The argument for more reliance on private insurance and/or direct payment by patients in funding health care is thus linked to the underfunding/overfunding issue. It underfunding is a problem on either equity grounds—health care workers, and particularly physicians, deserve higher incomes relative to the rest of society—or efficacy/efficiency grounds—the benefits to patients of more care would justify its resource cost—then private funding is a possible response.

The equity issue is, given the imperfections of health labour markets, largely a political value judgement, on which providers' arguments have yet to be widely accepted. And the extensive evidence of both inefficacious and inefficient servicing in health care suggests more effort to improve the use of current resources before expanding present funding levels.

If health care were underfunded, however, why privatization? The same results could be achieved by increasing hospital budgets, raising physician fees, or in the UK, raising the NHS budget.

Challenging the legitimacy of the State

Proponents of privatization generally argue that the public sector is unwilling or unable to fund health care at appropriate levels, that government fails to represent the social interest in either equitable treatment of providers or adequate provision of services. But the naive argument that governments 'cannot afford it' is clearly fallacious. Governments draw their resources from the rest of society. We all pay for health care through taxes, public or private insurance premiums, and out-of-pocket payments, the total burden is not changed by passing through one route rather than another.

More interesting is the implicit direct challenge to the legitimacy of the political process—providers know better than governments what ought to be done. If governments refuse to accept professional advice, then privatization is a way of giving greater effect to providers' judgements as to appropriate income and expenditure levels, and circumventing governmental constraints.

Such an argument is quite consistent with professional ideology. The fundamentally elitist concept of professional authority, 'doctor's orders', is not confined to the individual provider/patient contact. Self-regulation through delegated state authority represents a similar transfer of control from the state to the profession collectively (47). The 'underfunding/privatization' argument merely extends this claim of special professional expertise to include funding as well.

It does not appear consistent, however, for a government to accept, much less to advocate, a shift in funding sources on this ground. Governments *have* the power to expand public spending. If they reject the underfunding diagnosis, then they presumably must reject the private funding therapy. If they accept it, then they are hard put to explain why the public sector is not expanded. Governments cannot challenge their own legitimacy, or responsibly argue their own irresponsibility.

To this generalization, however, there are two qualifications—pre-commitment and distribution. A government might agree that spending should be increased, yet fear its successors. It might then view the development of a private system as much more difficult to reverse than a simple expansion of public budgets. The enormous difficulty, and apparent total failure, of the US in trying to develop a public health insurance programme in the face of the myriad of well-vested private provider and insurer interests, who are able to use the profits generated by their present system to great political effect, certainly suggests that moving to more private funding may be a one-way street.

Secondly a government advocating, or at least accepting, shifts in funding patterns might be less interested in global patterns of expenditure and effectiveness than in distributional issues. Its concern might take several forms.

Distribution issues: incomes, costs, and care

Most simply, a government might wish to effect a financial redistribution, independently of changes in patterns of care use, which it felt to be politically unacceptable if carried out overtly. A redistribution of income in favour of physicians, for example, might generate popular opposition or have expensive repercussions on other health workers' demands if passed through public fee schedules or budgets. Private funding would achieve the same result more quietly. Or a government might wish to redistribute the burden of public expenditure less progressively across income classes, yet feel limited in displaying overt inegalitarianism through the general tax system. Reducing the share of health expenditure supported from general revenue in favour of private funding would serve, given the relation between income and care use, to redistribute the costs of health care away from upper and back to lower income groups.

On the other hand, various schemes have been proposed for privatization without regressivity of expenditure burden across income classes, ranging from price discrimination by physicians to income-related co-insurance and deductible structures. Assuming these could in fact be workable, they would permit a government, by expansion of private funding, to redistribute income, not from poor to rich in general, but from ill to well, on the basis of actual (direct charges) or expected (private insurance premiums) care use. In addition, it would be able to redistribute utilization, making it more sensitive to willingness/ability to pay in addition to, or instead of, patient or provider perceptions of need. Total utilization might or might not be affected, however, as noted above this depends on provider reactions.

The traditional argument for public funding has been that differentials in care use correlate *negatively* with well-being, because use correlates with illness. At any given level of income, the highest users of care are on average least well-off, and the economic burdens of care merely exacerbate the direct burdens, physical, mental, and economic, of illness. This viewpoint, expressed as the desirability of a more equitable sharing of the burden of illness, was fundamental to the establishment of the Canadian health insurance programmes. Because information about individuals' health status is imperfect and costly, compensating redistribution takes the form of 'free' care, not direct financial subsidy (48).

Furthermore, the imperfections in consumer information plus the social interest in individual health and well-being make it appropriate for utilization to be linked to need, not to willingness to pay. The Canadian insurance system was intended to 'reduce the barriers to care', i.e. needed care. In practice, again because of incomplete information, this criterion is applied by observing the distribution of utilization across people in different income classes, geographic regions, age-sex groups, or symptom-disability complexes, with the idea that a 'good' system would show utilization varying with indicators believed related to need—age/sex class, symptom/disability complex, but not to those unrelated—geographic region, or (except as correlated with need) income (9,13). On these criteria the Canadian health insurance scheme scores reasonably well, while such limited 'privatization' as has occurred, opting out and extra billing, does appear to have impeded use by lower income people (49,50).

But treatment of care as an economic commodity tempts one to neglect its connection with illness, and to think of the recipients of care as in some sense privileged. The evidence that, at the population level, health care has only a limited impact on health can be misinterpreted to justify ignoring the predominant role of illness in care utilization at the individual patient level, with similar effect. If health care is viewed as a commodity which people choose to use, or not, like toothpaste, or if health status is viewed as the result of informed and deliberate choices (about drinking, smoking, exercise, etc.), then a government might wish to tie financial burdens to use patterns, and use patterns to willingness/ability to pay. But given the strength of the evidence counter to these views, it might not wish to be seen to do so—hence privatization (51).

But if it feels good, why not buy it?

There is, however, a broader perspective on distributional issues which suggests a much stronger case for the private sector, and which can be described in terms of efficacy and 'flat-of-the-curve' medicine. Suppose the curve in Figure 2 is not flat but very gently sloped. This is a technical question, and cannot be determined *a priori*. Moreover evidence of flat or declining curves in some sectors of health care does not prove that the envelope of all such curves is flat. There may exist efficacious but unexploited interventions, even after all current resources are most appropriately redeployed.

Alternatively, even if the overall curve *is* flat, in terms of clinical efficacy or health status narrowly defined, there may be a welfare or amenity payoff to more resources devoted to health care even in the absence of clinical effect. The process of receiving care may become more comfortable, pleasant, and convenient.

In either of these situations, the social resource-rationing mechanisms of whatever form will have to cut-off resources allocated to health care at a point such that their marginal payoff is still positive. In the first case, there will be some level of unmet 'need' in the sense that more resources would have a positive impact, however small, on someone's health. In the second case, of zero marginal clinical pay-off, more resources might still improve the quality of the care experience, make the patient feel better, reduce queuing times, etc. In either case, private funding would permit individuals to buy benefits additional to the publically supplied level.

Both of these arguments for 'sloped', rather than 'flat' curves can be found in the literature. Discussions of overutilization, particularly of diagnostic tests, are frequently posed in terms of an uncertain environment, in which each successive test adds a declining but still positive amount of information and thereby increases the probability of an effective therapeutic outcome (52). The increase in probability may become vanishingly small; but does not actually vanish. In rebuttal, it must be noted that testing is costly in clinical as well as economic terms, involving interventions, discomfort and anxiety, false positives, and iatrogenic effects. Moreover, in practice the testing behaviour of clinicians suggests that the curve is, in fact, flat (40).

Anxiety and illness: the limits of need

Anxiety occupies a middle ground between clinical measures of health status and amenity dimensions pure and simple. Acute anxiety is clearly not a state of health, though some degree of anxiety may be a normal and indeed highly functional characteristic. What then of the test or intervention, the routine annual physical examination, for example, which has no detectable effect on mortality or morbidity but reduces anxiety? There seems no avoiding the proposition that on a broad definition of health, such anxiety reduction represents efficacious care. One may argue that, for a variety of reasons, such care should not be publicly funded. But 'flat-of-the-curve' medicine clearly requires us to take a narrow, and in this respect incomplete, view of health.

The broad view has, however, some awkward consequences. If anxiety is illness, then anything which accentuates anxiety is deleterious to health—by definition. This includes a significant amount of so-called preventive activity, both advertising and advice. Anything which makes people more conscious of and concerned about their health status, including the activities of physicians and other health personnel, is a source of sickness. Consistent reliance on a definition of health which includes anxiety would require one to suppress a number of health care activities—preventive, diagnostic, and therapeutic,—on the grounds that they induce more anxiety than their clinical effectiveness, even if positive, can justify. If one is not prepared to accept that implication, then 'anxiety reduction' looks more like an excuse for current activities of dubious effect.

Going private for comfort, not care: the UK context

The amenity dimension pure and simple, however, raises no such problems of consistency. If people value the effects of more resources, then such effects are valuable, even if they have no clinical dimension. Thus it is suggested that in the UK people seek private care in order to get a choice of physician, general practitioner, or specialist, and if hospital care is needed to avoid queues, to be able to schedule care when convenient, and to have access to private accommodation. If such subsidiary characteristics of treatment are valued, and there is every reason to believe they are, then it is perfectly rational for individuals to be willing to pay something, over and above NHS contributions, to get them.

It is similarly argued, on much less secure grounds, that in Canada people choose to go to opted-out or extra-billing physicians in order to enjoy the advantages of perceived higher quality, perhaps less rushed and more personalized care. Such arguments, however, come only from physicians. All expressions of public attitudes seem to be vigorously against extra-billing (17,18), and indeed public statements by its advocates occasionally emphasize the importance of all physicians acting together so that patients *cannot* choose. Choice of an extra-billing physician has no implications for hospital access (unless a group of extra-billers has taken control of the medical staff), and there is little evidence that the patient 'buys' a significantly different style of ambulatory care. He just pays more, (37).

But in the UK context, private versus public payment does seem to be associated with significantly different amenity levels. And if therapeutic equivalence of care is assured, why should not people who wish to do so buy extra levels of amenity when they are patients, just as when they buy automobiles, or food? If the public at large, or the State, are able or willing to supply health care only of a certain limited amenity level, then permitting individuals to supplement this level with private purchases will, *ceteris paribus,* make those individuals better-off without making anyone else worse-off. The result may well be, probably will be, both an increase in health care spending and an increase in the share of health care (weighted by or including its amenity dimension) received by those most willing to pay, by reason of either wealth or preferences. But so long as the standard of care received by those who do not choose private care is unaffected, secured by the assumption of *ceteris paribus,* then how the rich or hypochondriacal spend their spare change need not and should not concern the state.

The argument is an important one, which bypasses many of the distributional concerns raised in the previous section. It rests on two very powerful assumptions or sets of assumptions: (i) that the *ceteris paribus* pound is indeed secure, and the choosers of privately funded health care do not make others worse off by their choice, and (ii) that those who choose to buy in the private or semi-private health care market will in fact be made better-off as a result. The latter depends, *inter alia,* on the pattern of state or self-regulation which persists in any nominally 'private' component of the health care system, and the former on how the relationship between the private and public sectors is regulated.

Public amenities without private payment: the Canadian experience

Before examining the twin pillars of the argument in more detail, however, we should note that some of the principal advantages, in terms of amenities, alleged for the private sector of care in the UK, are in fact available to everyone under the Canadian funding system. Free choice of physician, either GP or specialist, is available to all in provinces such as Quebec or B.C. where extra-billing and opting-out are effectively non-existent; in other provinces ones chosen physician may bill directly above the provincial fee schedule but even in Ontario only about 15 per cent do so. Preferred accommodation in hospitals is available at a surcharge to the patient. Scheduling of hospitalization is negotiated between patient and physician, subject, however, to the availability of space. The policy of trying to curb unnecessary hospital use by restricting bed-population ratios is alleged to have created problems in some areas in scheduling elective admissions, but the magnitude of the problem is unknown. There is no evidence, however, that patients would be willing to pay full costs for more convenient access. The more serious problem is that of making better use of currently available information on alternatives to inpatient care.

Thus some, at least, of the alleged short-comings of NHS versus private care in the UK are not an inevitable result of cost restraint. One can have restraint, as in Canada, in a payment system which has various free-choice dimensions, so long as one maintains sole-source funding. If it were possible for private insurance companies acting in conjunction with physicians and private hospitals to 'cream-off' low risk groups in Canada, it is highly unlikely that expenditures could have been contained during the 1970s. The public monopoly on the insurance and reimbursement is the critical control lever.

Nor does it seem that the ability of Canada to combine choice with expenditure constraint is due to higher levels of income per capita. It is true that 7 per cent of GNP is a good deal more money in Canada than in the UK. But since expenditures in health care are primarily wages, salaries, and professional fees, the real resource costs of health care in the UK should be lower as well. This would not be true, if relative incomes of health care workers are higher in the UK, but rather casual impression suggests the reverse.

Public consequences of private choices

The most obvious source of failure of the twin pillars is what may be called 'moral hazard' at the level of government. If the private sector begins to grow, there is an obvious temptation for a fiscally hard-pressed government to cut its own contributions. Those who continue to rely on the public system will then find service quality deteriorating, and will be worse-off than if the private sector had not developed.

Underlying this argument is an implicit theory of political behaviour. Hirschman has described 'exit' and 'voice' as alternative, but contradictory, forms of feed-back mechanisms for maintaining performance levels in social institutions (53). If the performance of, say, the NHS is viewed as unsatisfactory, people may 'exit' to private care, or exercise political 'voice' to secure improvement. But the more potential for exit, the less the remaining voice. And those most likely to exit are the wealthy, the well-informed and articulate, the politically most influential—the loudest 'voices'.

This behaviour is well illustrated by US approaches to health care cost control. The Reagan Administration is able to slash funding for social programmes, including Medicaid, because its beneficiaries are a minority of the population— poor, black, and generally voting Democratic if at all. By contrast a reduction of public support for the Canadian insurance programme affects every member of society, and generates much more intense political interest and scrutiny. When we are all in the same boat, the boat is maintained more carefully.

In addition to placing undue temptation in the way of governments, private funding may, depending on its form, create pressures on physicians and other providers to manipulate the supply of care. Physicians with interests in both public and private medicine are in a position to direct patient choices in a way which is virtually impossible to regulate. In the early days of Medicare in Ontario, opted-out physicians were able to engage in 'practice-streaming'—dividing their patients and seeing some as opted-in. The effect was to permit the physician to discriminate in price setting, according to his/her judgement of patient ability to pay. Discretionary extra-billing yields the same advantage. 'Practice-streaming' was forbidden in Ontario in November 1971, except for physicians with teaching appointments, among whom opting-out remains common (37).

Early experience with pre-paid group practices in the US showed similar problems of divided loyalties with physicians working only part-time for the group practice. Physicians gave time and attention preferentially to their private practices. Thus full-time appointments became the rule (54). Similar allegations have been made about the NHS in the UK, that physicians are in a position to manipulate hospital access and waiting times so as to encourage patients who can afford it to 'go private'.

Without trying, from a distance, to guess at the validity of such claims, one can say that absence of such behaviour, in a dual system, would be very surprising. And the regulation of provider behaviour, in an environment which creates strong incentives for them to encourage private use, is likely to be very difficult if not impossible. It may be necessary to set up parallel systems, public and private, side by side. This has been the approach adopted by the Saskatchewan Dental Service, for example, faced with intense hostility from the private profession (35). Any joint provision of services would merely provide an opportunity for the private practitioner to denigrate the public service and draw patients away. 'Separate but (therapeutically) equal' systems create continuing political tension, as it is obviously advantageous for private providers and (to a lesser extent) their patients to try through the political process to reduce public programme funding or competitive appeal.

Finally, there is a rather fuzzy but very important effect from the marketing of private care as in some sense 'better'. In a field as value laden as health, in which access to care is often perceived, rightly or wrongly, as critical to life itself, the explicit recognition of two- or multi-class medicine may weaken the social fabric in a way in which multi-class transportation, e.g. does not. The idea that one person's life and limb is more valuable, more worth saving, than another's, on the basis of his/her ability to pay, comes rather close to denying a fundamental 'cherished illusion' of equality which underlies our political and judicial system. A society in which people come to see themselves as fundamentally different, as unequal, becomes if not ungovernable, at least very costly to uphold. People with no perceived stake in the social order do not strive to maintain it.

All of which is rather apocalyptic and speculative. There is rather more to South-side Chicago than the inadequacy of the US health care funding system. Nor is Brixton a result of threats to the NHS. But it is true that Canadians (of both languages) see the country's health care system as a fundamental expression of social unity. This sense is not only political rhetoric, it is a genuine perception of equal status in confronting the common experience of illness and death. Such benefits are totally beyond quantification, but cannot be ignored.

In theory this issue might be dealt with if one could assure that private sector health care differed only in the amenity dimension. There would be only one therapeutic class of medicine, however many amenity classes the state and the market between them might provide. In practice, however, the creation of an impression of therapeutic difference is an essential part of the private sector marketing process. The private supplier does not say—my services are no more effective than anyone else's but the pile on my rugs is deeper, so I charge more. Rather he attempts, for abundantly obvious reasons, to blur the efficacy/amenity distinction and to suggest a general superiority. Nor is this activity in any way surprising or nefarious. Marketing is part of the law of life in the private, competitive market sector; and its participants operate under powerful incentives, rewards and penalties, encouraging sales growth. More or less subtle disparagement of the competitor's product, and praise of ones own, is inevitable. In such an environment, there is no way of keeping the efficacy/amenity distinction clear in the mind of buyer or seller.

Who benefits from private choice?

We are now in the area of perceptions as much as empirically demonstrable 'reality', and it is of course perceptions which govern both behaviour and satisfactions. This leads to consideration of the second pillar of the argument for a voluntary private sector; do such private transactions actually make the buyer better-off?

If differences are as straight-forward as waiting times and scheduling of elective procedures, the answer is obviously 'yes'. Free choice of physician is a bit more ambiguous, depending on the behavioural incentives it creates for physicians, but in general consumer sovereignty seems a reasonable guide here as well. Serious issues arise if the technically most competent physicians are the most widely sought after and go private, selling their services to the highest bidder. One might well prefer that exceptional technical competence be allocated to the most difficult problems, not to the wealthiest patients. But so long as patients' judgements of relative competence are, as they appear to be, on average rather poorly informed, then choice of physician is a matter of personality and style. *De gustibus* . . .

Questions arise, however, in the marketing of specific interventions—diagnostic tests, e.g. or surgical procedures. If the patient is fully informed as to the probable consequences, positive and negative, of the intervention, then the private sector argument goes through without difficulty. Informed buyers only purchase things which make them better-off. They may make mistakes, but not systematic ones. But if buyers of health care were fully informed about the consequences of its use, the regulatory structure which surrounds its provision in every developed society would never have arisen. The whole point of professionalization, self-regulation, delegation of public authority to provider associations, subsidized non-profit hospitals, relief of health care institutions from private market competition generally, is precisely to protect ill-informed buyers from the perceived harmful consequences of acting without professional protection. One can, of course, argue that this regulatory response to imperfect information is all a mistake, and that the supply of health care should be thrown wholly open to the private marketplace. But it is radically inconsistent, though depressingly common, simultaneously to accept the whole supply-regulation structure and then to assume that consumers/patients are necessarily better off when making their own choices in health care (46).

The practical import of this is that the private patient faces not only choices about when to have an operation, or how long to wait, but whether to have it at all. In this decision he relies on the physician's advice. Similarly patients accept diagnostic interventions, not on the basis of the carpet-pile or musical background of the clinic, but because they are told the tests are 'needed'. The critical dimension is perceived efficacy. And the clinician very rarely, if ever, goes into the complexity of possible results and probability of benefit, even if he understands such issues. He makes a judgement, on the basis of experience and training;—in such and such a situation, such tests are needed,—and instructs the patient accordingly (55).

But different professionals respond very differently to the same set of clinical circumstances, and their responses are conditioned *inter alia* by their own economic situations. The shift of the US clinical laboratory industry from professional to corporate for-profit ownership has been associated with the development of a number of different techniques for inducing clinicians to order more tests, including direct financial incentives (56). 'Best practice' standards are sufficiently loose as to permit a wide range of testing propensities, with very different financial implications for physician and laboratory (57).

In the US for-profit hospitals compete with not-for-profits by setting similar per day charges, but charge significantly more for 'ancillary' drugs and supplies, lab and radiology services, and use of operating and recovery rooms. They also supply significantly larger amounts of ancillary services per day—encouraging their physicians to prescribe drugs and tests (58). In a private, for-profit setting, sales promotion is a means to greater profit. The match between service and clinical need is of significance only insofar as it may relate to future sales (or lawsuits).

Thus one cannot lightly assume that the services which a patient agrees to buy are necessarily those which will make him better-off, either at all or enough to justify their cost. For some classes or dimensions of service, about which the patient may reasonably be or hope to become informed, the assumption is plausible. For others, one is relying on the professional ethics of the provider to discourage inappropriate care. Such ethics can in fact sustain a substantial burden of conflict with economic self-interest; otherwise fee-for-service medicine would have collapsed long ago. But the severity of the conflict can be substantially moderated or exacerbated by the structure of the funding process (26).

TO EVERY COMPLEX QUESTION THERE IS A SIMPLE ANSWER. BUT IT'S WRONG.

The dimensions of health system outcomes

Canada's experience with universal public health insurance has pointed more sharply to the basic questions which any society faces, consciously or unconsciously, in developing its health care system. Rhetorical flourishes of 'cost spirals' and of 'underfunding' are equally beside the point. Levels of funding are means, not ends in themselves. Similarly the institutional structure of delivery, funding through public or private budgets, insurance or service, more or less regulated public or private delivery, is a framework or a set of mechanisms for achieving certain outcomes or effects.

These outcomes can be classified under three heads. Most important, from a health perspective, are outcomes in terms of types of health services and goods produced, in what amounts, and to whom provided. These utilization or volume-mix-distribution issues are the principal focus of debate over health care organization and funding, though the traditional emphasis on how to provide more, and more equally (or at least more related to need) has now in many quarters shifted to less, and (in some) less equally.

Second, and of increasing interest, are the technical issues surrounding how particular services are produced, with what mix of different types of labour and capital. There is an obvious collective interest in efficient, minimum cost, production of whatever services are to be provided, but the incentives and constraints established in most countries by a variety of current regulatory and funding systems do not encourage and often actively discourage or prohibit technical efficiency. The social interest is not in general shared by providers.

Finally, there are outcomes in terms of distribution, not of services, but of economic burdens and benefits. Organization and funding mechanisms determine the distribution of expenditures over the population, they define the nexus between burden and such characteristics as income level, expectation of illness, or actual experience of illness, according to whether the system is financed by taxes, (private) premiums, or user charges. But they also influence the distribution of income/wealth between providers, users, and everyone else: the relative income status of providers, for any level of provision and real resource input, is very different under different funding systems. And these distributional issues, between providers and everyone else, seem to take up an inordinate amount of policy (and public) attention.

Alternative Canadian strategies for the future

Future directions for Canadian health policy can be grouped into four basic strategies, which also represent strategies which other countries have followed or might adopt. These we can characterize as, *first,* 'sitting on the lid', or continuation of present global control of expenditure; *second,* more active public intervention, by research, education, regulation, and perhaps direct provision, in the process of health care delivery; *third,* deregulation, and a move toward more reliance on competitive market forces to govern health care delivery, and *fourth,* reduced public intervention and a retreat to a pseudo-market in which public oversight and influence is withdrawn but competition is foreclosed by self-regulation, oligopolistic supply, and other forms of collusion and information management.

Canadian strategy has until now been to *sit on the lid.* Utilization issues—who gets what services—have been settled by providers within the constraints of public decisions over manpower, capital investment, fee schedules, and budget-setting. The only incentives to technical efficiency are pressures on conscientious providers to 'do more' with limited resources—these have had some limited success in the hospital area (e.g. the expansion of day-care surgery) but none at all in manpower use (mid-level practitioners).

The longer run viability of this form of macro-control, however, is open to doubt, in large part because of its distributional impact. While the distribution of the economic burden of care over the population, following that of the tax system, is almost universally approved, the impact of public insurance on provider incomes is leading to increasingly bitter conflict. Whatever the merits of current arguments, it is clear that one cannot reconcile global expenditure control, a steady (though much slowed) rise in the physician/population ratio, and constant (much less 'catching-up') physician relative incomes. The same dilemma exists in the hospitals— global cost constraint confronts income aspirations and great pressure for technological advance, or at least extension. The severity of this confrontation is showing up in several provinces in hospital strikes, work-to-rule and selective service withdrawal by physicians, threats to abandon the insurance system entirely, and where governments will permit it, direct billing of patients.

Thus far, provincial governments' positions in such conflicts have been very strong. Physician efforts to win public support either for their income demands or for changes to the public insurance system have been largely ineffective. Medicare remains the most popular public programme in the country. But a policy of cost constraint which relies on the increasing immiserization of physicians cannot continue indefinitely. Indeed, in two provinces, Ontario and B.C., governments have recently resolved extended confrontations with fee schedule awards which will substantially increase physician relative incomes once again—despite apparent absence of public support for physicians. The lid is slipping.

The control of hospital spending in the face of technological hypertrophy elsewhere is also becoming increasingly difficult. Partly this is because so little effort has been put into evaluating what interventions are efficacious, as well as for whom and under what circumstances. Unsupported arguments for expansion, on the basis of 'professional judgement', have not been met with hard evidence on need, or its absence, and must be turned aside with pleas of poverty. And this poverty is worsening, as physicians strive to expand their share of health spending.

In this environment, it will become increasingly difficult to maintain both cost restraint and universal access. It may not be too harsh to suggest that Canadian governments have wasted ten years of grace during which the substantial issues of 'What is to be done?' could have been addressed. The present political climate is a good deal less favourable to direct public management, but the task remains.

One could, of course, simply sit on the lid more tightly. One could effectively prohibit practice outside the plan, as Quebec has done, by ruling that neither physician nor patient will be reimbursed if the physician bills the patient directly. One could close medical school places until the physician/population ratio stabilized, and set fee schedules to hold physician relative incomes constant over time, similarly freezing hospital personnel establishments, and linking budget adjustments to the general economy. This would permit stable expenditure ratios for the indefinite future, while perhaps defusing the income problem. In such a lock-step system, current forms of inefficiency, and ineffective patterns of servicing, would presumably persist.

The more constructive, but now perhaps even more politically difficult, strategy would involve *more direct intervention in medical practice*. The descriptive data generated by the present insurance systems represents an enormous, and virtually untapped, resource. It would be possible to go through this data, identifying on the basis of current evidence the effective and ineffective practices, encouraging the former, and weeding out the latter. An energetic reimbursement agency would investigate the wide and persistent variations in surgical rates across regions, or the large differences in lengths of stay for e.g. uncomplicated delivery Canada (five days) and California (two), or myocardial infarct Canada (about two weeks) and Duke University Medical Center (one), or the steady escalation of laboratory testing. The 'shopping list' would be long and detailed, but in total most rewarding.

In the limit, active intervention could lead to direct supply. The Saskatchewan Dental Service, a public delivery system for children, has had great success in coverage, efficacy, and efficiency (59), and this model might be extended.

The opposition to such a management strategy is obvious, as Figure 3 emphasizes, expenditure control by whatever route, including improved efficacy or efficiency, implies reduction of incomes as well. Industry spokesmen therefore advocate instead *more private funding, through a well-controlled pseudo-market,* with direct billing relations between provider and patient, and a return to private insurance as supplement to or substitute for public insurance.

In this environment, physician fees could be lifted well above current reimbursement levels, while public capital constraints could be circumvented by the opening of private, physician or corporate-owned hospitals, catering for the less ill and more affluent, and reimbursed by private insurance. Patterns of care use would become very different by income class and insurance status.

The effects of such a pseudo-market are well understood from US experience—escalation in total costs, through both price and utilization increases, higher profits for private corporations selling health-related goods, services, and insurance, increased problems of inefficacious servicing as well as unmet needs, no gain in technical efficiency, a redistribution of burden from well to ill,—and higher incomes for physicians.

A more limited form of the pseudo-market would leave hospitals under public budgetary control, but free physicians to bill patients directly, over and above the provincial reimbursement schedule, in whatever amounts they choose. Alberta has accepted such a scheme, as of 1982, but as yet no clear picture of its scope, or of the Federal government's response, has emerged. It amounts to a privately administered tax on the sick, enforced by control over access to public facilities, which is used to supplement physicians' incomes. As long as the prohibition on private health insurance competitive with the public plans is maintained, however, the economic feasibility of extending 'privatization' to hospitals or the bulk of medical care is doubtful. But over the longer run, if direct billing spreads this prohibition will probably come under increasing attack.

More interesting, though less relevant politically, are proposals for *a genuine competitive market in health care*. These have been developed in most detail by US analysts, where the distinction between the 're-privatized' pseudo-market and truly unregulated free enterprise seems more widely appreciated, in theory at least. Such proposals form two strands. The more radical approach would simply remove the public regulatory framework, including legislative support for self-regulation, and all public subsidy, from the health care industry (60). More plausibly, the advocates of a system of competitive health maintenance organizations (HMOs) accept that health care as a commodity displays a number of special characteristics which may make unregulated private markets both inefficient and dangerous in its allocation. They argue, however, that free competition would be effective among larger organizations—prepaid group practices or HMOs. In the US, these groups of physicians and other medical staff offer enrollees a package of all needed health care, as determined by the HMO, for a fixed payment per time period. They own or contract for their own hospital space, including this in the fixed charge. Such groups obviously face economic incentives both to avoid inefficacious care and to minimize technical inefficiency, under competitive pressures from other HMOs who might bid away their enrollees (61). Their success in limiting hospital use and employing physician substitutes has been extensively documented (62,33).

The special characteristics of health care—collective or selective regulation

Support for the completely free market is ideological, rather than empirical, and is largely confined to the US. The special characteristics of health care, the asymmetry of information between provider and patient, the uncertainty of incidence of illness and its at best limited insurability, and the distributional consequences of ill-health, are obvious even to economists. The radical response, to ignore such problems as unimportant or to postulate that private institutions would develop to meet them, is a pure statement of faith. The extensive structure of regulation of health care which has evolved in every developed society is not just an unfortunate accident, a stupid mistake, or a cunning plot by suppliers.

But the form and scope of this regulation *is* questionable. In some areas of health care there does appear to be scope for deregulation and increased competition. Where commodities are concerned—pharmaceuticals, opthalmic goods, and health appliances—there is both analysis and empirical experience to suggest that an open, competitive market combined with product inspection and certification, not licensure, of providers, might significantly enhance efficiency and lower costs (63,64,65). Competition is not self-maintaining; public policy would have to protect against monopolies as in any other market. Particularly in pharmaceuticals, the complex links between manufacture, prescribing, and dispensing would require public intervention at several steps in the chain. But there seems no reason why dispensing charges (as opposed to ingredient costs) for drugs should not be freely set and advertised by competitive pharmacies (35).

Dentistry likewise presents an opportunity for significant deregulation. Competition between dentists and denturists in Canada has had the usual benefits of lower prices for the public, with no evidence of quality deterioration. These benefits could be greatly enhanced by removal of existing restrictions on price advertising, ownership of dental practices, and use of auxiliaries. The evidence of large potential benefit in this field is very good, and the risks from more competition small. At the very least the licensure of intermediate professionals competitive with dentists (denturists being the model) would open up the market substantially (35,66).

A question of judgment

The present Canadian insurance system blocks such changes by its universal coverage and uniform reimbursement. But the areas of most deregulatory promise, outlined above, are largely outside the national programmes. If the Supreme Court removes self-regulatory bodies' powers to restrict or prohibit price advertising by members (currently *sub judice*), some test of competition may occur automatically. The extent of deregulation required for a full test, however, requires substantial additional restraints on the powers of professional bodies to police their members' conduct (26), and these do not appear to be on the political cards.

The Canadian insurance system also inhibits the development of US-style HMOs. Such organizations have long existed in Canada, but they are not growing, because they cannot recruit members by offering savings in costs, or police members' use of outside services by direct charges. One current focus of policy analysis in Canada is how to modify the terms of the programme for such groups and their enrollees so as to encourage their growth. A variety of alternatives competitive to conventional private fee-for-service medicine, within the context of the universal insurance programme, might significantly improve efficiency and effectiveness. To date, however, this is not a major policy thrust in any province.

Nor is it obvious that competitive HMOs would be a panacea. Though growing rapidly in the US, they have yet to deal with several serious concerns. It is obviously advantageous for them to select away from the very ill, and it is well established that a large proportion of health costs is generated by identifiable chronic high users (67). Without either direct regulation or a very detailed matching of reimbursement to patient characteristics, and possibly even with them, the most ill will be left out. So far, the growth of HMOs has been primarily among the well, and there is anecdotal evidence of selectivity. Moreover, while less costly than private counterparts, they are alleged still to display both inefficiency and ineffective use, especially in primary care. Much better performance is possible; present competitive forces are not strong enough. Yet a highly competitive market dominated by for-profit HMOs would raise very serious questions of both selection bias and quality control.

In any case, from the Canadian perspective, a bird in the hand is worth two in the bush. The potential of competitive market forces is sufficient to justify experimentation in some areas of health care but their problems are sufficiently serious that dismantling the present insurance system in order to move in this direction would be unwise in the extreme. Their appeal is obviously much greater in the US, where the present situation is felt to be so unsatisfactory that there is much less to lose.

Moreover, as is widely appreciated by providers, a shift to competitive markets with improved efficiency and efficacy of care would significantly lower provider incomes. Any serious deregulatory strategy will come under strong, perhaps irresistable, pressure to divert it to a pseudo-market strategy. This appears to have happened in the US; in the spring of 1982 the Reagan Administration has apparently abandoned the competitive approach under pressure from the threatened interests. The alternative will probably be some mix of 'disintervention', the privately controlled pseudo-market, plus regulation to limit the federal government's share of costs. In Canada, provincial governments have shown little or no interest in deregulation even in areas such as dentistry or pharmacy, where the risks are least and the benefits best documented.

Even if an ideal competitive system were politically feasible, however, for the very sick, the poor, or those insufficiently informed to make (or disabled from making) their own care decisions, the market will never function. 'Your money or your life' is not a market offer. And given the cost and complexity of modern health care, this group with inadequate personal resources of wealth and information will at various times take in all of us. Their, our, care will be collectively financed, or not at all, and will be directed by others. The key question is, by whom, and to what ends? The most attractive option seems to be to build on the present Canadian system, not to dismantle it, with perhaps more competition around the fringes, but much more, and much better informed, public management of the main core of hospital and medical services. The nature of the task is apparent; the failure of political will is difficult to justify. If the challenge is not taken up, the Canadian performance of the 70s will be very difficult to maintain.

REFERENCES

1. NEWHOUSE, J. P. (1977). 'Medical care expenditure: A cross-national survey', *J. Human Resources,* **12**(1), Winter, 115–25.

2. MAXWELL, R. J. (1981). *Health and Wealth.* (Lexington, Mass: D. C. Heath).

3. CANADA, DEPARTMENT OF NATIONAL HEALTH AND WELFARE (1963). *Expenditures on Personal Health Care in Canada, 1953–1961.* Research and Statistics Division, Health Care Series Memorandum 16. (Ottawa: DNHW).

4. HEALTH AND WELFARE CANADA (1979). *National Health Expenditures in Canada, 1960–1975,* Information Systems Branch. (Ottawa: HWC).

5. Unpublished recent and historical material supplied by Health and Welfare Canada, Health Information Division.

6. COOPER, B. S., WORTHINGTON, N. L., and McGEE, M. F. (1973). *Compendium of National Health Expenditure Data.* Office of Research and Statistics, Social Security Administration, DHEW (SSA)73-11903. (Washington, D.C.: DHEW).

7. GIBSON, R. M. (1979). 'National health expenditures, 1978', *Health Care Financing Review*, 1(1), Summer. (Washington, D.C.: DHEW).

8. ——, and WALDO, D. R. (1981). 'National health expenditures, 1980', *Health Care Financing Review*, 3(1), Summer. (Washington, D.C.: DHEW).

9. ADAY, L. A., ANDERSEN, R., and FLEMING, G. V. (1980). *Health Care in the U.S.: Equitable for Whom?* (Beverly Hills: Sage) pp. 82–3.

10. BIRNBAUM, H. (1978). *A National Profile of Catastrophic Illness.* NCHSR Research Summary Series, DHEW #(PHS)78-320. (Washington, D.C.: DHEW).

11. BARER, M. L., *et al.* (1982). *Income Class and Hospital Use in Ontario.* Ontario Economic Council Occasional Paper 14. (Toronto: OEC).

12. BECK, R. G. (1973). 'Economic class and access to physician services under public medical care insurance', *Int. J. Health Services*, 3(3), Summer, 341–55.

13. BOULET, J. A., and HENDERSON, D. W. (1979). *Distributional and Redistributional Aspects of Government Health Insurance Programs in Canada.* Economic Council of Canada Discussion Paper 146 (mimeo) (Ottawa: ECC).

14. MANGA, P. (1978). *The Income Distribution Effect of Medical Insurance in Ontario,* Ontario Economic Council Occasional Paper 6. (Toronto: OEC).

15. McDONALD, A. D., *et al.* (1974). 'Effects of Quebec medicare on physician consultation for selected symptoms', *New Eng. J. Med.*, 293(13), 26 Sept. 649–52.

16. SIEMIATYCKI, J., RICHARDSON, L., and PLESS, I. B. (1980). 'Equality in medical care under national health insurance in Montreal', *New Eng. J. Med.* 303(1), 3 July, 10–15.

17. HALL, E. M. (1980). *Canada's National-Provincial Health Program for the 1980's.* Report of Health Services Review '79, commissioned by Health and Welfare Canada. (Saskatoon, Sask.: HSR '79).

18. CANADA, HOUSE OF COMMONS (1981). *Report of the Special Committee on the Federal-Provincial Fiscal Arrangements* (Breau Committee). (Ottawa: The Queen's Printer) Chapter 4.

19. THUROW, L. (1974). 'Cash versus in-kind transfers', *Amer. Econ. Rev.* 64(2), May, 190–5.

20. HAVIGHURST, C., and HACKBARTH, G. M. (1979). 'Private cost containment', *New Eng. J. Med.* 300(23), 7 June, 1298–1305, and POSNER, R. (1974). 'Theories of economic regulation', *Bell J. Econ. & Man. Sci.* 2(1), Spring, 335–65.

21. EVANS, R. G. (1982). 'The fiscal management of medical technology', forthcoming in D. BANTA, (ed.) *Resources for Health: Technology Assessment for Policy Making.* (New York: Praeger).

22. GORECKI, P. (1981). *Regulating the price of prescription drugs in Canada:*

Compulsory Licensing, Product Selection, and Government Reimbursement Programmes. Economic Council of Canada Technical Report 8. (Ottawa: ECC).

23. CANADA, HEALTH AND WELFARE CANADA (1982). 'Increases in the schedules of benefits for physicians' services under the Federal/Provincial Medical Care Insurance Plan', (mimeo). Health Information Division. (Ottawa: HWC).

24. EVANS, R. G. (1976). 'Beyond the medical marketplace: Expenditure, utilization, and pricing of insured health care in Canada', in R. ROSETT, (ed.) *The Role of Health Insurance in the Health Services Sector,* (New York: Neale Watson).

25. LEFEBVRE, L. A. (1976). *Public General and Allied Special Hospitals in Canada.* Statistics Canada, Health Division Research Paper. (Ottawa: S.C.), and STATISTICS CANADA. *Hospital Statistics* annual issues, Cat. #s 83–217, 227, 232. (Ottawa: SC).

26. EVANS, R. G. (1980). 'Professionals and the production function: Can competition policy improve efficiency in the licensed professions?' in S. ROTTENBERG, (ed.) *Occupational Licensure and Regulation.* (Washington, D.C.: AEI) pp. 225–64.

27. CANADA, HEALTH AND WELFARE CANADA (1981). *Canada Health Manpower Inventory, 1980.* (Ottawa: HWC), and *Health and Welfare Services in Canada, 1970.* (1970). Research and Statistics Directorate (Ottawa: HWC).

28. —— (1980). *Salaries and Wages in Canadian Hospitals.* (Ottawa: HWC).

29. BARER, M. L., EVANS, R. G., and STODDART, G. L. (1979). *Controlling Health Care Costs by Direct Charges to Patients: Snare or Delusion?* Ontario Economic Council Occasional Paper 10. (Toronto: OEC).

30. NEWHOUSE, J. P. (1981). 'The demand for medical care services: A retrospect and prospect' in J. VAN DER GAAG and M. PERLMAN, (eds), *Health, Economics, and Health Economics.* (Amsterdam: North-Holland).

31. —— et al. (1982). *Some Interim Results from a Controlled Trial of Cost Sharing in Health Insurance.* RAND R-2847-HHS. (Santa Monica, Cal.: Rand).

32. OWENS, A. (1981). 'How's inflation treating you?', *Medical Economics,* 28 Sept. 173–85.

33. RECORD, J. C. (1981). *Staffing Primary Care in 1990: Physician Replacement and Cost Savings.* (New York: Springer).

34. SPITZER, W. O. (1978). 'Evidence that justifies the introduction of new health professionals' in P. SLAYTON and M. J. TREBILCOCK, (eds) *The Professions and Public Policy.* (Toronto: University of Toronto Press).

35. EVANS, R. G., and WILLIAMSON, M. F. (1978). *Extending Canadian National Health Insurance: Policy Options for Pharmacare and Denticare.* (Toronto: University of Toronto Press).

36. WOLFSON, A. D., EVANS, R. G., and LOMAS, J. (1980). *Physician Incomes in Canada,* background study prepared for E. M. Hall (17).

37. ——, and TUOHY, C. J. (1980). *Opting Out of Medicare: Private Medical Markets in Ontario.* (Toronto: University of Toronto Press).

38. BANTA, H. D., and THACKER, S. B. (1979). *Costs and Benefits of Elec-*

tronic Foetal Monitoring: A Review of the Literature. NCHSR Research Report Series, DHEW (PHS) 79-3245. (Washington, DC: DHEW).

39. ALTMAN, S. H., and BLENDON, R. (eds) (1979). *Medical Technology: The Culprit Behind Health Care Costs?* NCHSR, DHEW (PHS) 79-3216. (Washington, DC: DHEW).

40. MARTIN, A. R., *et al.* (1980). 'A trial of two strategies to modify the test-ordering behaviour of medical residents', *New Eng. J. Med.*, **303**(23), 4 Dec. 1330-36.

41. McNEER, J. F., *et al.* (1978). 'Hospital discharge one week after acute myocardial infarction', *New Eng. J. Med.*, **298**(5), 2 Feb. 229-32.

42. ROOS, N. P., and ROOS, L. L. (1981). 'High and low surgical rates: Risk factors for area residents', *Amer. J. Pub. Health*, **71**(6), June, 591-600.

43. EVANS, R. G., and ROBINSON, G. C. (1980). 'Surgical day care: Measurements of the economic payoff', *Can. Med. Assn. J.*, **123**, 8 Nov. 873-80.

44. ——— (1982). 'An economic study of cost savings on a care-by-parent ward', *Medical Care* (forthcoming).

45. STOCKMAN, D. A. (1981). 'Premises for a medical marketplace: A neoconservative's vision of how to transform the health system', *Health Affairs*, **1**(1), Winter, 5-18.

46. PAULY, M. V. (1969). 'A measure of the welfare cost of health insurance' *Health Services Research*, **4**(4), 281-92, and FELDSTEIN, M. S. (1973). 'The welfare loss of excess health insurance', *J. Polit. Econ.* **81**(2), pt. 1, 251-80.

47. TUOHY, C. J., and WOLFSON, A. D. (1977). 'The political economy of professionalism: A perspective', in M. TREBILCOCK, (ed.), *Four Aspects of Professionalism.* (Ottawa: Consumer Research Council Canada).

48. KRASHINSKY, M. (1981). *User Charges in the Social Services: An Economic Theory of Need and Inability.* (Toronto: University of Toronto Press).

49. BECK, R. G. (1974). 'The effects of co-payment on the poor', *J. Human Resources*, **9**(1), 129-42, and BECK, R. G. and HORNE, J. M. (1978). *An Analytical Overview of the Saskatchewan Copayment Experiment in Hospital and Ambulatory Care Settings*, a Report for the Ontario Council of Health, reproduced in R. F. BADGELY and R. D. SMITH, (1979), *User Charges for Health Services.* (Toronto: Ontario Council of Health).

50. STODDART, G. L., and WOODWARD, C. A. (1980). *The Effect of Physician Extra-Billing on Patients' Access to Care and Attitudes Toward the Ontario Health System*, Background study prepared for E. M. Hall (17).

51. TESH, S. (1981). 'Disease causality and politics', *J. Health Politics, Policy and Law*, **6**(3), Fall, 369-90.

52. NEUHAUSER, D., and LEWICKI, A. M. (1976). 'National health insurance and the sixth stool guiac', *Policy Analysis*, **2**(2), Spring, 175-96.

53. HIRSCHMAN, A. O. (1970). *Exit, Voice, and Loyalty: Responses to Decline in Firms, Organizations, and States.* (Cambridge, Mass.: Harvard University Press).

54. MacCOLL, W. A. (1966). *Group Practice and Prepayment of Medical Care.* (Washington, D.C.: Public Affairs Press).

55. McNEIL, B. J., WEICHSELBAUM, R., and PAUKER, S. G. (1978). 'Fal-

lacy of the five-year survival in lung cancer', *New Eng. J. Med.*, **299**(25), Dec. 21, 1397–1401.

56. BAILEY, R. M. (1979). *Clinical Laboratories and the Practice of Medicine.* (Berkeley, Cal.: McCutchan).

57. SCHROEDER, S. A., and SHOWSTACK, J. A. (1978). 'Financial incentives to perform medical procedures and laboratory tests: Illustrative models of office practice', *Medical Care*, **16**(4), 289–98.

58. LEWIN, L. S., DERZON, R. A., and MARGULIES, R. (1981). 'Investorowneds and nonprofits differ in economic performance', *Hospitals: J.A.H.A.*, **55**(13), 1 July, 52–8.

59. LEWIS, D. W. (1981). *Performance of the Saskatchewan Health Dental Plan, 1974–1980.* (mimeo), Department of Community Dentistry, University of Toronto.

60. FREIDMAN, M. (1963). *Capitalism and Freedom.* (Chicago: University of Chicago Press).

61. ENTHOVEN, A. (1980). *Health Plan: The Only Practical Solution to the Soaring Cost of Medical Care.* (Reading, Mass.: Addison-Wesley).

62. LUFT, H. (1981). *Health Maintenance Organizations: Dimensions of Performance.* (New York: John Wiley).

63. CANADA, CONSUMER and CORPORATE AFFAIRS (1978). *The Ophthalmic Products Industry in Canada,* Report of the Restrictive Trade Practices. Commission (Ottawa: CCA).

64. BENHAM, L., and BENHAM, A. (1974). 'Regulating through the professions: A perspective on information control', *J. Law & Econ.*, **18**(2), October, 421–47, and BEGUN, J. W., and FELDMAN, R. D. (1981). *A Social and Economic Analysis of Professional Regulation in Optometry,* NCHSR Research Report Series, DHHS (PHS)81–3295. (Washington, D.C.: DHHS).

65. CADY, J. F. (1975). *Drugs on the Market.* (Lexington, Mass.: D.C. Heath).

66. BLACKSTONE, E. A. (1980). 'Dentists and Denturists: the Development and Consequences of Competition in Dentures', *The Antitrust Bulletin*, **25**(4), Winter, 751–76.

67. ZOOK, C., and MOORE, F. D. (1980). 'High-Cost Users of Medical Care', *New Eng. J. Med.*, **302**(18), 1 May, 996–1002, and SCHROEDER, S. A., SHOWSTACK, J. A., and ROBERTS, H. E. (1979). 'Frequency and clinical description of high-cost patients in 17 acute-care hospitals', *New Eng. J. Med.*, **300**(23), 7 June, 1306–9.

Unscrambling the omelet
Public and private health care financing in Australia

J. S. DEEBLE

JOHN S. DEEBLE

Dr John Deeble B.Com., Ph.D (Melbourne) is Head of the National Health and Medical Research Council's Health Economics Research Unit at the Australian National University, Canberra. He has written extensively in the economics of health and medical care, with particular reference to financing. After experience as a hospital administrator, he was Senior Research Fellow in the Institute of Applied Economic and Social Research, University of Melbourne; and Senior Lecturer in Economics at Monash University. From 1973 to 1975 he was Special Adviser to the Minister for Social Security, and Deputy Chairman of the Australian Health Insurance Commission. Prior to joining the Australian National University in 1977, he was Economic Adviser to the Commonwealth Department of Health.

Unscrambling the omelet
Public and private health care financing in Australia

ABSTRACT

This paper examines Australian health care financing over the decade to 1980, a period in which a voluntary private insurance system was replaced by a short-lived universal compulsory scheme (1975–6) and subsequently reinstated almost completely by a series of legislative steps to 1981. Experiences with respect to expenditure, service usage, and provider incomes are examined, together with some evidence of the effects of the different systems on service distribution, patterns of delivery, and the degree of public regulation involved.

The main conclusions are as follows. First, expenditures bore no clear relationship to financing systems. Two-thirds of the large increase in the proportion of GDP devoted to health arose from 'excess' price and wage inflation, rather than increased real resource use. Hospital use did not rise at all relative to population, and the considerable rise in medical care consumption appears to have been primarily related to doctor supply, not financing arrangements. Second, the offer of free public care under universal insurance appears to have had little effect on consumer preferences for public or private treatment, although restrictions on public supply make this conclusion somewhat tentative. Provider incomes have, on average, increased more rapidly than other incomes in the community, but this has been a function of the Australian wage-fixing system on the hospital side, and of fee-for-service reimbursement insurance on the medical side, not the degree of public or private management. Finally, the extent of government regulation appears to have been just as great in the 'private' as in the public insurance system, mainly because purely competitive outcomes are unacceptable on social welfare grounds. Private insurance has been extremely successful as a revenue raising device outside the formal public sector, but the coverage of disadvantaged people and the regressive incidence of flat-rate premiums remain problems. Also, diffusion of responsibility raises doubts about the private system's ability to cope with cost-expanding pressures.

427

INTRODUCTION

Like many aspects of Australian life, the health care system has features of most of the major systems overseas. Over the last decade, it has undergone more change—or at least more appearance of change—than any comparable system elsewhere. It is also not entirely uniform throughout the country, so that the effects of various policy measures have been different in different places. Australia is therefore a quite useful case study of differences in the mix of public and private activity, particularly financing, both cross-sectionally and over time. This chapter is concerned mainly with the period from 1972 when a government committed to some apparently radical changes in financing came to office. From 1975 to 1981 the course of policy was, to say the least, erratic and included the establishment of, probably, the shortest lived national health insurance scheme in history. The current situation is relatively clear, however, and a brief review of experience over the past few years may suggest some conclusions of value to policy makers generally.

The paper is in three parts. The first part provides some background to health service policy in Australia, the structure of health services, their financing and the changes of recent years. The second part analyses, as far as is possible, the effects of these changes on the use of services, costs and their distribution. The third part suggests some conclusions which may be relevant to the overall theme of this book.

BACKGROUND

Several historical factors are basic to an understanding of the structure of Australian health services and their financing. The first is the constitutional position. Australia is a Federation of six States and two Territories, with all of the divided and overlapping powers which a Federal system implies. The Constitution grants the Commonwealth Government powers over certain specified activites, all other authority vesting in the States, although in practice the ceding by the States of the major revenue source—income tax—together with the central government's ability to make grants to them on such terms as it thinks fit, widens the Commonwealth's influence considerably. Health was not one of the areas over which powers were granted to the Commonwealth in 1901, but a Constitutional Amendment in 1946 provided sufficient spending authority for it to influence policy significantly. It is widely believed that this Amendment prevents any National Health Service in Australia because it contains a specific prohibition of anything which would involve 'civil conscription'—a clause inserted at the behest of the medical profession. The proposition is doubtful, but the threat and the obvious need to decentralize administration in a country as large as Australia, have been sufficient to limit the Commonwealth's intervention to the use of its financial powers (1).

The second is that the systems originally developed by the States have always mixed public and private service delivery, and public and private finance. Public health services apart, the accepted role of government has generally been to provide the capital and organizational infrastructures within which the private health professions operate. Governments have certainly accepted an obligation to care for the poor which was satisfied by the public hospital systems, but because Australia never developed the community hospitals of the United States or the old municipal hospitals of the UK, the State public hospitals have also provided subsidized care to most of the community. By the time the Federal government entered the financing of personal health services in the 1950s, the public/private mixture was well set. Then, as now, the delivery of out-of-hospital services depended almost entirely on private sector activity, but widespread public subsidization was thoroughly accepted.

The Australian system is therefore an amalgam of the British and American arrangements. Though links with the founding British institutions remain strong, medical practice is organized along North American lines. The predominant mode is fee-for-service private practice. Of the approximately 28,000 physicians in the country in 1980—nearly 1·9 doctors per thousand of population—about 21,000 were involved in some private fee-for-service work and about 18,000 of these were exclusively engaged in private practice (2). General practice has been maintained at a fairly high level —over half of all private practitioners—and the proportion is currently rising after years of increased specialization. This practice is relatively uniform throughout the country but specialist medicine varies slightly with the different hospital systems of the States. They are all predominantly 'public'— nearly 80 per cent of beds are in publicly subsidized insitutions—but in most states the majority of admissions in fact relate to 'private patients' who contract separately for medical care with their own doctors and pay uniform, state-regulated, hospital fees of only about half the average operating cost. The exceptions are the States of Tasmania and Queensland—which has had a free public hospital service with salaried doctors (mostly part-time) for nearly forty years. In the largest states, relationships between hospitals and doctors are more like those in North America, and the current programmes to care for the aged and the needy are conceptually quite similar to Medicare and Medicaid. However, the predominantly public ownership of hospitals and the control over both capital and operating budgets exercised by State Health Commissions inject elements not present to the same degree in North America.

General hospitals and medical services account for nearly 60 per cent of all Australian health expenditures. The remaining large items are psychiatric hospitals, nursing homes, and out-of-hospital prescribed drugs. Psychiatric hospitals are almost entirely state owned and provide free care. By contrast, long-term care in nursing homes is provided largely by private organizations (of which about half are profit-seeking), supported by a Federal government subsidy scheme which pays daily benefits and/or budget subsidies to approved homes. Since over 90 per cent of nursing home patients are of pensionable age, the scheme is really an extension of the age pension system. Prescribed drugs are covered under a Federal government programme similar to that in the UK, which provides nearly 95 per cent of all out-of-hospital prescriptions at a uniform fee of $3.20 per prescription to the patient (3). The balance of a government negotiated price is paid by the government to the supplying pharmacist, so that the financial impact of high-cost drug utilization is greatly reduced so far as the consumer is concerned. Apart from concern over the high aggregate cost of nursing home care, none of these programmes are controversial and they have changed little over the last decade.

Most controversy has been over the financing of hospitals —in which both the States and the Commonwealth are involved—and out-of-hospital medical care in which the States play little part. The latter has been a Federal government function which until 1975 involved:

(a) the subsidization of cash benefits to people who contributed to approved, non-profit health insurance funds, and

(b) the provision of free services to aged and invalid pensioners through agreements with the Australian Medical Association with respect to GP services, and with the state public hospitals with respect to inpatient and specialist outpatient care.

These Federally supported schemes began in 1952 and by 1975 covered about 85 per cent of the population. The uncovered 15 per cent included low-income earners (despite attempts to locate and subsidize this group), certain national minorities—particularly recent migrants from Southern Europe—but also included an unknown number of young, healthy, people for whom insurance was unattractive. The non-profit insurance organizations operated on a relatively small scale in each state, incurred high administrative expenses, and accumulated considerable reserves despite close government control (4). As a consequence, there was considerable public disquiet in the late 1960s and early 1970s over both efficiency and the failure of the voluntary insurance system to achieve universal coverage, particularly of the most disadvantaged groups. Linked with these concerns was a growing dissatisfaction with programmes for the aged and the poor which required categorization and the stigma which many people believed to be attached to it.

A second criticism of subsidized private insurance was the quality of the medical cover it offered. Up to 1971 the system followed, in principle, a 'one-third' formula first enunciated by its founding Minister for Health—one-third of the doctors fee to be covered by a Commonwealth Benefit, one-third by the private health fund and one-third borne by the patient.

While most services were provided by GPs charging traditional, stable fees, these proportions could be maintained, but specialization produced increasing divergences. In the absence of a formal fee schedule or procedures for setting and adjusting fees, both the government and the insurance funds were reluctant to increase their benefits in the (correct) belief that it would simply induce further rises. By the early 1970s the distribution of benefits was quite perverse—coverage was highest for the inexpensive and relatively predictable GP services, lowest for expensive and episodic specialist treatment.

The response of the government of the day was to restructure the medical insurance system by increasing Commonwealth subsidies combined with, in 1971, the offer of higher and more certain benefits for expensive specialist services. It involved establishing, for the first time, a formal schedule of 'most common fees' and the recognition of differential fees for specialists. For insured people, the uncovered portion of the fee had fallen to an average of 19 per cent by 1972/73, and the proportion was much lower for the more expensive services. This did not satisfy the opposition Labor Party, however, which had adopted a policy of compulsory insurance in 1968. National Health Insurance was a major plank in its platform when finally elected in 1972, but it was not the only Labor health initiative. To counter increasing specialization and to, hopefully, co-ordinate health and welfare services, a Community Health Program was established, together with a Hospitals Development Program designed to correct the maldistribution of resources in the States but which actually began with a substantial building programme.

National Health Insurance, Mark I

The Labor Government's programme had been set out in some detail before the 1972 election. It involved;

(i) The establishment of a single Health Insurance Fund to finance medical and hospital benefits to which the whole population was entitled.

(ii) Medical coverage, based on benefits calculated at 85

per cent of the fees in a schedule negotiated with representatives of the medical profession. The maximum difference between fees and benefits was five dollars for any one service. Doctors could bill the fund direct, in bulk, and accept the benefits in full settlement, or bill their patients with the benefit then payable to the patient.

(iii) Free hospital treatment in standard ward accommodation, without means test, under agreements negotiated with the States. Treatment included medical care provided by doctors appointed by the hospital. Outpatient treatment was also available without means test and without charge. Doctors providing services to 'hospital' patients were to be remunerated by salaries and sessional payments. Public hospitals continued to admit private patients at fees agreed between the governments, and the private health funds were free to offer insurance against them.

(iv) Funding of the Health Insurance Fund by a 1·35 per cent levy on taxable incomes, with a matching Commonwealth government subsidy.

The programme therefore offered the prospect of care free at the point of service, but could not guarantee it in the absence of (a) agreements with the States covering free hospital care (which had in turn to negotiate agreements with doctors), and (b) the acceptance by doctors of bulk billing. Indeed, in the absence of fee adherence (even without bulk billing) the government could only guarantee a specified coverage of *schedule* fees, not the actual fees charged. But this was also true of the earlier voluntary system, and in the medical area the new scheme really differed from the earlier one only in paying slightly higher benefits to all. Changes were more fundamental on the hospital side in the removal of means tests and other restrictions on access to public hospital care, and the preference for salaried payment of doctors. From the patient's viewpoint, the major impact was simply the replacement of flat-rate premiums with income-related contributions, but there were several subsidiary objectives on the supply side. Bulk billing was certainly seen as a form of indirect medical-fee fixing. Through its control over hospital posts, a salaried medical service was intended to divert resources from the larger city hospitals and affluent areas to the relatively underserviced country and suburban-industrial regions; from specialist practice towards primary care; and from 'private' treatment to public. These were the first overt instrusions of the central government into such areas (5). They were also policies which ran counter to all existing trends, and which threatened to restrict both the income prospects of some doctors and the range within which they could choose the type and location of their practice. Not surprisingly, they met with strenuous opposition.

After several years of acrimonious debate, the rejection of the necessary Bills by the Senate (an upper house elected on a quite different procedure to the Houses of Representatives and which the Government did not control), a dissolution of Parliament and a general election, National Health Insurance finally became law in July 1974 and came into operation a year later. Through a legal technicality, the Senate was able to prevent the imposition of a levy, so that funding was entirely through general taxation. The scheme was operated by a statutory Health Insurance Commission and was known by the title of Medibank.

National Health Insurance, Mark II

The original Medibank scheme had been in operation for less than six months when the Labor Government was defeated in December 1975. The incoming government had promised to maintain Medibank but had vigorously opposed it when in opposition, and the promise was short-lived. Reforms were introduced in October 1976. Under the new arrangements, a Health Insurance Levy was applied at the rate of 2·5 per cent of taxable income with a maximum amount applying at just under the average earnings (6). Every Australian citizen was liable for the levy, which entitled him to exactly the same benefits as in the original Medibank scheme. However, any taxpayer could claim exemption by showing that he subscribed (or had subscriptions paid on his behalf) to an approved private insurance policy which provided:

(a) medical benefits identical to those in the government schedule, and

(b) hospital benefits which fully covered the charges for at least shared-room accommodation as a private patient in a public hospital.

Further insurance was available (for single-room or private-hospital accommodation) but without subsidy and had to be offered as a separate policy additional to the basic package conferring exemption from the levy. Private insurers were required to apply community rates within each state (i.e., they could not vary premiums according to age, occupation, past health experience, or any other factor affecting the risk) and to accept all applicants without discrimination. As compensation, all were compelled to participate in a government-subsidized reinsurance pool covering high-use members. Formally, they were free to set premiums and conduct their business subject only to government surveillance of their financial viability, but in practice the 'approved' rates were quite closely controlled.

These provisions had the not-surprising effect of creating a fairly narrow band of private insurance rates for 'standard' cover, so that the individual's choice was relatively simple. The 'opting out' programme, as it was known, preserved the major objectives of the original Medibank system, and offered a choice of insurer, although the practical effect of the latter was really little different to the earlier, simpler plan. Insurance was universal and compulsory, the main effect of the opting-out provision being to offer the higher-income groups private in-hospital care at a somewhat lower cost than would otherwise apply, and so induce them to take out wholly private cover. Reduction in the size of the public sector was a major objective of the incoming government, and the revised health insurance system provided a set of psuedo-market signals to achieve a distribution of business along essentially income lines. Because the levy rate and the private insurance premium together determined the income level at which opting-out became cheaper than public cover for those desiring private, fee-for-service medical care in hospital, the system was obviously manipulable. In fact, it was designed to produce about a 50:50 division of business between the public and private insurance sectors, and this was almost exactly achieved despite the variety of factors in addition to income which influenced each individual's choice.

Medibank Mark II, as it was popularly known, operated from September 1976 to October 1978. It certainly reduced total Commonwealth payments, though it is clear that retention of the original scheme with a (lower) levy would have actually reduced the Commonwealth government *deficit* by more. Concurrent with these changes, there was a scaling-down of the community health programme in real resource terms, and moves to merge the hospital development programme with the general capital works programme of the states. Mark II proved workable, although its administration was often unnecessarily complex and there was criticism of the association between income and the choice of private insurance encouraging dual standards of health care. Its termination was motivated by a desire to reduce Commonwealth responsibilities and to take advantage of a quirk in the way in which health service charges enter calculation of the Consumer Price Index then used for wage indexation. Given the importance of wage adjustment in macro-economic policy, some disruption to the health services financing system was apparently judged a small price to pay.

Further amendments

From November 1978 the health insurance levy and the compulsion to insure were abolished. The Commonwealth government would henceforth provide medical benefits of 40 per cent of schedule fees (with a maximum gap of $20 per service) without the need to insure and payable either directly to uninsured people or through the benefit funds to those who chose to take additional private cover. Benefits at the Medibank I level (85 per cent of schedule fees) were retained for old age pensioners, and for disadvantaged people the government paid benefits equal to 75 per cent of schedule fees, provided that doctors agreed to direct bill the Department of Health and accept benefits in full settlement of their accounts (7). Access to public hospital treatment without charge or means test, which had been introduced in Medibank I, was also retained. Despite the government's protestations, the system was conceptually similar to Medibank I except that the level of general benefits was lower, methods of payment were different, and the image of contributory national insurance was abandoned with abolition of the levy.

The problem with this third variation was that it actually increased the Commonwealth government's outlays a little, so that the system was changed yet again, from November 1979, by replacing the general benefit of 40 per cent of schedule fees with a government subsidy—again paid directly or through the private funds—of all the excess over $20 per service up to the schedule fee. Higher benefits for pensioners and the 'disadvantaged' remained, and access to free public hospital treatment was retained under the Federal-State agreements, at least until their review in 1981. However this programme had some distinctly uncomfortable implications for the government's long-term aim. While access to free public hospital care remained, and a public 'catastrophe insurance' scheme operated for all private medical fees, good-risk people found private insurance increasingly unattractive. Between March 1979 and March 1980 the number of people who were privately insured fell by about 10 per cent and by early 1981 only about half of the population held medical or hospital cover. The insurance funds were threatened with substantial premium increases as the selection of risks became steadily less favourable to them, and the demand for free public hospital care rose.

Withdrawal

Following a prolonged 'softening-up' period (including the establishment of a government inquiry into 'inefficiencies' in the public hospitals), the Federal government announced in April 1981 its intention effectively to withdraw from any detailed health policy formation and any direct financing of services. From 1 September 1981, responsibility for hospital financing reverted to the States. Those public hospital cost-sharing agreements which were due for review were terminated and Federal funds absorbed into overall tax-sharing arrangements, but with a reduction of central funding based on the requirement that States would substantially increase hospital inpatient fees, impose fees on outpatient services, and limit free public care to old age pensioners, recent migrants, the unemployed, and low-income earners qualifying under a Federally-administered means test (8). Only about 20 per cent of the population are eligible for these programmes, any extension being at the expense of the States. On the medical side, the position has reverted to pre-1975 conditions, with Federal benefits being limited to old age pensioners, the unemployed, migrants, and those who privately insure (85 per cent of scheduled fees for the first three groups, 30 per cent for the latter). Tax deductibility of private health insurance premiums has been restored on a flat-rate basis, but financed by the withdrawal of tax 'indexation', a system whereby personal income tax rates had been adjusted for inflation so as to maintain relatively constant real tax collections. The policy has been justified on the basis of 'user-pay' principles, and is designed to substantially reduce Commonwealth expenditures, partly by shifting them to the States and partly by boosting private health insurance membership through the withdrawal of universal public benefits. With one exception (Queensland), the States have certainly responded in the required way. Free care has been limited and fees imposed at levels which, in some cases, exceeded the Commonwealth expectations. Private insurance membership has risen (to about 70 per cent of the population) but because tax concessions indirectly subsidize this insurance, the initial shift between *all* public and *all* private sources of funds may be quite small—perhaps 2 per cent of total health care costs in 1982. The process will accelerate, however, and in the meantime the style of administration has certainly changed. Operation of the system has been shifted firmly to the private sector.

RESULTS

Much has been made of the effects of these changes on health service expenditures, costs, and use, mostly from *a priori* bases. Those opposed to collective financing attribute virtually all of the cost expansion of the 1970s to the profligacy of public programmes and the weakening of incentives to cost minimization which they are supposed to produce.

Those in favour point out that the realistic alternative is not a free market system but private insurance which may be restricted in its coverage, inequitable in its distribution of costs, indifferent to resource allocation, and even less effective in cost containment than its public counterpart. In fact, the available material throws little light on these issues. None of the five financing systems lasted long enough to show clear-cut effects, and the collection of policy-relevant data was not a major operational priority.

So far as measurable expenditure, financing and utilization information are concerned, the main changes are shown in Table 1, which brings together data from a variety of sources and includes some estimates for 1981-2 (9). As can be seen, health expenditures as a proportion of Gross Domestic Product (GDP) rose steadily throughout the period with the largest increases occurring at, and just before, the introduction of National Health Insurance in 1975-6. However the figures are somewhat misleading, firstly because the relationship of health expenditures to GDP depends as much on the growth of GDP as on that in health service spending; and secondly because price and cost inflation in the health care industry was significantly higher than in the rest of the economy. The increase in real resource use was much less than the crude statistics would suggest.

Figure 1 compares the health service sector's share of GDP in current prices with the same concept measured in constant 1966-7 prices. The large increase in the current-price GDP proportion is shown to have been largely due to price effects; in constant prices, health expenditures rose from 5·1 per cent to only 5·8 per cent of GDP, so that about two-thirds of the current-price rise was due to 'excess' wage and price inflation. The course of changes over time is shown in Figure 2 where annual increments in constant-price expenditures and constant-price GDP are compared. Apart from the first year movement (which may reflect measurement errors), the increments in health service spending bore no clear relationship to the financing system operating at the time. The relationship with real GDP movements was very much closer, but with a lag of approximately one year—not a surprising result given the way in which public hospital

Table 1. *Health services use and expenditure statistics Australia, 1969–70 to 1981–82 (selected years).*

Year ended 30 June	Financing system	Expenditures Current as per cent GDP	Service use per person		Private medical services	Financing total funds per cent			
			General hospital days			Government		Private	
			Public	Private		Direct	Total	Insurance	Users
1970	Private insurance	5·1	1·38	0·26	4·39	54	64	14	22
1973		5·6	1·39	0·26	4·92	56	65	14	20
1975		6·5	1·38	0·27	5·39	61	73	16	11
1976	Medibank I	7·2	1·38	0·33	5·50	73	74	10	16
1977	Medibank II	7·3	1·37	0·32	5·70	65	67	17	16
1978		7·4	1·32	0·31	na	61	62	21	17
1979	Medibank III	7·4	1·31	0·30	na	60	61	20	19
1980	Medibank IV	na	1·31	0·29	6·58	na	na	na	na
1982 (est.)	Private insurance	7·5	1·30	0·29	6·80	52	59	22	19

Source: Appendix 1

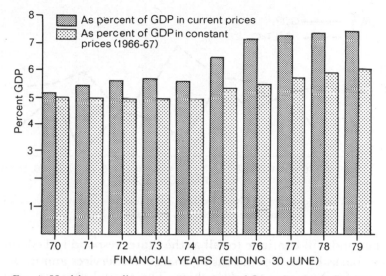

FIG. 1. Health expenditure as a percentage of Gross Domestic Product.

budgets are determined. The increments in health expenditure were consistently greater, however, and it is true that the increased real resource share of the health services apparently began with the imminent introduction of centralized public funding in 1975 (10). To 1979 at least, the rise had not been checked.

Financing

Changes in sources of finance are also shown in Table 1, the difference between 'direct' government expenditures and total public spending being the indirect subsidies provided through tax concessions on health insurance premiums and unrecouped medical expenses. As can be seen, the 1975 changes did not much alter the overall net shares of public and private finance; their impact was mainly distributional in altering the shares of the Federal and State governments, and the incidence of costs on individuals, mainly through converting tax concessions (which generally favoured the well-off) into direct benefits. The public sector share has fallen steadily since then (entirely in Commonwealth spend-

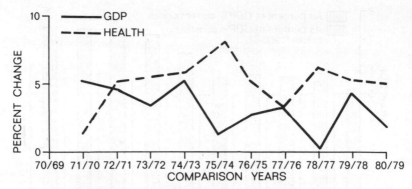

FIG. 2. Yearly changes in Gross Domestic Product in constant prices and expenditure on health in constant prices.

ing) and will continue to fall as the States respond to Federal cut-backs by further increasing charges for services and insurance funding rises to cover them. The overall changes were not as large as the rhetoric of governments or public controversy would lead one to believe, but they were still substantial. Since 1976, nearly $1000 million of health service costs have been shifted from the public to the private sector (11).

Service use

Figure 3 shows the use of general hospitals and private medical services over the decade. Hospital bed use has hardly changed at all, the slight decline towards the end of the period being largely explained by some administrative reclassification of hospital beds as nursing homes. The public hospital/private hospital balance has not changed either. Admission rates have increased (through a shorter average stay) but there is no evidence of any relationship between admission rates and financing systems.

Nor has the use of private medical services shown any such relationship. Average use per person was 4·39 services in 1970, had risen at an almost uniform annual rate to 6·58 services per person in 1980, and will probably reach 6·8 services per head in 1982. If anything, there was a slight pause in the first year of National Health Insurance in

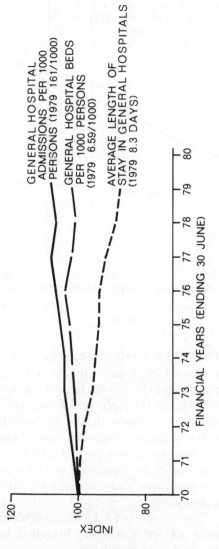

FIG. 3. Indexes of hospital bed numbers, admission rates, and length of stay.

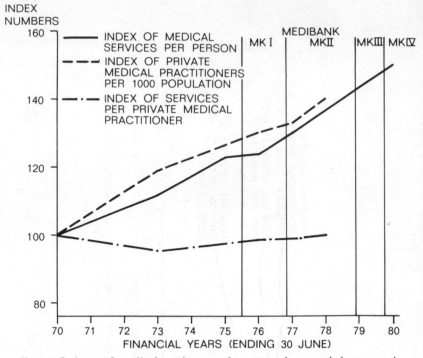

FIG. 4. Indexes of medical service use, doctor numbers, and doctor workload.

1975–6, associated with a small increase in the proportion of 'public' (non fee-for-service) inpatient care in hospitals which was subsequently reversed. These figures almost certainly overstate the real rise in the volume of care because of the continuing subdivision of items in the fee schedule and its use by doctors for income maximization. Doctor supply certainly seems by far the closest correlate of medical service use. Figure 4 shows, in index number form, the behaviour of service use, doctor numbers and the apparent average workload per doctor for as many years as reliable statistics are available (12). The apparent doctor workload has not changed, increased service use being matched by a similar proportionate rise in doctor numbers.

How did such increased service use arise? Some must be explained by a combination of higher insurance cover and increased government subsidies. In 1969-70, the average user charge for all private medical services was 37 per cent of the gross fee. By 1972-3, the proportion had fallen to 19 per cent, by 1975-6 to about 9 per cent and the user's share had only increased to 12 per cent in 1979-80, despite the fact that insurance was no longer universal (13). If we accept the highest plausible estimate of the price elasticity of demand (about −0·4), then about half of the increased consumption over the decade could reasonably be attributed to lower net fees. The remainder is not so easy to explain. Income increases are a possible explanation, but consumers' real incomes were almost static between 1974 and 1980. In any case, widespread insurance virtually removes the direct effects of income on demand. Higher quality, in the sense of improved outcome, could also have stimulated demand, but it is extremely difficult to demonstrate. In its absence, one is left with the conclusion that the main driving forces have been simply availability, and the treatment technologies which doctors have selected and patients have acquiesed in.

In-hospital care

One of the few significant changes in 1975 was the removal of fees for public hospital care and the abolition of means tests on access to it. Had this not been accompanied by increased subsidies to private in-hospital treatment, the relative price of private status would have increased considerably, but in fact the then Federal government felt unable to guarantee public care in the face of medical opposition and so continued to subsidize 'private' patients in both public and private hospitals so as to maintain the existing price differentials. Net fees were still significant however (equivalent to about $50 per day in public hospitals and $70-80 per day in private hospitals in 1982 values), so that the take-up of free hospital care provides some evidence of preferences at going prices.

Table 2 shows 'hospital patient' bed-days as a percentage of (a) public hospital bed-days and (b) all hospital bed-days over the period of major change, separating those States which prior to 1975 restricted access to public care by means test from those which did not. In a situation where universal insurance covered *all* medical fees, and the only advantage which private patient status in hospital conferred was the right to be treated by a doctor in fee-for-service practice, the initial effect was a shift towards public treatment of about 5 per cent of all hospital days in those states where access had previously been restricted. The subsequent movement was about 1 per cent per quarter. There was no change in the 'free access' states. After a year of the opting-out variant, the position had reverted to almost exactly that of 1974-5, not because of any restrictions on access or changes in relative price, but simply because the insurance package was presented in a different way. The proportion had varied only a little by 1981, but the stated aim of the Commonwealth's most recent policy is to achieve a shift of about 10 per cent in the proportion of patients treated privately with a minimum of 50 per cent private patient days within the public hospitals in each State.

How far might the earlier move towards public treatment in hospital have gone? Doctor opposition makes the initial figures misleading. Public care was not a practical option for many patients, whatever their legal entitlements, so that the only useful indicator is experience in the two states which had maintained open public hospital systems for many years. Table 3 shows the percentage composition of hospital bed use, by States, in 1975-6. Not surprisingly, the highest proportions of public care were in the two 'open' states, but even in these systems a significant number of patients chose private treatment at the going prices. The big differences were in private care within the public hospitals. The private hospital share was similar throughout and the actual use of private hospitals was remarkably consistent despite quite large differences in public hospital provision. The evidence is by no means conclusive, but what it suggests is that, under Australian conditions, the private hospitals serve a category of patients (and doctors) which is quite separate from those who use the public system; and that there is a further group of patients—10 to 15 per cent at least—whose demand for private status is unlikely to be much affected by costs so long as insurance facilities exist to cover them.

Table 2. *Hospital patient bed-days as percentage of public hospital bed-days and all hospital bed-days, 1974–5 to 1978–9.*

Period	New South Wales, Victoria, South Australia, Western Australia		Queensland, Tasmania	
	Public hospital days	All hospital days	Public hospital days	All hospital days
Year to June 1975	49·1	40·6	82·5	65·2
First quarter Medibank I (Dec. 1975)	54·5	45·0	82·6	65·3
Last quarter Medibank I (Sept. 1976)	56·8	46·9	82·9	65·5
Fourth quarter Medibank II (Sept. 1977)	49·5	40·8	80·6	63·0
Year ended 31 March 1979	50·1	41·4	79·4	60·3

Sources: Appendix 1

Table 3. *Percentage composition of hospital bed-days by patient status, 1975–6, by States.*

	New South Wales	Victoria	Queensland	South Australia	Western Australia	Tasmania
Public hospitals						
Hospital patients	42·5	42·0	62·4	47·0	56·5	76·8
Private patients	41·0	32·2	14·6	28·0	23·3	5·8
Private hospitals	16·5	25·8	23·0	25·0	20·2	18·4
	100·0	100·0	100·0	100·0	100·0	100·0

Sources: Appendix 1

Provider incomes

A common criticism of fee-for-service insurance is that it unduly enriches suppliers, and critics of public financing in Australia made much of the apparently high incomes earned by private doctors under universal cover. Data on private practitioners' net incomes are not easy to obtain. No surveys have been conducted and the taxation statistics which are next best source do not distinguish between specialties, between doctors engaged exclusively in private practice and salaried doctors with private practice rights, and also include income from sources other than medical practice. The most reliable indicator of change is the 'average gross business income' (gross fees) of doctors receiving at least some returns from private practice, on the assumption their net incomes move in a similar way.

Figure 5 shows, in index form, movements in the average gross fee income of private doctors, the average weekly earnings of all Australian employees, and the average salaries and wages paid to hospital staff. Contrary to popular belief, the disparate movement was in the average wage level of hospital employees, *not* in medical practitioner incomes. It is possible, of course, that the publicity given to apparently high doctor earnings raised the income expectations of other health service workers and so contributed to this result, but the timing does not support this hypothesis. The upward adjustment in hospital employee pay-scales predated the Medibank-induced concern with doctor incomes, and the differential rate of increase has persisted. It was achieved mainly in the public sector, within a compulsory arbitration system which takes almost no account of ability to pay and was quite unaffected by financing arrangements. The course of doctor incomes, on the other hand, has undoubtedly been influenced by financing systems, though in an indirect way. Doctors' average gross fee receipts have moved almost exactly in line with average earnings generally, a condition which required firstly that fees be adjusted quite precisely and secondly that service volumes rose in line with doctor numbers. Mechanisms exist for both types of adjustment. One consequence of publicly-regulated medical insurance is that

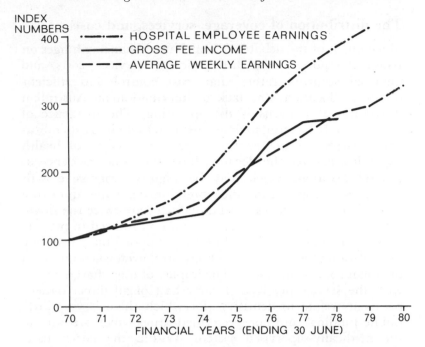

FIG. 5. Indexes of average gross fee income of private medical practitioners, earnings of hospital employees, and average weekly earnings.

the fees insured against need to be known, and the Australian system has developed a Medical Fees Tribunal to determine a schedule of fees which doctors are not compelled to charge, but to which in practice they adhere quite closely (14). At these Tribunals, the AMA has successfully argued for adjustments which would preserve medical incomes relative to others, *provided* that average doctor workloads remained constant; and the system has sustained such workloads in the face of steadily increasing doctor numbers. I have argued elsewhere that these fee-fixing methods have maintained fees and doctor incomes at a higher level than the market would provide, but *only* because an increased service use has been supported by more government subsidies and higher insurance benefits (15). Average *individual* incomes may not have increased unduly, but the profession as a whole has prospered.

The distribution of coverage, services, and costs

Since much of the debate on health care financing hinges on issues of equity in the distribution of services, costs, and financial security—rather than cost control and efficient resource allocation—the lack of information on Australian distributional patterns is disappointing. The incidence of costs can only be estimated approximately. Public expenditures—between 61 per cent and 73 per cent of all health expenditures over the decade—have the same incidence as general taxation, which may be slightly progressive with respect to income. Insurance premiums are not quite the equivalent of poll-taxes (all family rates are twice the single rate, so that families with children are subsidized in proportion to the numbers of children they support) but since they are flat-rate their incidence is regressive, even when modified by low-income concessions. The impact of user-charges varies with the service involved. Nearly half of all direct patient payments relate to dentistry (for which there is very little public funding) and non-prescribed drugs which are outside the medically-supervised system. Within the latter, user-charges are quite small—about 12 per cent for medical services and only about 3 per cent for hospitals—and the poorest people are, in principle at least, protected against them by a means-tested public programme. The overall income incidence of medically-supervised costs may at best be roughly proportional, whereas ten years ago it was distinctly regressive.

Almost nothing is known of the effects of the various financing systems on the distribution of services. The only purposeful attempt to assess the outcome of Medibank I was by Richardson and Phillips in 1976 from a survey of doctors similar to that conducted by Enterline, *et al.* in Quebec (16). There was some evidence that doctors *thought* that distribution had improved (17) and because changes in doctor behaviour were similar to those found by Enterline (and Beck and his associates in Saskatchewan), the tendency to generalize their other results was strong; that is, to assume that some redistribution of services towards the poor and disadvantaged groups resulted (18). Subsequent changes have produced anecdotal evidence of movements in the opposite direction, but neither claim has broad empirical support. Richardson found no significant relationship between service use and income (or any characteristics other than age and sex) in his study of private medical care usage in 1975-6 (19) and other workers using the 1977 Health Interview Survey of the Australian Bureau of Statistics have failed to establish any significant relationships with income in data from a later financing variant. However, the system of 1977 was still a universal one, and there is as yet no public data of behaviour since September 1981 when access to public treatment was restricted. Insurance membership certainly rises with income, so that financial security is apparently greater for the well-off; and usage also rises with the level of insurance, but self-selection based on known risk makes the apparent association of service use with income uncertain. About all that can be said is that whereas universal public funding tended to break down the association between delivery systems and income (public treatment for the poor, private for the rich) the current arrangements reinforce it.

CONCLUSIONS

Despite the special historical and institutional factors which it reflects, the Australian experience in health care financing may be of some relevance to other countries. Most interest will centre on the compulsory and voluntary versions of social insurance funding. For the latter is what the so-called private health insurance system in Australia has always been—the contracting-out of a basic social welfare programme. The benefit funds have been technically free to manage their affairs and to compete on the basis of different insurance options, but to qualify for subsidy they have had to offer specific forms of reimbursement insurance at uniform premiums for all, adhere to government-determined benefit schedules, impose no significant restrictions on payments (at least in their basic tables), and submit both their rules and their contribution rates for government approval. This regulation has been related to the social and public policy objectives of insurance, not merely its financial viability and, nominally at least, the objectives have been very little different under public or private operation—as high a level of membership as possible leading to as low an average premium as possible, with similar incentives and restrictions on consumers but rather less interference with suppliers in the private version. The insurance funds have *never* been policymakers in other than superficial matters. The various interest groups—doctors, hospitals, etc.—have always negotiated on policy issues with the Federal government, not the funds, and while the public view of these apparently private organizations is mixed, most people hold the government responsible for both the faults and virtues of the system. The organized medical profession supports voluntary reimbursement insurance through non-government organizations (with government subsidization of the poor and high-risk people) primarily because it preserves the private nature of the doctor-patient contract, but also because it places a buffer between doctors and the government, hinders the compilation of any centralized information and restricts the organizations' function to that of financial intermediary (although the Australian funds have never seen themselves in any other role). The States have tended to support it for similar reasons, and the diffusion of responsibility which it produces has been welcomed by a succession of Conservative Commonwealth administrations. Essentially, the Australian voluntary insurance system succeeded for so long because it offered advantages to all of the participating parties—the doctors, the Commonwealth government, the State governments, and the subscribers—without imposing binding obligations on any of them. Its importance as a revenue raising device is less significant than its support of a particular type of private health care delivery and a particular style of government.

As a revenue source outside the formal public sector but under close government control, private insurance has nevertheless been extremely successful. Since 1976, when a government came to office committed to reducing both public expenditures and the apparent influence of the central government, health care costs have been by far the easiest item of 'social' expenditures to shift. As pointed out earlier, about

12 per cent of all health expenditures were transferred from the Federal budget to the private sector between 1976 and 1981 and the current arrangements will ultimately shift a good deal more. Since they applied to short-term general hospitals and private medical care almost exclusively, the changes were much greater in those services and virtually all of the transferred costs were covered by insurance. That this was possible without any serious political consequences was due partly to the government's success in attributing health care cost increases entirely to centralized funding, but also to the pre-existence of an alternative financing system. No such systems exist in the broader field of social security or in services such as education in which any reduction in government funding leads directly to a reduction in service output. Where individuals have been able to insure, activity in the health services has not fallen at all; only where the States have been forced to cut back on uninsured activities (community health for example) have outputs and expenditures declined.

The base of this success is, of course, the extreme risk-aversion which Australians apparently feel with respect to health care costs. The latest statistics of insurance membership show that, in March 1982, 68 per cent of the population held medical insurance and 71 per cent held hospital cover (20). A year earlier the proportions were 58 per cent and 60 per cent respectively, which was before the universal entitlement to some Commonwealth benefit was withdrawn and before free public hospital care was terminated and fees substantially increased. In 1982, about 14 per cent were identified as entitled to free government benefits so that coverage was about 84 per cent of the population, and in the States where free public hospital services have been most severely restricted it was almost certainly higher. Not all of this response is rational. The few studies which have been carried out of health insurance buying behaviour in this country suggest that many people hold cover well in excess of the level which their health experience and expectations of service use would warrant (21), and there is also some evidence of confusion about the benefits which insurance actually conveys (22). For practical purposes, however, the fact is that most people can be induced to insure by the risk of large financial losses and that the higher are the charges for services the higher the level of insurance cover tends to be.

The issues are not as simple as this, however, because efficacy in revenue raising is not the only test of a financing system. In the first place, it can be argued that if people so fear health care costs that virtually everyone insures against them, then the insurance premium has many of the characteristics of a tax and must be judged accordingly. Supporters of the voluntary system would deny that any such thing as *de facto* compulsion could exist, but there are some logical inconsistencies in the criterion by which they, and the general public, judge the system's success—namely, the extent to which membership approaches universality. Equally important is the accessability of insurance to low-income people and the incidence of costs on them. This has always presented problems because flat-rate premiums have a regressive impact that can be modified by concessions to low-income earners only at the cost of great administrative complexity. At present, the combined family premium for insurance against medical fees and charges for basic accommodation in a public hospital represents 2·25 per cent of the income of a family with an income equal to the 'average weekly earnings' after tax concessions are taken into account (23). At an income just above the level where rights to free treatment terminate, the proportion is about 3 per cent, declining to less than 0·7 per cent for families with twice the average family income. With some rearrangement of existing government subsidies, a universal contribution of about 1·5 per cent of income would fund all current net payments through insurance, and the incidence would be slightly more favourable to lower income earners if the collection medium was general tax. Equity may not be an appropriate criterion on which to judge a purely voluntary programme, but when the system is an integral part of public policy its cost distribution is a legitimate subject of concern.

Other criteria

What of the properties of the various financing systems with respect to government intervention, cost control, and resource allocation? Here the Australian experience is again limited because all have been variants of the same fee-for-service reimbursement model, with almost identical incentive structures. Federal-State co-operation along Canadian lines has not flourished in Australia, except for the now terminated hospital cost-sharing agreements. Salaried medical services by other than trainee doctors are limited to the aged and the poor in public hospitals, and pre-paid plans (which once served a significant proportion of the population through the Friendly Societies) have almost disappeared. The organized medical profession is opposed to any extension of the former and is extremely suspicious of the latter. Prepayment *may* have some chance to develop now that access to public hospital treatment is no longer free, although it does not fit well with the structure of the state hospital systems, and the recruitment of doctors is still a problem.

Regulation

Within the standard reimbursement framework the degree of regulation has depended on the purposes which private insurance has been expected to serve. When it has been a major funding mechanism—as in the pre-1975 system and the present one—regulation has been as complete as in the public version, and has produced almost identical results. The basis for such regulation is, of course, that unrestricted competitive insurance is likely to produce results quite unacceptable on welfare grounds. Three main factors contribute to this probability. The first is 'moral hazard'—a situation where risks change with insurance against them. Health insurers are especially vulnerable to this condition, because they cannot normally verify the 'need' for services or the prices which should be paid for them. Delegation to physicians as agents is unavoidable, but physicians are also agents for their patients and, in Australia, entrepeneurs selling their own services for fees. To protect themselves against exploitation by either party, insurers commonly limit the range of services covered, offer fixed cash benefits only, and impose expenditure limits and/or significant co-insurance or co-payment provisions on extremes of use.

The second factor is that, whereas insurance deals only with unpredictable events, demands for health care are highly predictable for certain groups of people. In a competitive system differential pricing based on predictable risk-factors will soon draw the best risks away from any non-discriminating insurer, and in health insurance a great deal of the variation in service use is systematically related to such factors as age, sex, and health status. Thus 'experience rated' insurance will always be competitively superior to a 'community rated' (level premium) system as long as individuals can correctly assess their own health status and seek insurance which, at that particular time, is actuarially 'fair' to them. Such discrimination is technically unexceptionable, and unavoidable if good risk policy-holders are not to subsidize the bad.

Finally, there are the obvious properties of insurance with respect to the size and probability of losses. The coverage of highly predictable, small losses is relatively pointless, since the costs of administering and marketing insurance may raise the premium to equal or exceed them; whereas the gains from insuring against large but unlikely costs are considerable. 'Disaster insurance', offering indemnity against all costs in excess of a fixed amount, should therefore be a highly marketable commodity which has the additional advantage for the insurer of concentrating on medically-supervised procedures the 'need' for which can be most easily established. A competitive system would be expected to develop it.

The problem is that a programme which restricts the range of services covered, imposes reimbursement limits and co-payment requirements, and which charges the highest premiums to the old and sick, is not the kind of insurance the community wants. Many people regard as unjust any discrimination based on such characteristics as age, sex, and health status which are beyond the individuals' control, and hold coverage of the chronically-ill to be the *first* requirement of the system, not a risk to be avoided by exclusion. In fact, the equity criteria of social welfare actively *require* cross-subsidization between risk classes, on the basis of both income and health status. Other policy objectives may dictate a concern for resource allocation, whereas insurance as such is quite indifferent to it. Survival in a competitive climate will generally lead to more and more options of the amenities kind, leaving such 'uninsurable' services as preventive medicine and care of the chronically-ill to public programmes; and the implications of schemes like 'disaster' insurance may also be resisted by both administrators and suppliers (24). Insurance can provide the *mechanism* for risk-pooling in health but it may meet neither the allocative nor the distributional goals of social policy without conditions being imposed on it by government.

The Australian solution to these problems has been firstly to cover all the worst risks through public programmes (the aged, the mentally-ill, etc.), and secondly to use entitlement to government subsidies as a lever over the insurance funds. Direct subsidies are paid only to members of 'approved' organizations and only members of these funds qualify for tax concessions. 'Approved' funds are then bound, by law, to provide the type of non-discriminatory insurance which the government requires, and the subsidies payable directly and indirectly to their members are set at levels sufficient to make competitive commercial insurance unattractive. At present, nearly 50 per cent of all the monies passing through the health insurance funds are ultimately met from government sources—nearly 20 per cent in direct subsidies and about 30 per cent in tax concessions. Such a policy is undoubtedly effective, but it has nothing to do with the virtues of choice under competition usually advanced in support of a 'private' scheme. Its whole purpose is to *avoid* a competitive outcome.

Supplementary insurance

Where private insurance has been required only to provide supplementary benefits (as in Medibank I) the same problems of regulation have not arisen, although in practice a good deal of it remained. Where it was used in a competitive situation vis-a-viz public insurance (Medibank II) regulation was extreme (because benefits had to be identical in the two systems, though supplied at different prices), and both of the subsequent variants used regulation as their main policy weapon. Obviously however, the necessary regulation is not as great if welfare objectives are all achieved within the basic public system.

The main difficulty has been in defining what 'basic' and 'supplementary' are supposed to mean. There is a widespread, somewhat naive, belief that *a priori* distinctions can be made between 'necessary' and 'unnecessary' services, and that the problems of financing would somehow be solved if public programmes were limited to necessary treatment. Such distinctions are, of course, impossible to make. The only optional items which have been generally agreed upon are insurance for cash benefits above the standard level (relevant only when standard benefits are less than fees) and the right to 'private' status and/or superior accommodation in hospitals. Otherwise, services have been either wholly included or wholly excluded, not on grounds of efficacy but according to whether they are medically-supervised or not, doctors being regarded as the 'managers' of the system (25). Categorical exclusions of this kind seem unavoidable in public programmes. They could apply to classes of people as well as classes of services—the well-off for example—but they would be based on different policy considerations.

Cost-control and resource allocation

As suggested earlier, the aggregate statistics give no clear indication of the cost-controlling properties of the various financing systems. Since state public hospitals are by far the largest expenditure item, much has depended on the *total* funds available to the States, not only those specifically related to health. There is some evidence that in the very long run, the most 'public' hospital systems are the least expensive and that they allocate resources in a somewhat different way. Per capita, hospital and medical costs are below the national average in Queensland and Tasmania— about 20 per cent below in both cases for Queensland—with apparently somewhat lower surgical procedure rates (26). International comparisons suggest the same conclusions and their policy implications were one of the main reasons for encouraging 'public' hospital treatment under Medibank.

In the short period, however, the advent of centralized funding in 1975–6 probably raised costs by allowing the State public hospitals to expand some services more than they would otherwise have done. Other Federal government programmes also treated the States generously at that time and the fiscal regime was relatively lax. Although this was a problem of public finance generally, to which there were a number of general solutions, some change in hospital cost-sharing was probably desirable. Medical care costs were influenced by different factors. Superficially, the advent of National Insurance corresponded with the largest medical fee increases on record. Average fees rose by 22 per cent in 1974–5, the year preceding Medibank, and by 34 per cent in 1975–6, rates well above the total increase of 31 per cent in general consumer prices over the two years (27). Increases since then have been less than in the CPI and there is no doubt that political considerations influenced the vigour with which the AMA prosecuted its fee claims under the Labor Government. But they were granted by an independant Fee Tribunal using a formula established in previous hearings and represented a delayed response to inflation over a period when the AMA had, also for political reasons, restrained its claims. The subsequent reduction in increases was partly due to the profession's co-operation (no claim was made in 1977) but also to a change in the attitude of Fee Tribunals away from the mechanical adjustment of fees by selected cost indexes to a consideration of the incomes which those fees produce.

Changes in attitudes have, in fact, been the major outcome of the financing experiments over the last decade, and the main potential influence for cost control. Centralized financing concentrated attention on both the level and the distribution of health care costs because of their impact on *one* level of government. An immediate consequence was an intense popular interest in doctor incomes and the fraudulent exploitation of the system by some doctors. Fraud clearly existed, but its overall impact was overstated, and it was gradually realized that over-servicing was just as significant an issue; and that it may have been just as prevalent under the preceding system but had not been revealed until the Medibank statistical collections (based largely on Canadian models) accumulated sufficient data. Until then, no one authority had a sufficient interest to pursue the matter.

The result has been a complete change in the position of the medical profession. From a policy of bitterly opposing any review of medical work under Medibank I, the AMA has come to an acceptance and a grudging but growing support of peer review. The original Medibank system established Medical Service Committees of Inquiry to investigate allegations of fraud and over-servicing by doctors under the bulk-billing system. The majority of their members were to be practising doctors, but the AMA initially refused to nominate any representatives to them. This prohibition was relaxed in 1976 after the Labor Government had fallen. In May 1976, the Association accepted a substantial grant from the Commonwealth government to investigate peer review systems after the Minister for Health had pointed out that if the profession did not establish effective review mechanisms within a period of three years, the government would consider action. Neither result actually eventuated, but the AMA has continued to promote the programme despite the reluctance and even hostility of its more conservative members (28). In early 1982, figures compiled by the Department of Health suggesting that fraud and over-servicing by doctors accounted for medical benefit payments of at least $100m—about 6 per cent of the total—were actually *announced* by the AMA, which promised its full support for legislation strengthening both the investigative powers of the Department and the penalties available to it. While the motives for this AMA move are not entirely clear—anxiety over possible government action may have been just as important as dissociation from the less reputable minority of doctors—the fact remains that the present attitudes of organized medicine would have been unthinkable a decade ago.

Prospects

The Australian financing system is still not stable. The present arrangements, like their pre-1975 antecedents, meet the current Federal government's budgetary targets very well and have none of the self-destructive tendencies of their immediate predecessors. Unrestricted access to public hospital treatment, inpatient, or outpatient, is simply not compatible with voluntary insurance as a major and reliable source of funds as long as the public alternative is 'free'. Good-risk people do not insure under these conditions. In every financing variant between Medibank I and the present system, use by people other than pensioners was significantly higher amongst those with insurance than those without, and the higher users chose the highest cover. Premiums were therefore under constant pressure, but the higher the premium level the more that healthy people—particularly single people —tended to rely on public facilities and government benefits, even when the rates of benefit were low (29). Restriction of this option to the aged and the needy is an obvious solution to the problem of instability in the insurance market. As far as cost control is concerned, the prospects are uncertain. On the one hand the financial and administrative systems introduced in 1981 diffuse responsibility in much the same way as their predecessors of pre-1975, with incentives to cost containment correspondingly reduced. On the other, new patterns of behaviour have been set. Most of the centralized statistical collections will remain, incomes' have been admitted as the basic factors in fee adjustment, and peer review accepted as contributing to both quality assurance and protection from abuse. In these respects, the *status quo* has not returned.

Political considerations may well be more important, however. The opposition Labor Party is committed to a return to universal insurance almost identical to Medibank 1, with a renewed emphasis on public care. Its arguments are based largely on equity, but also on the contention that private insurance is inherently cost-expanding, and that the only restrictive elements—Commonwealth influence over State hospital budgets, centralized medical-fee fixing and utilization review—all originated in the universal scheme. Labor has reasonable prospects of election in 1983 so that the experience of 1973–5 may be repeated with only minor modification. Whether it would lead to the same degree of confrontation remains to be seen.

NOTES AND REFERENCES

1. See R. G. PALMER, 'Commonwealth/State Fiscal Relationships and the Financing and Provision of Health Services', in P. M. TATCHELL, (ed.) *Economics and Health 1981,* Health Research Project, Australian National University, 1981, p. 3.

2. The balance were salaried doctors with part-time private practice rights.

3. No charge for old age pensioners or veterans.

4. No discriminatory pricing was permitted and the subsidy system effectively excluded commercial competitors.

5. Previous Commonwealth subsidies, by favouring those States which charged fees, were just as intrusive, but their operation was slow and their objectives unstated.

6. Ironically, exactly the same impost, at about half the rate, had been refused by the same parties in opposition.

7. The definition of 'disadvantaged persons' was left vague and at the doctors' discretion, but was broadly intended to cover the unemployed and non-aged social service beneficiaries.

8. In two States, formal cost-sharing agreements of 10 years currency could not be terminated, but arbitrary reduction in Commonwealth government payments has had the same effects.

9. Sources are shown in Appendix 1.

10. Apparently, because the promise of cost-sharing led the States to change their accounting systems to attribute to hospitals many services previously costed to general revenue. The real position cannot now be known.

11. For a detailed analysis of financing changes to 1978, see R. B. SCOTTON, in *Public Expenditures and Social Policy in Australia,* SCOTTON and FERBER (eds.), Institute of Applied Economic and Social Research, University of Melbourne, Vols. 1 and 2, 1978, 1980.

12. Figures for doctor numbers and apparent workloads are not available for 1978–9 because of changes in the taxation statistics on which they are based.

13. Because of the high proportion of people taking insurance for '100 per cent cover' and their relatively high use.

14. Although 32 per cent of patient-billed services were charged at more than scheduled fees at June 1979, the value of over-billing was only 2·4 per cent of total fee receipts.

15. 'Medical Fees Under Insurance' in P. M. TATCHELL, (ed.) *Health Economics, 1981,* Health Research Project, Australian National University, 1982, p. 24.

16. J. R. J. RICHARDSON, and T. PHILLIPS, *Report of a Survey of Sydney Medical Practitioners Before and After Medibank,* Macquarie University, School of Economic and Financial Studies, Research Paper No. 109, 1977.

17. 23 per cent of GPs and 35 per cent of specialists thought that patient access had improved, over three times the proportions who thought that crowding-out was a significant problem.

18. R. G. BECK, and J. M. HORNE, *An Analytical Overview of the Saskatchewan Co-payment Experiment in the Hospital and Ambulatory Care Settings,* Report to the Ontario Council of Health, Ottawa, 1978, and PHILLIP E. ENTERLINE, *et al.,* 'Effects of free medical care on medical practice—The Quebec Experience', *The New England Journal of Medicine,* May 31, 1973, pp. 1152–5.

19. J. R. J. RICHARDSON, 'The inducement hypothesis: That doctors generate demand for their own services' in J. VAN DER GAAG, and M. PERLMAN, (eds.), *Health, Economics, and Health Economics,* North Holland, Amsterdam, 1981, p. 189.

20. AUSTRALIAN BUREAU OF STATISTICS, *Health Insurance Survey, March 1982,* (Preliminary), table 3.

21. See C. BURROWS, and K. BROWN, 'Health insurance decision making: an exploratory study', in P. M. TATCHELL, (ed.) *Economics and Health, 1980,* Health Research Project, Australian National University, 1981, p. 100.

22. Some apparently believe that uninsured people will not be treated, which is of course wrong, but an attitude fostered by some suppliers (including some public hospitals).

23. Strictly, 'Average weekly earnings per employed male unit', a statistic which weights male and female earnings by the composition of the workforce.

24. Because of its cost increasing tendencies (low-cost services have a high marginal price to users, high-cost services a low one) and because it underwrites the incomes of some suppliers more effectively than others.

25. The only non-hospital exceptions are refraction services by optometrists, which were added in 1975 after years of dispute with the opthamologists.

26. See *Report of the Commission of Inquiry into the Efficiency and Administration of Hospitals* (The Jamison Report), AGPS, 1981, Vol. 2; J. R. J. Richardson, and J. S. Deeble, *Statistics of Private Medical Services in Australia, 1976,* Health Research Project, Australian National University, 1982.

27. Deeble, *op.cit.,* p. 30.

28. A good deal of work has actually been done, including the publication of a regular series of case study reports.

29. Under the 'opting-out' variant, this had no serious financial implications, because the levy was high enough to more than finance the extra public spending, but preservation of the private sector share *per se* was an equally important policy consideration.

APPENDIX 1

Statistical sources

Table 1
DEEBLE, J. S. *Health Expenditures in Australia, 1960-1 to 1975-6.* (Health Research Project, Australian National University, Canberra, 1978).
—— and SCOTTON, R. B. 'Health Services and the Medical Profession' in K. A. Tucker (ed.) *Economics of the Australian Service Sector.* (Croom Helm; London, 1978).
COMMONWEALTH DEPARTMENT OF HEALTH. *Australian Health Expenditure 1974-5 to 1978-9; an Analysis.* (Canberra: AGPS, 1981).
COMMONWEALTH DEPARTMENT OF HEALTH. *Annual Reports.*
Taxation Statistics. Supplement to the *Annual Report of the Commissioner of Taxation.* (AGPS, various issues).
HEALTH INSURANCE COMMISSION, *Annual Reports.*

Figures 1 and 2—deflators derived from:

For institutional care
TATCHELL, P. M., 'Rising Wage Costs in Victorian Hospitals', *Community Health Studies,* **3**(3), 1979.
SCHAPPER, P. R., *Measurement and Analysis of Australian Hospital Expenditure, 1970-1 to 1978-9.* (University of Western Australia, 1980).

For medical and other professional services
DEEBLE, J. S., 'Medical Fees Under Insurance' in P. M. Tatchell (ed.) *Economics and Health, 1981.* (Health Research Project, Australian National University, 1982).
SCOTTON, R. B., *Medical Care in Australia: An Economic Diagnosis.* (Sun Books: Melbourne, 1974).

For drugs
COMMONWEALTH DEPARTMENT OF HEALTH, *Annual Reports* (average cost per prescription).

For other items
AUSTRALIAN BUREAU OF STATISTICS, *Australian National Accounts,* implicit price deflators for government expenditures on health and social security.

Figures 3, 4, and 5
COMMONWEALTH DEPARTMENT OF HEALTH, *Annual Reports;* HEALTH INSURANCE COMMISSION, *Annual Reports; Report of The Commission of Inquiry into the Efficiency and Administration of Hospitals* (AGPS, 1981); DEEBLE, J. S., 'Medical Fees Under Insurance', *op.cit.*

Table 2
HEALTH INSURANCE COMMISSION, *Annual Reports;* COMMONWEALTH DEPARTMENT OF HEALTH, *Annual Reports,* 1978-9, 1979-80.

465

PART
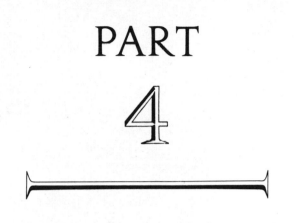
4

Finale

PART

4

Finale

Reviewing the evidence

The preceding essays on the public/private mixes in the European, North American, and Australian environments have demonstrated that despite the great variety in the arrangements of health care finance and provision, many of the policy problems are common across all health care systems. The ubiquitous nature of the concerns about cost containment, efficiency in the use of resources and equity in the distribution of services at present tend to lead to policy innovations which are poorly constructed and ineffectively implemented.

The purpose of this section is to bring together the more relevant of these regulatory experiences and draw some conclusions from them for policy formulation in all health care systems in the future. The chapter on regulation by Maynard emphasizes that superficial concerns derived from naive ideological perspectives, both socialist and liberal, have wasted scarce intellectual resources and prevented careful evaluation of the improvements in health care systems, public and private.

There is no substitute for reading all the essays for relevance but the final essay draws together the lessons to be learnt from altering the public/private mix and analyses some of the implications of increasing the size of the private sector. In addition some policy initiatives are set out, together with a series of questions drawn from the essays, which could form the basis of an ambitious but desirable research agenda, within a coherent strategy so that the present inefficiencies and inequalities of health care systems, public and private, can be reduced and the optimum use made of resources.

469

The regulation of
public and private health
care markets

ALAN MAYNARD

ALAN MAYNARD

Alan Maynard is a Reader in Health Economics at the University of York, England and Director of the Graduate Programme in Health Economics in the Department of Economics and Related Studies at York. He has been a visiting lecturer at the University Institute of European Studies, Milan, Italy; the Department of Economics, University of Otago, New Zealand; the Institute of Public Finance, University of Genoa, Italy; and the Department of Economics, University of Gothenburg Sweden. He is an examiner for the Faculty of Community Medicine of the Royal College of Physicians of the United Kingdom and a member of the York Health Authority and the York Family Practitioner Committee. He has worked as a consultant for the Commission of the European Community, the Organization for Economic Co-operation and Development, the World Health Organization, and for governments and industry.

He has written widely in books, academic journals, and elsewhere and one of his main interests for the past ten years has been the economics of the organization and regulation of health care systems. His conviction is that the nature of the health and health care policy choices, and their associated problems, are similar wherever you may go on this planet!

The regulation of public and private health care markets

ABSTRACT

The thesis elaborated in this chapter is that policy problems in health care systems, whether they are of an efficiency or a distributional nature, are similar across the Western world. Differences in institutional structure do not remove the need for decision-makers, public and private, to regulate prices, and the quantities and qualities of services provided in health care systems.

After a general introduction which outlines the similarity of policy problems across different countries, the nature of the ideology of the 'marketeers' and the 'collectivists' is elaborated. A common ideological liberal or market 'strain' of literature is described and the characteristics of the alternative ideologies is set out. This analysis indicates that the proponents of the different ideologies seek different goals and prefer different means to achieve these ends.

The characteristics of the health care market are elaborated: monopolistic, non-competitive markets, the primacy of the doctor in making decisions about resource allocation, and the imperfection of both private and public funding arrangements.

This analysis is followed by an investigation of the necessary conditions which have to be met if the market is to work in a competitive manner. It is pointed out that the abolition of the monopoly power of the professions will be difficult to implement—because it will involve the substitution of cheaper labour inputs, creating unemployment and reduced incomes amongst professionals. Furthermore the effects of patient co-payments will affect the utilization of health care, particularly outside the hospital, and this may not be consistent with distributional goals. The effects of 'market' incentive schemes, for instance fee-per-item of service payments, may induce expenditure inflation and may make budget limitation difficult to attain. Much of this analysis of the market is hypothetical, i.e. the evidence to refute competing assertions about

473

outcomes is incomplete. However the evidence that is available indicates that a competitive market would be difficult to create and sustain: to acquire and maintain the market would require government regulation.

This is not to say the collective alternative is flawless. In fact it has many of the problems of its market 'twin'. The mechanisms to achieve the ends of the collectivists have not been developed. Nationalization of the UK health service did not change the fundamental nature of the health care market: it merely changed its finance and ownership but it did not alter the poor incentives for decision-makers to strive for efficiency and equity.

The conclusion reached after the discussion of the market and the NHS alternatives in health care is that both are defective because of the lack of definition of policy objectives and the absence of incentives which induce decision-makers, largely doctors, to strive after the efficient use of resources and distributional justice. Both types of organization, the market and the NHS, must develop mechanisms which ensure that decision-makers are induced to achieve policy goals. Such mechanisms, always and everywhere, imply regulation of prices, quantities, and qualities by public and private institutions: the problems of BUPA, Blue Cross/Blue Shield, and the NHS are very similar.

INTRODUCTION

Policy-makers in health care systems throughout the world are facing similar problems and their attempts to grapple with these problems are leading to a sharper definition of the universal policy issues and the alternative ways of dealing with them. The principal issues of health care in the 1980s seem to be cost-containment, best subsumed into the general problem of efficiency, and distributional equity.

Once it is recognized that the historical role of health care in the reduction of disease levels and death rates has been limited and less important than improvements in nutrition, water supply, and sewerage (McKeown, 1977, 1979), and that the majority of health care therapies in use today have not been evaluated in a scientific fashion and hence may lack efficacy despite their high cost (Cochrane, 1972), the true magnitude of the problems involved in evaluating competing health care policies can be seen. It is difficult to identify and eradicate existing inefficient practices and it is difficult for policy makers to oppose the introduction of new therapies. The tradition of the medical profession and policy makers has been to assume that innovations are efficacious and to commit large amounts of resources on the basis of faith rather than on the basis of evidence of relative advantage in outcomes and costs.

The design of health care systems, both 'socialized' and 'private', has tended to reduce the price barrier to consumption to the patient, care is provided free or at a highly subsidized price, and has ensured that the cost constraints on producers, in particular doctors, are minimal: the costs are borne by insurers, sickness funds, or the taxpayer, i.e. the third-party pays. Thus health care systems encourage patients to maximize consumption regardless of costs, and producers (doctors) to maximize, within the constraints of their ignorance about efficacy, benefits regardless of costs. Both demanders and suppliers have no incentives to compare and trade-off the costs and benefits of health care at the margin.

The behaviour of demanders and suppliers has inevitably led to a rapid escalation in the costs of health care, and the adoption of cost containment policies. These policies, usually quite naive and concerned with the limitation of increases in expenditure and not with the effects of such policies on the price, quality, and quantity of health care delivered, have been adopted in a variety of guises in a majority of countries. In West Germany the Concerted Action programme (see Dr Beske's chapter) has sought to limit budget expansion by mutual agreement between producer, financer, and beneficiary interests. In Belgium cost inflation has led to the discussion of radical changes in public provision and the development of private provision. Similar developments have taken place throughout the European Community (Abel-Smith and Maynard, 1979), in North America (e.g. see Schweitzer (ed.), 1978) and in Australasia (e.g. see the Jamieson Report, 1980).

Some of these measures have been discussed with remarkably little attention being paid to the need for more micro-evaluation (cost-benefit and cost-effectiveness analysis) and for the development of incentive systems which induce decision makers, both patients and doctors, to take action to minimize costs and maximize benefits. The lack of such incentives has contributed to the rapid escalation in costs and expenditures in health care, and to the situation where many of the therapies in use remain of unknown or dubious validity (Cochrane, 1972; Bunker, Barnes, and Mosteller (eds), 1977).

Any discussion of cost-containment and efficiency is usually complicated by the propensity of policy-makers to introduce, often implicitly, distributional issues. These take a variety of forms. Most health care systems are characterized by explicit policies to secure advantages to particular geographical areas and socio-economic groups.

Geographical inequalities in the provision of health care facilities have led to policies to equalize either financial capacity or more directly, the provision of facilities, especially beds. In 1970 the first resource allocation formula was introduced in England, and since then a variety of formulae have been evolved for the constituent parts of the United Kingdom (Maynard and Ludbrook, 1980a). In 1971 the French adopted the 'health map' which is a mechanism used to direct hospital bed resources to underprovided areas. In 1972 the Germans began to provide Federal funds for hospital beds, provided new construction reduced geographical inequalities in provision. More recently the Italians, the Dutch, and the New Zealanders have begun to discuss RAWP-type (Resource Allocation Working Party—Department of Health and Social Security, 1976) formulae (e.g. Department of Health (NZ), 1980) and similar attempts to control the geographical allocation of resources have been implemented in North America.

Whilst the degree of government financial involvement in the provision of health care varies across countries, all developed countries provide some subsidies to give special support to poor groups: although the magnitude of involvement varies, no country has failed to recognize that some groups, usually the poor, the aged, and the chronic sick (here used as a collective term to cover the mentally ill, the mentally and physically handicapped, and those with long-term illnesses such as cancer and TB), require special treatment which is bound to involve special funding. This concern manifests itself as Medicare and Medicaid in the United States, Federal and State finance of health care for the 'needy' in Australia, the comprehensive 'heavy risks' insurance programme in the Netherlands, and many similar programmes elsewhere. The experience of these countries is that a substantial section of the community is unlikely to be able to buy health care insurance coverage in the market, and that as a consequence the State must offer substantial subsidies of one form and another. With such subsidies comes government concern about 'value for money' (efficiency) and access (distribution). This concern seems to generate inevitably further State regulation of the health care market.

It is against this international background of common problems and the similarity of policy responses in nations with very different health care systems, that this chapter is written. The current debate about health care policy, wherever it takes place, is set against a background of severe public expenditure constraints, little knowledge about the efficiency with which health care is produced, and ill-defined (and usually unevaluated) distributional goals. Because of these background characteristics, in particular because of the numerous, generally perverse incentives which do not induce economical behaviour in decision-makers, the State has sought to increase its regulation of this market place, or divest itself of some of its responsibilities by allocating them to the private sector.

Whether health care is provided and financed publicly or privately, these problems are ubiquitous. If the response of the State is to regulate it will seek to use existing and develop new policy instruments to affect the prices, quantities, and qualities of health care services. This task is fraught with difficulties because of our ignorance of the nature of the input/output link and because of the economic power of many of the groups demanding and supplying health care.

If the State fails in its efforts to regulate the public sector's provision and finance of health care, it can divest itself of these functions i.e. they can be privatized. However whilst such policies may reduce public expenditure, the overall effect on total (social) expenditures on health care is unlikely to lead to economy, as the fundamental problems involved in the delivery of health care remain. The private financers and providers will ultimately face the same pressures that are generated in a public system, as can be seen in the United States. They will respond to these pressures by self-regulation i.e. the private insurers will seek to control the prices, quantities, and quality of health care.

So whether the State or private agencies finance and provide health care, the fundamental problems of this market are similar and regulatory activity, defined as action by financers and providers to manipulate prices, quantities and quality, is unavoidable and ubiquitous (Maynard and Ludbrook, 1980b).

This thesis will be developed below. After a discussion of ideology, which demonstrates how much of the contemporary debate about health care is dominated by values, the nature of the health care market will be elaborated. This is followed by a discussion of the nature of the liberal/market and collectivist/socialist options in health care and the development of the thesis that regulations in the health care market are ubiquitous and unavoidable.

THE IDEOLOGY AND THE OBJECTIVES OF THE REFORMERS

A consistent ideological position characterizes those who, over the last twenty years, have sought to reform, or even to, abolish the National Health Service. This section will summarize these arguments and then compare and contrast the competing ideologies in an attempt to identify the objectives of the reformers and the defenders of the NHS.

The first carefully articulated critique of the NHS by a member of the reformers group was published in the early 1960s and written by Dennis Lees (1965). Lees argued that the market was a superior mechanism (to the ballot box) for registering consumer choices and that the most efficient means of providing care was in a competitive market which created incentives for decision-makers to take appropriate action to minimize costs rather than in a State monopoly where there were limited incentives. He argued that patients could be subsidized if necessary and that the State 'would retain a special responsibility for the mentally ill and the chronic sick' (Lees, 1965 p. 77). Lees argued that because of the insensitivity of the vote mechanism, health care had been underfinanced in the NHS and he advocated the common Institute of Economic Affairs preference for decentralized rather than centralized decision making.

The 'Jones' Report (1970) also asserted that the NHS was underfinanced, although it offered no means of determining what this term meant in any exact sense. The writers of the Report argued that additional finance could not be acquired from taxation and that the bulk of everyday health care for the normally healthy should be financed out of private insurance. This insurance would be compulsory for all to some (government determined) national minimum but consumers would be free to purchase cover over and above this level. The premia of these policies would be related to costs and the Report emphasized the need for State regulation of the insurance industry to prevent cost escalation (Jones, 1970 p. 156). Those unable to pay the compulsory premiums would be subsidized via the tax system: the poor, the aged, and the chronic sick would be credited with compulsory insurance cover, and their family income subsidies would decline *parri passu* with income increases until they paid the full cost of the premium. These subsidies would be financed out of government taxes.

The more recent reformist literature on the financing of the NHS tends to be more polemical and generally less carefully articulated. Two books in this literature (Goodman, 1980, Lindsay, 1980) are written for American audiences as contributions to the debate about national health insurance in the USA, and seek to demonstrate the weaknesses of the NHS. This they do in a highly imperfect manner; the Royal Commission on the NHS (1979) provides a much more analytical approach to the Service's defects than is available in the limited, and sometimes inaccurate, work of Goodman in particular.

Goodman and Lindsay contribute to the Litmus papers

(Seldon, 1980). The style of these papers is polemical and very superficial. No serious issues are discussed and over twenty authors offer often emotive and always very short 'pyrotechnics' on disparate issues. The themes which come out of these papers are familiar: rejection of the 'monopoly bureaucratic power' of the NHS, a preference for 'choice', decentralization, and private insurance, and an assertion that the NHS is a more inefficient and inequitable health care system than some of its private and insurance financed rivals.

Many of these preferences are consistent with what, following Donabedian (1971), we might call the market ideology. The implications of this ideology, and its collectivist alternative, are discussed in the context of health care in Culyer, Maynard, and Williams (1982). Following the framework used there it is possible to distinguish between the two ideologies in relation to their beliefs about personal responsibility, social concern, freedom, and equality:

Personal responsibility
Market view. Personal responsibility for achievement is seen as very important, and this is weakened if people are offered unearned rewards. (e.g. 'free' health care). Furthermore, such unearned rewards weaken the motive force that assures economic well-being (e.g. incentives to work to save and to take risks). The weakening of the motive force which generates economic growth also undermines moral well-being, because of the intimate connection between moral well-being and the personal effort to achieve.
Collectivist view. While accepting the desirability of some personal incentives to achieve, economic failure is not equated with moral depravity or social worthlessness.

Social concern
Social Darwinism dictates a seemingly cruel indifference to the fate of those who fail in the economic system. A less extreme position is that charity, preferably expressed and carried out under private auspices, is the proper vehicle to meet social concern. Charity however needs to be exercised under carefully prescribed conditions, for example such that the potential recipient must first mobilize all his own re-

sources, and when helped, must not be in as a favourable position as those who are self-supporting (the principle of 'lesser eligibility'). Without such provisions, incentives, economic growth and moral well-being will be reduced

Private charitable action is rejected, and is seen as potentially dangerous morally (because it is often demeaning to the recipient and corrupting to the donor) and usually inequitable. It seems preferable to construct social mechanisms that create and sustain self-sufficiency, and are accessible according to precise rules concerning entitlement which are applied equitably and explicitly sanctioned by society at large.

Freedom

Freedom is to be sought as a supreme good in itself. Compulsion attenuates both personal responsibility and individualistic and voluntary expressions of social concern. Centralized health planning and a large governmental role in health care financing are seen as an unwarranted reduction of the freedom of clients (patients) as well as of health professionals (providers), and private medicine is therefore viewed as a bulwark against totalitarianism.

Freedom is seen as the presence of real opportunities of choice, and although economic constraints are less openly coercive than political constraints, they are none the less real, and often the effective limits on choice. Freedom is not indivisible, but may be sacrificed in one respect in order to obtain greater freedom in some other. Government is seen not as an external threat to individuals in the society, but the means by which individuals achieve greater freedom of choice (that is, greater real freedom).

Equality

Equality before the law is the key concept, with clear precedence being given to freedom over equality wherever the two conflict.

Since the only moral justification for using personal achievement as the basis for distributing rewards, is that everyone has equal opportunities for such achievement, then the main emphasis is on equality for opportunity, and where this cannot be assured, the moral worth of achievement is thereby undermined. Equality is seen as an extension to the many of the freedoms actually enjoyed only by the few.

The detractors of the NHS have a strong preference for freedom as elaborated in the market ideology, and from this prime objective it is possible to identify their preferred means to attain this goal:

Selectivity

Health care is part of the reward system of society and the well-being of society depends on this reward system. As a result access to health care is to be determined largely by ability and willingness to pay. Those without the ability to pay would be guaranteed some minimal level of access to health care. Thus this approach regards inequality as efficient: it is the engine of economic growth and the guarantee of freedom. Also it implies private (insurance) finance of health care.

Private ownership

Freedom requires decentralization and private (usually non-profit making) ownership of the means of production (e.g. hospitals) with only minimal government control of finance and resource allocation.

Rewards

Providers of care (e.g. doctors) to be directly rewarded according to market forces, usually with a fee-per-item of service system of remuneration for doctors and *per diem* fees paid to hospitals.

Those rejecting this ideology (e.g. the defenders of the NHS) regard equality of access to health care and of health status as their prime objectives. The means by which this goal can be attained are:

Universality

Health care is not part of the reward system and should be allocated on the basis of need or the patient's capacity to benefit from care regardless of their willingness or ability to pay. Universality implies public finance of health care.

Public ownership

Equality requires centralization and public ownership of the means of production (e.g. hospitals) with extensive government control of finance and resource allocation.

Rewards

Providers of care will be rewarded by the outcome of bureaucratic bargaining procedures between monopoly providers (e.g. doctors) and monopsonistic financers (the NHS).

The goals of 'freedom' and 'equality' are imprecise. The means by which these goals will be attained are generally asserted to be efficient. Usually health care systems have goals whose nature is imprecise and even where some degree of precision is attained in goal-setting, the efficiency of the means is an area of supposition rather than of fact. The contending ideologies contain empirical statements whose verity could and should be tested. Unfortunately at this level of argument such scientific rigour is noticeable by its absence and, as a consequence, we have, through time, the recurring advocacy of privatization or socialization. Whilst such advocacy may be the stuff of politics, it guarantees, by its dominance and use of scarce intellectual and policy making talent, that policy formulation is superficial and that scarce resources in policy analysis are wasted.

The naive pyrotechnics of the contending ideologists must be set aside. All parties, whatever their ideological predilections, must recognize the precise nature of the health care market and the ramifications for policy, public and private, of the imperfections of this market.

THE NATURE OF THE HEALTH CARE MARKET

Monopolistic non-competitive markets

The advocates of the market solution recognize that a major obstacle to the smooth running of a competitive market is monopoly power, or the ability of the sellers of health care services to influence (to their advantage) the prices of their services. As Adam Smith (1776) observed over two hundred years ago:

People of the same trade seldom meet together, even for
merriment and diversion, but the conversation ends in a
conspiracy against the public, or in some contrivance to
raise prices. Smith (1776), Everyman edition (1910),
book 1, chapter 10, page 117.

Thus the health market is not competitively organized: it
is highly imperfect and characterized by powerful monopolies which inhibit the free play of the competitive 'hidden'
hand of the market.

The market for health care is characterized also by uncertainty: the patient does not know when he will be ill, and the
patient may be relatively inefficient in determining the appropriate diagnosis and treatment. Generally the comparative knowledge of doctors may be greater and society, in
order to protect its members from 'quacks' and uncertainty
has created social institutions, professional regulation, to
ensure that doctors are 'expert' in their trade and do offer
efficacious health care. (see Arrow, 1963).

The counter argument to this position has been set out by
Friedman (1962) who argues that professional regulation is
used to further the interests of the profession. Citing US
experience, he argues that the profession by controlling entry
into medical schools, has restricted the supply of doctors, and
inflated their wages. Furthermore it is argued that professional control has permitted discrimination of a racial, sex-
ual, and colour nature, and that the profession has inflated
the 'quality' of doctors (measured in terms of duration of
training) regardless of its costs and in the absence of scientific
evidence that the quality of physicians (measured in terms of
their impact on the health status of patients) is adequate.

Whether the Arrow or the Friedman position is adopted, it
is clear that the State, in all Western countries, has given the
medical profession considerable monopoly powers to influence the quantity and quality of its services and its own
remuneration. The evidence available about the effects of
this seems to indicate that the profession has used its power
both in public interest and in its own self-interest (see e.g.
Frech, 1974 and Leffler, 1978). Thus professional organizations use their power to influence their remuneration and

hence all such organizations will seek to protect health care expenditure as it is their income!

The uncertainty associated with health care which led to State enforcement of professional power, creates additional problems. The individual patient is typically quite poorly informed about diagnostic techniques and treatments. Although it is generally an individual patient decision to make the first contact with the health care system, after that much of the demand decision-making may be delegated by the patient to the doctor. Thus the patient uses the doctor as his agent to make health care demand decisions for him and it can be argued that the supplier of health care (the doctor) is the demander rather than the patient. (For a summary of the literature see US Department of Health and Human Services, 1981).

If this agency relationship is used neutrally by the doctor, that is in the interests of the patient only, there may be limited implications for the efficient use of resources. The doctor may however use this relationship non-neutrally, e.g. to increase his income by raising the demands for his services, by increasing the size of his 'empire', and by pressing for other ends which are not conducive to efficiency. This theory of physician-induced demand, that doctors can create demand for their services, has been tested imperfectly. Some of the evidence that is available (e.g. Fuchs, 1978) seems to substantiate this hypotheses in part anyway, e.g. Fuchs finds that a 10 per cent increase in the supply of surgeons, all else held constant, leads to a 3 per cent increase in surgical activity. Other evidence indicates that not only can physicians generate demand for their own services, they may also be able to raise their fees as their number increases. (US Department of Health and Human Services, 1981).

The effects of professional power and the agency relationship cannot be ignored in any discussion of the supply of health care in particular and health care policy in general. Professional power has given doctors control over their training and a strong influence over the supply of doctors and their earnings. This power has led to increases of inputs (training time) in training but little evaluation of this training and little investment in managerial and economic skills, or in scientific evaluation, despite the fact that doctors are managers of scarce resources. Furthermore monopoly power may be used to create demand for doctors services. Thus the existing market for doctors is highly imperfect (i.e. non-competitive) and this fact cannot be ignored in policy discussions.

Not only is the market for doctors services characterized by monopoly, there are also severe restrictions on competition elsewhere in the health care market. The pharmaceutical companies are highly regulated by the State and have been given monopoly powers by it, e.g. patent legislation. The hospital sector is either State owned, at local or central level, or run by private non-profit-making bodies. The incentives to seek out cost-effective practices in both the State sector and the private non-profit making sectors may be similar and weak: in both types of organization the managers get no direct reward in any cost savings so why should they seek them out? Not only are incentives weak, there is also scope for 'producer agreements', often protected by State legislation, which may limit competition in the market for hospital beds.

Thus the supply side of the health care market is characterized by a lack of competition and powerful, well established, State supported monopoly power. It is not surprising that in this environment we know little about the efficiency with which resources are used. Efficiency, in economic terms, means that resources are used in a way which ensures the least cost production of these goods and services which are most highly valued by society. In the context of the health care market the doctor may regard a procedure as 'efficient' (=clinically effective) if it is the most effective therapy available to improve the health status of the individual suffering from a particular complaint: often evidence to reach this conclusion will be absent due to the lack of evaluation of practice. A procedure may be cost-effective if it is the cheapest way of achieving a given therapeutic end, with the value of this end (outcome) being unquestioned. A procedure is economically efficient if cost is minimized, outcome benefit is maximized, and the services provided are those most highly valued by society. In the health care market, the supply side forces which induce the achievement of this outcome, the efficient use of resources, are limited. Clinical freedom and professional power have led to a failure to create mechanisms which ensure that practitioners evaluate clinical outcomes and their cost implications. Such behaviour is not only inefficient but it is also unethical: resources used inefficiently are not available to treat those who are in the queue and who could potentially gain more, in terms of health status, if they were treated.

Doctor demands, not patient demands

The effects of these 'supply side' failures in the market mechanism, have been compounded by demand side institutions. The effects on the demand side of the NHS and private insurance-type institutions is similar. The NHS is tax financed and removes the price barrier to consumption. With the demand for health care infinite, and supply finite and fixed by Government fiat, the NHS inevitably manifests excess demand, *i.e.* waiting-lists. Scarce resources (supply) are allocated amongst competing demanders by doctors according to imprecise notions of 'need' (see Williams (1978)), e.g. scarce kidney-machines are allocated in the NHS to young married people rather than single, elderly people.

The insurance system allocates resources according to willingness and ability to pay. Insurance coverage may remove the price barrier to consumption just like the NHS. Excess demand is, however, rationed in this system by prices (co-insurance). Prices reduce the demands of the poor more than the rich, and of the less ill more than the severely ill (see Cairns and Snell (1978), Maynard (1979) and Newhouse *et al.* (1981)). Prices remove waiting-lists, those unable to finance care can be left in pain and/or to die without benefit of treatment in due course! Those who can pay the price of the co-insurance and the insurance premiums can enter the market, and subject to the agency relationship, will get access to care.

In both the NHS and insurance system the doctor has a crucial role as an allocator of resources. In the NHS he decides who will be treated or not treated, and how. In the insurance system, subject to willingness and ability to pay (which may induce some limited competition by doctors for customers), the doctor decides who will be treated or not treated, and how. The doctor is the 'guardiăn' who determines treatment patterns. Because of the ethic, which dominates his training, to provide the best care for the patient in his charge, the doctor seeks to maximize the benefits of health care regardless of cost. In the NHS, the State meets the cost of care. In the insurance system, the insurance fund or company meets the cost of care. In neither régime does the doctor have to evaluate costs and benefits at the margin. The demand and supply sides of the health care market contain muted and limited devices to persuade doctors and patients to be efficient users of society's scarce health care resources: the bill is picked up either by the long suffering tax-payer or by the insurance company, the third-party (not the supplier or demander of care) pays.

The many imperfections of the health care market

Those people who have adopted the market idealogy tend to believe that markets will be more efficient than governments in allocating resources because the competitive process rewards those who wish to minimize costs and provides incentives for decision-makers to behave efficiently. This paradigm may however be defective in the health care sector. Significant market imperfections, professional power, the agency relationship, and the nature of the insurance mechanism, blunt the competitive system considerably, making it likely that the outcomes of the market will be uneconomic and not necessarily superior to those of alternative institutions such as the NHS. The superiority, if it exists, of the market has to be identified and quantified, not merely asserted as a matter of faith rather than scientific fact.

THE CHARACTERISTICS OF THE ALTERNATIVE SCENARIOS

The market and collectivistist ideologies identify objectives and associated means which could be used to design a health care system. However, at the level of generalized ideology, such designs are imprecise and beg greater definition and careful analysis.

The market alternative

The market ideology is held and articulated by many members of the Thatcher Conservative Government. For instance Sir Geoffrey Howe is convinced that high public expenditure is financed by high tax-rates which 'stifle incentives and inhibit economic growth' (Howe, 1981, page 10). He favours the development of the private sector and the possible wider use of charges in the NHS to make patients aware of the costs of care. All these arguments are consistent with the views expressed by the 'Jones' Report (1970) of which Howe was a member. They have been reflected by Leon Brittan, Chief Secretary of the Treasury, in a speech to the Institute for Fiscal Studies (Brittan, 1982) in which extensive privatization of, *inter alia* the NHS, was advocated.

The creation of competitive conditions

The efficacy of the private health care market depends on reform and the development of new institutions and incentives which would make the market work in a competitive rather than a monopolistic fashion. The achievement of competition could not be acquired without some cost.

As Milton Friedman argues 'there is no such thing as a free lunch', what would you have to pay in order to achieve the Friedmanite Nirvana of competition and consumer sovereignty? The first necessary reform as set out by Friedman, (Friedman, 1962, chapter 9) would be the abolition of professional licensure as it exists in the UK, the USA, and Europe today. Friedman argues that professional power has been used to raise professional incomes above their market rates, and to inhibit the exploitation of substitution possibilities: although we know nurses could do many of the tasks of doctors, and dental assistants could do many of the tasks of dentists equally well and cheaper (see e.g. Reinhardt, 1975), such substitution of cheap inputs for expensive inputs is not permitted. Indeed the British Government, advised by the dental profession, has just closed the only training school for dental assistants!

If the barriers to specialization and cost minimization were removed by the abolition of professional licensure, health care might be provided more efficiently but doctors' incomes significantly reduced. This outcome would arise from competition and substitution reducing doctors' fees and reducing their opportunities for employment. Thus the implication of Friedman's radical policy proposal is potentially severe income losses for powerful professional groups.

Let us assume that Geoffrey Howe and Leon Brittan are sincere in their wish for privatization and competition, and that they are prepared to accept as a necessary cost of achieving this goal, a reduction in the affluence of some powerful health care professionals. If monopoly power is mitigated, can the market work efficiently?

Only a theoretical answer can be given to this question since evidence is lacking. In theory it could however work over time. The first reform after the abolition of professional power would be the adoption of the use of the price mechanism as a means of allocating scarce health care. This allocation method, which is regarded as functional by liberals as it creates incentives which, it is alleged, are the engine of efficient resource use, would require private financers of health care to use co-payments to limit demand.

Co-payments—cost-sharing

At present the UK provident companies (see Maynard, pp. 00) are not fully developed insurance carriers in that their monitoring and rationing of demand is limited and unsophisticated. In the present, limited UK market for private health care, BUPA and its rivals generally meet all expenditure and the financial burden on patients, apart from contributions, is minimal. The absence of a price barrier to consumption may induce increased utilization, what the Americans term 'moral hazard', where the cost of marginal units of health care may exceed their value. If the market for private health care expanded, and insurers carried a wider burden of risks, escalating expenditure would lead to the use of co-payments as a device to ration the demands of patients.

The effects of such co-payments, co-insurance (paying a percentage of the bill) or deductibles (paying a given lump sum) in the jargon, on the demand for health care by patients seems to be quite clear and consistent with the predictions of economic theory: a rise in price will reduce the quantity demand and the magnitude of this effect, the price elasticity of demand, will depend on the extent of the price rise and the nature of the service which is being priced (e.g. the demand for essential emergency care is less likely to be reduced by a price rise than cosmetic surgery). The results of studies of price elasticities are surveyed in Cairns and Snell (1978) and Maynard (1979).

These results were however generated by experiments and statistical analysis of events which were imperfect in scientific design and execution. In an attempt to improve the available data about elasticities and, in particular, to determine the nature of the utilization-health status link, the United States Government financed a study by the Rand Corporation. This work consisted of multi-centre trials with varying co-insurance rates and in varying geographical locations. This work shows that expenditure per person does respond to variations in cost-sharing, it is 50 per cent higher with no cost-sharing compared to 95 per cent co-insurance up to a maximum of $1000, and that as cost-sharing declines patients seek more care. Furthermore this study shows, contrary to earlier ad hoc studies, that the poor (the bottom one-third of the income distribution) and the rich (the top one-third of the income distribution) respond to cost-sharing in similar ways. However the response of the poor would have been greater than that of the rich if the cost-sharing arrangements had not been income related. Hospital utilization does not appear to be affected by co-insurance.

Thus the Rand study shows that some health care cost inflation can be contained by cost-sharing, that for situations where cost-sharing is related to income the utilization effects on rich and poor are similar, and that hospital cost inflation cannot be contained by co-payments. These utilization effects tell us nothing however about whether changes in use affect, adversely or beneficially, the health status of the patient. A familiar argument in the UK and the USA is that many patients present 'unnecessarily'. This argument has led to the joke that a person who presents to a doctor with nothing wrong, should go and see a doctor i.e. the definition of an 'unnecessary' presentation by the doctor may not coincide with the patient's definition of his problems. The use of cost-sharing to reduce 'unnecessary' demands may in fact reduce the demand for care of people who have identifiable illnesses. To what extent does cost-sharing (co-payments) reduce the demands for care of people who are ill and whose delayed treatment may lead to greater ill-health and higher health care 'repair' costs in the long run? The Rand study is capable of answering this question but as yet the data have not been analysed. Previous ad hoc studies in California have shown that prices do reduce the health care consumption of people who have identifiable illnesses which could be treated. (For a summary of this material see Cairns and Snell, 1978). The health status evidence from the Rand Study is urgently needed if this element of the policy debate is to be clarified.

The effect of co-payment is that utilization patterns are affected. The patient faces a price and has an incentive to economise in the use of health care services. He can either decide to reduce his consumption or seek out cheaper alternative forms of health care provision. This latter impulse will generate demands for the substitute (to doctors and dentists for instance) practitioners and develop the fruits of the Friedmanite destruction of professional monopolistic power.

Alternative insurance plans

Another effect will be that the patient will be faced in a competitive market by a choice of alternative insurance plans. These plans will offer varying degrees of coverage at various prices. The patient will shop around to identify and select the policy of his choice. The insurers will have an incentive to market policies for which there is a demand at a price which the patient is prepared to pay.

In order to compete for the custom of the cost-conscious consumer, the insurer will have an incentive to minimize costs. One way of achieving this goal is to evaluate health care provision and rigorously monitor the practice and fees of the providers. Thus the insurers will create information systems, evaluate provision, establish practice norms for practitioners, monitor behaviour, and develop incentive systems to control deviant behaviour, and ensure practitioners are efficient users of scarce resources. Such behaviour can be seen in some United States hospitals already where administration costs are high, and used in order to police with great care the operation of the hospitals budget. It can be seen also in the United Kingdom, where BUPA has now recognized that some providers (e.g. Hospital Corporation of America) are high cost. In an effort to reduce costs, BUPA seems at long last to be embarking on the different process of evolving cost and quality control mechanisms which are commonplace in North America (see *Financial Times*, 1982).

Yet such intervention is likely to raise administrative costs The Organization for Economic Co-operation and Development (1977) have shown that the NHS is cheap to run: its administrative costs were 2·6 per cent of total health care expenditure in the mid 1970s compared to 10·8 per cent in France, 10·6 in Belgium, 6·5 in the Netherlands and 5·0 in Germany. These costs contain two elements: revenue collection and resource management. The costs of revenue collection for the NHS are small as the tax system is cheaper than an insurance system. It is difficult to separate out resource management costs from these figures but it is likely that they would be higher in an insurance system with duplication. Whether the resources available to finance management are used effectively and are adequate is unlikely.

The reintroduction of the price mechanism gives the patient an incentive to seek the lowest cost method of providing efficacious care (i.e. substitution possibilities are exploited) and the lowest cost provider of insurance cover. Price searching (the seeking of the lowest price) by consumers gives the providers and the insurers an incentive to compete and to minimize costs. The predicted effect of the competitive process is that prices will reflect costs at the margin and the surplus profits of inefficient and monopolistic providers and insurers will be dissipated.

All these conclusions are theoretical statements based on the famous economic assumption of *ceteris paribus*: other things being equal. The things which are being held equal are no monopoly power (i.e. a reduction in income for existing powerful professional groups, and no cartel-type behaviour by insurers), the exploitation of substitution possibilities (i.e. reduced employment opportunities for some providers), and the availability of alternative and competing providers and insurers for consumers (i.e. choice is available and sustained).

These conditions require a radical change in the existing medical care market. Friedman is clearly aware of this as are, no doubt, the politicians. The political costs of disturbing the *status quo* should not however be underestimated: powerful producer and financer groups will not take kindly to their members income and jobs being destroyed by the competitive process.

Furthermore it is debatable whether this competitive Nirvana is attainable. The quotation from Adam Smith above indicates that capitalists are the enemies of capitalism. Capitalists can gain, in income and in a quieter life, by rigging the market, covertly or explicitly, and acquiring monopolistic powers. If capitalists manage to acquire such powers they destroy the competitive process because they obtain the ability to fix prices and to determine outputs and the quality of care. In any market the forces of competition and monopoly are in continual conflict. The monopolist rigs prices to his advantages and acquires profits from his action. These profits provide an incentive for a competitor to enter the market place and compete for these profits. This process does however take time and the monopolist can create many barriers to prevent new firms entering the market.

Two important conclusions can be drawn from this analysis. Firstly it is theoretical and its validity has to be demonstrated with evidence from operating markets. As Culyer argues the correspondence between the predicted outcomes and the evidence of the market place indicates that health care markets do not conform to the competitive ideal.

Indeed in the United States the main thrust of reform is to 'make the market work' (e.g. see Enthoven, 1980) and conform more closely to the competitive ideal. However, many Americans are recognizing the difficulties involved in this approach and it seems unlikely that the political will necessary for its adoption in any significant way will be present.

The second conclusion is that the competitive market even if it could be attained, would have to be sustained by considerable government intervention. The natural inclination of a competitive market is for it to become monopolistic. Thus Enthoven (1980) *advocates legislation* to ensure that consumers are offered an effective choice of insurers annually. Similarly Friedman's advocacy of the removal of licensure would almost certainly be challenged by the self interest of professionals. Would the competitive market survive with the removal of licensure alone or would it need to be evaluated and monitored continually by anti-trust bodies? The liberal-marketeers admit a role for the State as the 'policeman of the market place' who protects the competitive process. It is likely that this role would be substantial and executed with some difficulty in the health care market.

The nature of outcomes of the competitive process and the need for government supervision of the market are conjectural: the evidence from competitive markets is absent and many liberals doubt whether politicians could take on and survive a conflict with vested monopoly interests. Let us however assume that politicians were men of principle, that they could convince their electorates that these principles were advantageous, and a competitive market was somehow created and sustained, what other problems arise with the liberal alternative in health care?

Competition and distribution

The competitive market is unlikely to create a distribution of income and wealth that conforms with the distributional goals of any Western society. The liberal response to this problem is not to abolish the market but to let it operate freely and redistribute income directly by the tax system.

Unfortunately redistributing financial capacity to buy goods and services from the rich to the poor will not necessarily lead to greater equality in health care consumption or even perhaps health status. Such redistribution of cash if it is to be effective, must be spent on health care and this health care must be the more efficient means of reducing the inequalities in health which society wishes to mitigate.

The fear that people might spend cash on the 'wrong things', such as alcohol and tobacco which may worsen health status, has led liberals such as Lees (1965) and Seldon (1977) to advocate redistribution by vouchers. Vouchers would tie redistributed resources to health care: they represent a judgement by liberals that in the short run, at least, paternalism is necessary although the liberals hope that, in time, the consumers will learn to be responsible, value health care appropriately, and be given cash rather than tied (voucher) resources.

The use of the voucher is not only a deviation from the 'pure' liberal-market position, it is only tied to health care and this may not be the most efficient way of improving health status. As has been argued in economic theory (Grossman, 1972; Muurinen, 1982) and in the historical-epidemiological literature (McKeown, 1977, 1979), there is good reason to believe that many inputs, of which health care is only one, affect health status and that higher income, better nutrition and public health measures which induce environmental and behavioural change may be more productive than medical care in improving the quality and length of life of individuals. Cash redistribution would, perhaps, be more efficient in these circumstances.

Another complication in the liberal-market model is that it regards incentives as the engine of economic growth and moral well-being. Any redistribution by fiscal measures will reduce the incentives to save, to work and to take risks. The more significant the redistribution that takes place the more the liberals enter into conflicts with their own ideology and have to face problems similar to their collectivist colleagues. Clearly the preference for redistribution among liberals varies considerably (as can be seen from the inspection of output of the Institute of Economic Affairs) from the relatively limited (Friedman) to the more substantial (Peacock and Wiseman).

The liberal would not favour redistribution through institutions, rather he prefers redistribution to individuals. Thus rather than adjust the existing budget allocation formulae, e.g. the formula devised by the Resource Allocation Working Party (RAWP) as suggested by Klein the typical liberal, for instance Friedman, would prefer direct redistribution to individuals by a negative income taxation. Within a competitive market system with private production of health care this may have many attractions but in a mixed public-private system the administrative costs may be substantial and the problem of devising a sensible and sensitive method of redistribution might be considerable as Klein notes.

The preference of the liberal for the private production of health care and decentralized decision making is likely to make the competitive market difficult to regulate with regard to distributive goals. The logic of the liberal position is for cash redistribution and private production of health care.

Whether such arrangements would enable society to achieve its distributive goals is a moot point. As liberals have been the first to note (e.g. Tullock, 1976), the motivation of bureaucrats and politicians is such that the achievement of the goals of social policies are often frustrated. The radical reforms and limited redistribution envisaged by Friedman are likely to injure many powerful pressure groups and their response may be to oppose measures which improve efficiency and permit the effective pursuit of distributional goals. The risk is that we may get some form of uncompetitive market and no effective redistribution because of these pressures. Such an outcome, like all the liberal arguments, is theoretical and awaits empirical verification.

Incentives, producer behaviour, and expenditure inflation

An important aspect of the market mechanism is the effect of incentive structures and the behaviour of producers. Co-insurance (prices) causes consumer behaviour to alter. What is the effect of remuneration systems on the behaviour of producers? In many health care markets and in the minds of many liberals, incentives should be determined by the 'competitive process'. This process, influenced, if not determined by powerful professional influences, usually results in doctors being paid on a fee per item of service basis (piece rates) and hospitals being financed by *per diem* payments.

It is generally accepted amongst economists that both theory and evidence leads to the conclusion that a system of payment on a fee-per-item of service basis has some unattractive features. If we assume that the doctor is an individual concerned with maximizing his income and if he is paid on an item-of-service basis, it is predictable that he would maximize the number of items-of-service delivered to the patient. Thus the payment system induces the doctor to maximize quantity, perhaps with little regard to quality. The testing of these predictions has not been precise but arguments have been put forward to the effect that surgical acts are more numerous, more prescriptions are written, and many other indicators show a comparatively higher level of activity than in health care systems without such payment rates.

Such an outcome raises questions about 'clinical necessity': is the higher level of surgical activity in the Eastern United States indicative of greater illness in the United States or is it due to the fact that there are more surgeons than in England and these surgeons are paid fees per item-of-service? (Bunker, 1970). Because of the lack of evaluation no sensible conclusion can be drawn about the quality of care in both diagnosis and treatment, in regimes where such payment schemes exist. There is a belief on the part of government in Britian that piece-rates affect behaviour, after all such payments were introduced into the remuneration of general practitioners in order to induce them to provide preventive services such as vaccination, immunization, and ante-natal care.

Fees-per-item of service may induce doctors to work longer hours and to produce more medical 'acts' (for which they are paid). Such inducements must however be introduced with caution when we know so little about the efficiency of the services provided. Also such activity leads to greater expenditure. Clearly doctors do not have an infinite desire for income, they value leisure too. Yet fees per item-of-service may make leisure more expensive, in terms of fees foregone, and the effect on overall health expenditure may be inflationary.

The payment of hospitals on a *per diem* (or patient daily rate) basis guarantees income for the hospital provided they can keep their beds full. The predicted effect of this from that dismal scientist the economist is that the hospital would have an incentive to keep its beds full and that bed stocks would be high and lengths of stay longer. Why should the hospital administrator seek to use his bed stock efficiently if, by removing patients from hospital quickly, he is left with empty beds and no *per diem* income? Once again we have a perverse set of incentives which may induce hospital managers to use scarce resources inefficiently.

In health care markets using fee per item-of-service and *per diem* payment systems, the financers (the insurance companies) of health care are often price-takers i.e. they accept the usual, customary and reasonable rates (UCR) set by the providers. The inflationary pressures on expenditure created by the perverse incentives inherent in these payment schemes, have led to the financers of care to question the UCR principle and, instead of taking prices as given by providers, seek to regulate fees by using their buying power. The literature on these developments is vast but the success of the insurance companies in regulating this market place is limited.

The failure of the insurers to curb expenditure inflation, the incentives which induce providers to increase their utilization and bills, and the fact that co-insurance is used generally only in a limited way, means the existing market arrangements are characterized by cost inflation. By and large, health care systems other than the NHS, cost more and their expenditure is growing more rapidly. Perhaps the main cause of this is that providers and consumers have little incentive to economize, and the financers have been slow to implement effective means of evaluating the prices, quantity and qualities of the health services whose costs they meet.

In summary the market alternative is concerned with altering the incentive structure in the health care market so that producers, consumers, and financers are rewarded for behaviour which is efficient and the 'hidden hand of the market' produces an optimal allocation of resources. These alternative incentive structures are not without their costs. Co-payment means that patients pay part of the cost of care. This has known effects on utilization and little known effects on health status. Some schemes of co-payments, particularly if they are not related to income, lead to utilization reductions which may be larger amongst the poor, a group which typically has an inferior health status. Before co-payments are used it is necessary that policy goals be identified clearly. Otherwise it may be found that the outcomes produced by such incentives are unwanted: if a market health care is rationed with reference to willingness and ability to pay, patients, in clinical need of care, may not be able to get access to it because of the price barrier.

Such distributional outcomes could, according to the liberals, be rectified by redistribution directly to the individual. Whether this redistribution would be in cash or vouchers, and whether it would be very substantial are matters of heated debate. This debate is based on the images in competing crystal-balls rather than on evidence.

The marketeers have failed to resolve the obvious problems created by the perverse effects of incentives on providers. The incentive for doctors to carry out too many medical acts and perhaps have too little regard for the quality of their work is an inevitable outcome of payment by fees per item-of-service. The payment of hospitals on a *per diem* basis also leads to inefficient use of resources.

The market mechanism in health care is fine in theory. In fact it works in a highly imperfect manner. To get it to work more efficiently requires radical reforms (e.g. the removal of professional power), the use of co-insurance with its uncertain attributes, and the reform of perverse market incentives which encourage providers to be inefficient. To the extent that liberals have remedies for these problems they are usually radical, untested, and will require if introduced, to be maintained by much private and perhaps public regulation of the health care market-place. Such characteristics should make potential innovators very cautious about implementing the privatization proposals: good evidence is required that private incentives (regulation) of the market produce better outcomes than public regulation of the market.

The collective alternative

The preceding criticisms of the liberal Nirvana do not imply that the alternative to the market, collectivist or socialist organization, is not without defects, sometimes of a serious nature. These defects are similar to those in the private market place and have survived often because of the failure of the public regulators to monitor and evaluate their regulatory activities.

Allocation according to need

The collectivist seeks to allocate scarce health care resources on the basis of need rather than on the basis of willingness and ability to pay, But what is need? Need may be a demand or a supply concept as Williams (1978) has pointed out. The patient may need care according to his own evaluation. An agent of the patient, for instance the doctor, may demand care on his behalf. These needs may be very different. A supply concept of need would concentrate on the productivity of health care as seen by the professional for the individual patient. It is perhaps this latter concept that is in the mind of some collectivists. Competing patients are to be appraised in the light of the potential productivity of health care allocated to them. The scarce resource, health care, is to be allocated on the basis of the maximum possible gains in outcomes, improved health status.

Even if this view was accepted, it contains certain difficulties. How do we measure outcomes? There are no good health status measures in use today. The intellectual problems associated with these measures seem to have been overcome but they have not been tried in operational conditions. The lack of outcome measures together with the lack of evaluation of health care means that little is known about the efficiency of competing therapies for a given illness let alone the relative values of therapies for different illnesses

(e.g. does a heart by-pass operation give greater benefits in health status than an operation for varicose veins?)

As a consequence the allocation of care is governed by principles that are implicit and imprecise. Thus the feeling of solidarity inherent in the collectivist ideology means that care may still be given to the terminally ill without adequate reference to cost. This care might be radical surgery which has little or no effect on life's length and possibly negative effects on its quality, or nursing care in a hospice. No rules have been established to allocate resources effectively in this or most other cases. Often the allocation is based on past practice, the supply of surgeons or hospice beds, and random chance. It does not and cannot conform with the collectivist ideal because of ignorance about the benefits of competing therapies. Until such information is available it will not be possible to detect whether resources are allocated in a manner consistent with the collectivist ideal: according to capacity to benefit from care regardless of the individual's resources.

Collective allocation, public ownership, and planning

If the technocrat's dream was fulfilled and it was possible to identify outcomes and those patients who would benefit most from the use of the scarce collectively provided resources that are available, the attainment of this collectivist Nirvana would require careful regulation of the means of production. Despite the fact that the ideology of those who created the NHS was collectivist, there was little attempt to devise regulatory devices and monitor their efficiency in relation to the goals of greater equality of access to health care and greater equality of health status. The transfer of the ownership of hospitals to the State and the institution of tax finance in 1948 changed some of the fabric of the 'health care shop' but it did not immediately lead to a radical change in the production or distribution of the wares of that shop.

The removal of the price-barrier to the consumption of health care in 1948 did not mean that health care was provided comprehensively at zero cost to consumers. Significant non-price cost-barriers remained, in particular time-costs and costs associated with work income-losses related to with the use of the NHS. These costs are likely to affect income groups in different ways. The worker at Rowntrees Chocolate factory who consults his GP may lose income and have to use slow public transport to get to his doctor, the pharmacy, and the hospital. The academic at a University will lose no income and have access to a car which reduces the time costs of consumption. Location of new hospitals and clinics in 'green field' suburban sites tend to accentuate these cost differentials and explain, in part, different health care consumption patterns.

To overcome such cost-barriers requires careful research to identify the cost-characteristics of the alternatives and effectively control capital information in the NHS. Such controls are noticeable by their absence. Only recently (1981–2) has the Department of Health refined investment appraisal techniques (Capricode) and suggested that capital decisions take account of the full social costs (including time-costs) and benefits of the alternatives.

This lack of control of capital expenditure is parallelled by the relative lack of control of revenue expenditure. Until the early 1970s the NHS revenue budget was allocated on the basis of the following criteria: what was needed last year *plus* an allowance for inflation *plus* a small growth allowance *plus* a residual item related to public scandals (usually in the mental illness sector) which were covered by the media! During the 1970s explicit revenue allocation formulae were devised for each of the constituent parts of the United Kingdom (DHSS, 1976b; Maynard and Ludbrook, 1980a). These sought to equalize the financial capacity to provide health care by allocating monies in relation to need, adjusted by population weighted by standardized mortality rates. Whilst the NHS had positive growth rates in total resource levels, territorial redistribution of resources was possible without much trouble. With the tightening of cash-limits however this first attempt to systematically equalize resources is running into increasing opposition when significant inequalities in geographical financial capacity remain.

Attempts to meet need, observed however crudely, by shifting resources out of acute care and into care of the

504 *Finale*

elderly, the mentally ill, the physically and mentally handicapped, and the chronic sick, has proved also to be difficult
to implement (DHSS, 1976a). Despite regular reiteration of
this 'priorities' policy, the system has been relatively unre-
sponsive to these statements and the moral persuasion of the
Department of Health. The Department's influence is not
improved by the relative autonomy of the Regions and the
casual way in which Regions have traditionally monitored
the Districts (and until recently the Areas).

The activation of the Department of Health in 1982, in
terms of a decision to attempt to establish 'performance
indicators' and call each Region to account each year, is
novel, naive, but well intentioned. The Ministers wish to
determine whether they are getting 'value for money' and
whether priorities criteria are being followed but this is
impossible to know with much certainty because of the
NHS's ignorance and unwillingness to monitor and evaluate
what it is doing. The risk is that an admirable venture
will fail because of optimism about the ease of the task
and hope for quick payoffs which will prove impossible to
attain.

Thus the paradox of the collective alternative, in the form
of the NHS, is that public ownership of the means of
production and public finance has not led to the achievement of collective goals. The Black Report (DHSS, 1980)
and Le Grand's work (Le Grand, 1982) has demonstrated
seemingly that significant inequalities continue to exist
nearly 35 years after the creation of the NHS. Planning,
monitoring, and evaluation have hardly been tried in the
NHS! The socialization of the health care system has not
brought the collective Nirvana much closer and the NHS,
like all other health care systems, has not resolved the
problems associated with the achievement of efficiency or
equality.

Collective allocation and incentives

The failure, or relative absence, of 'top-down' planning from
the centre has been supplemented by an unwillingness to
develop 'bottom-up' incentives by accepting that decision

makers respond to inducements and that care has to be used in designing and evaluating appropriate incentive systems.

The effects of the NHS on producer and patient incentives are very similar to those produced by private insurance systems. The patient consumes health care and the price at the point of consumption is usually zero (except for the few items such as prescriptions, dental care, spectacles, and some appliances for which there are charges): he has no incentive to economize. The main decision maker on the supply side, the doctor, has no incentive to economize either, especially as he has no idea of the cost of his decisions anyway. Thus whether it is believed that the patient or his agent, the doctor, is the demander, neither has an incentive to economize. Thus all decision-makers have little incentive to be careful in their use of society's scarce resources.

Indeed not only are the incentives inadequate they are, as in the insurance system, sometimes perverse. Some elements of doctor remuneration may induce less than efficient responses. For instance *per capita* payments to general practitioners may give doctors an incentive to economise on their use of their time because, whilst they cannot increase their income, they can increase their leisure with such a payment system. The fact that GPs give average consultations of four minutes duration may be the outcome, in part at least, of the way they are paid. Similarly hospital doctors are paid a fixed salary. This means their income is not affected by their work rate and if they prefer 'on-the-job leisure' to do research or private practice, they may press for more appointments, particularly juniors who do not compete for private practice and can carry out their NHS functions for them.

These outcomes are predicted and the causal evidence available does not seem to refute them. It is clear that any payment-system, salary, piece-rate, or capitation, may have effects on behaviour. These effects require evaluation continually in order that the payment systems can be 'tuned' to generate behaviour consistent with the objectives of policy: we need to pay the piper appropriately if we are to get the tune that is wanted!

Possible reforms

The reform of the collective allocation system on health care is not about changing institutional structures (e.g. reorganizing the NHS), the usual pre-occupation of politicians. Such policies change the facade outside the NHS 'shop' but do not affect behaviour within the shop. At present the NHS is probably under-managed (i.e. inadequately regulated) and the meagre management resources are badly trained and ill-informed.

In the NHS there is no information about speciality costs, there is little evaluation of the process of providing care or the outputs, if any, of the caring process, and the idea of quality evaluation is regarded as novel and radical. For a trader to use resources efficiently in a market such information is essential: imagine an oil company that did not know the cost and quality of the oil and petrol it sold! Such a situation is unlikely in the oil market but commonplace in the health care industries of most countries including Britain.

The basis minimum for any collective system to be efficient and for it to meet its distributional targets, is that it collects, manipulates, and evaluates information about costs, quantities, and qualities. Such information is required at a specialty level so that it is possible to identify which actors are least cost, quantity, and quality maximizers, and which doctors use resources inefficiently. The costs of collecting and using this information will be considerable but efficiency can be bought only at the price of using scarce resources.

The production of such information will enable all health care actors, doctors, nurses, physiotherapists, and others, to establish explicit professional standards of practice. The establishment of standards or norms of practice would enable the professions to use peer review and medical audit systems to ensure that professionals adhered in their everyday practice to the standards of their trade.

The problems associated with standard setting is that it tends to be conservative. It thus needs to be reviewed continually, and even if deviants are identified, they may not always be prepared to alter their practice. This latter effect has to be substantiated by research but if it is a major problem then 'sticks and carrots' would have to be devised to induce decision makers to behave efficiently. The most obvious, but contentious, method of doing this would be to make decision-makers budget holders.

One example of such an arrangement is the Health Maintenance Organization (HMO). The literature on this subject is vast (see e.g. Luft, 1981) but the idea is simple. Patients pay a lump-sum annual contribution. This could be paid by the individual (as in the USA) or by the State (the NHS), to a 'firm' of doctors who promise to provide a comprehensive range of health services for the contributor and his family. The firm's income is the fees. Its costs are determined by its activities. The firm retains surpluses for redistribution to its members as income and for use in developing the firm. Thus the managers (doctors) of the firm have an incentive to economize, they get cash rewards. They buy in hospital care and monitor its use and they provide ambulatory (primary care) themselves. It seems that such HMOs use less hospital time, have lower costs, and that the quality of their care is not inferior. Such organizations, essentially labour managed firms on the Yugoslav model, could be developed in collective health care systems to encourage efficiency in resource usage.

Such reforms must however proceed slowly. There are no 'instant' solutions to these problems and all innovations require careful evaluation. Progress will be slow and will be costly to achieve: as Friedman has argued 'there is no such thing as a free lunch'.

To summarize this brief discussion it seems clear that the collectivistic alternative indicates clearly that, as it manifests itself in Britain and elsewhere, is far from perfect in the efficiency with which it uses resources and of its achievement of distributional goals. The regulatory devices that have been used have been few in number and introduced only recently after the rediscovery of defects which the Service was created to remedy.

Existing collective health care systems have been reluctant to develop means to analyse efficiency and the distributional goals have not been monitored effectively. The means to remedy these defects are difficult to identify and there is an apparent unwillingness to experiment. Until experiments are implemented and evaluated in Britain, the NHS will continue to use resources inefficiently and will fail to achieve the distributional goals which have been set. Principle and practice in the socialist system like principle and practice in the market, bear all too little relation to one another.

CONCLUSION

To assert that the market is more efficient than the National Health Service is naive and unhelpful. Both the market and the NHS have severe limitations and the achievement of the objectives of liberal freedom and socialist equality is obstructed by similar forces: monopoly power, lack of evaluation of costs and benefits, and perverse incentives for providers and demanders. It is inappropriate to judge the NHS in the light of market objectives or the market in the light of collective objectives but it is necessary to be aware of the characteristics of each of the alternatives, both in terms of the goals and the means by which these goals can be attained.

It is doubtful whether the market could achieve the objectives of its liberal architects. The power of the monopoly interests and the income losses these interests would suffer if competition existed, make it likely that any market for health care will be dominated by monopolies. Such concentrations of power inhibit freedom as much as a large public sector and it is likely that to protect freedom, the State would have to regulate the monopolies and actively try to sustain competition. Whether the State could do this, when the frustration of monopolies will cost votes, is a contentious subject.

It is unlikely that a market, as set out in the liberal paradigm, could achieve collectivist ends. Although economists in the past (e.g. Lange and Taylor, 1936) have believed that all that is necessary is to set out goals, adjust prices, and then set the market to work, this economic theory of socialism has been shown not to work in practice.

The socialist model is fraught with difficulties which arise from the same problem that exists in markets. The removal of health care from the private market does not remove the problems of inefficiency and inequality. Active intervention (planning) and the creation of new incentive structures consistent with the goals of policy are necessary. However in the NHS these challenges have been ignored until recently and even now the efforts in these areas are feeble.

The definition of efficient policy, whether the market is 'better' than the NHS, begs the definition of objectives. If social objectives are being redefined away from collective action, the changed public/private mix will raise many new regulatory problems for the State and private institutions. If objectives are static, then the existing public/private mix awaits effective regulatory action to improve performance of both its constituent parts. Probably the problems of the health care market are insoluble whether publicly or privately organized. However whatever organization exists and whatever the policy goals, regulation, by which is meant intervention by public and private interests to determine the price, quantity, and quality of health care, is unavoidable.

REFERENCES

ABEL-SMITH, B. AND MAYNARD, A. (1979). *The Organisation, Financing and Cost of Health Care in the European Community*, Commission of the European Communities, Social Policy Series, No. 36, Brussels.

ARROW, K. (1963). 'Uncertainty and the Welfare Economics of Medical Care', *American Economic Review*, **liii**, December.

BRITTAN, L. (1982). 'Health service pressure point', *Guardian*, 11 May, page 20.

BUNKER, J. P. (1970). 'A comparison of operations and surgeons in the United States and in England and Wales', *New England Journal of Medicine*, 136–43 (15 January).

— —, BARNES, B. A., AND MOSTELLER, F. (1977). *The Cost, Benefits and Risks of Surgery*. (Oxford University Press: New York).

CAIRNS, J. AND SNELL, M. (1978). 'Prices and the Demand for Health Care', in CULVER, A. J. AND WRIGHT, K. G. (eds.), *Economic Aspects of Health Services*. (Martin Robertson).

COCHRANE, A. L. (1972). *Efficiency and Effectiveness: random reflections on health services*. (Nuffield Provincial Hospitals Trust).

CULYER, A. J., MAYNARD, A., AND WILLIAMS, A. (1981). 'Alternative systems of health care provision: an essay on motes and beams', in

OLSON, M. (ed.), *A New Approach to the Economics of Medical Care.* (American Enterprise Institute: Washington D.C.).

DEPARTMENT OF HEALTH (NEW ZEALAND) (1980). *Funding for Health: An Allocation Formula,* Special Report No. 58. (Wellington).

DEPARTMENT OF HEALTH AND SOCIAL SECURITY (1976a). *Priorities for Health and Personal Social Services in England: a consultative document.* (HMSO: London).

— — (1976b). *Sharing Resources for Health in England: report of the resource allocation working party.* (HMSO: London).

— — (1980). *Inequalities in Health: a report of a research working group,* (The Black Report). (HMSO: London).

DONABEDIAN, A. (1971). 'Social responsibility for personal health services: an examination of basic values', *Inquiry,* **viii,** 2, 3–19.

ENTHOVEN, A. C. (1980). *Health Plan.* (Addison Wesley).

Financial Times (1982). Some hospitals to be ruled out for BUPA cover by R. SNODDY, 12 May, page 7.

FRECH, H. E. (1974). 'Occupational licensure and health care productivity: the issues and the literature', in RAFFERTY, J. (ed.), *Health Manpower and Productivity.* (Lexington).

FRIEDMAN, M. (1962). *Capitalism and Freedom.* (University of Chicago Press).

FUCHS, V. (1978). 'The supply of surgeons and the demand for operatives', *Journal of Human Resources,* **xiii,** Supplement, 35–6.

GOODMAN, J. (1980). *National Health Care in Great Britain: Lessons for the USA.* (The Fisher Institute: Dallas, Texas).

GROSSMAN, M. (1972). *The Demand for Health: a theoretical and empirical investigation.* (National Bureau of Economic Research: New York).

HOWE, G. (1981). *Health and the Economy,* speech to the Royal Society of health. (mimeo).

JAMIESON REPORT (1980). *Report of the Commission of Inquiry into the Efficiency and Administration of Hospitals,* three volumes (report).

JONES, I. M. (1970). *Health Services Financing.* (British Medical Association: London).

LANGE, O. and TAYLOR, F. M. (1938). *An Economic Theory of Socialism.* (University of Minnesota Press).

LEES, D. (1965). 'Health through choice', in *Freedom or Free for All?* (Institute of Economic Affairs: London).

LEFFLER, K. B. (1978). 'Physician Licensure: competition and monopoly in American medicine', *Journal of Law and Economics,* **xxi**(1), 165–86.

LE GRAND, J. (1982). *Strategy for Equality.* (Allen and Unwin: London).

LINDSAY, C. M. (1980). *National Health Issues: the British Experience.* (Hoffman La Roche: New York).

LUFT, H. S. (1981). *Health Maintenance Organizations: dimensions of performance.* (Wiley: New York).

MAYNARD, A. (1979). 'Pricing, insurance and the NHS', *Journal of Social Policy.*

— — AND LUDBROOK, A. (1980a). 'Budget allocation in the National Health Service', *Journal of Social Policy,* July.

— —, — — (1980b). 'What's wrong with the NHS?', *Lloyds Bank Review*, October.

McKeown, T. (1977). *The Modern Rise of Population*. (Edward Arnold).

— —, (1979). *The Role of Medicine*, 2nd edition. (Blackwell).

Muurinen, J. M. (1982). 'Demand for health: a generalised Grossman model', *Journal of Health Economics*, **1**(1).

Newhouse, J. E., *et al.* (1981). *Some Interim Results from a Controlled Trial of Cost Sharing in Health Insurance*. Rand Corporation, Health Insurance Experiment Series, R-2847-M.MS.

Organisation for Economic Co-operation and Development (1977). *Public Expenditure on Health*. (Paris).

Schweitzer, S. O. (ed.) (1978). *Policies for the Containment of Health Care Costs and Expenditures*. (US Department of Health, Education and Welfare, Government Printing Office: Washington).

Seldon, A. (1977). *Charge!* (Temple Smith: London).

— — (ed.) (1980). *The Litmus Papers: A National Health Dis-Service*. (Centre for Policy Studies: London).

Smith, A. (1976). *An Inquiry into the Nature and Causes of the Wealth of Nations*. (Everyman editors: London).

Tullock, G. (1976). *The Vote Motive*. (Institute of Economic Affairs: London).

United States Department of Health and Human Services (1981). *Physician Induced Demand for Surgical Operation*. (Health Care Financing Administration: Washington D.C.).

Williams, A. (1978). 'Need: an economic exegesis', in Culyer, A. J. and Wright, K. G. (eds.), *Economic Aspects of Health Services*. (Martin Robertson).

The public/private mix in health care

The emerging lessons

GORDON McLACHLAN AND ALAN MAYNARD

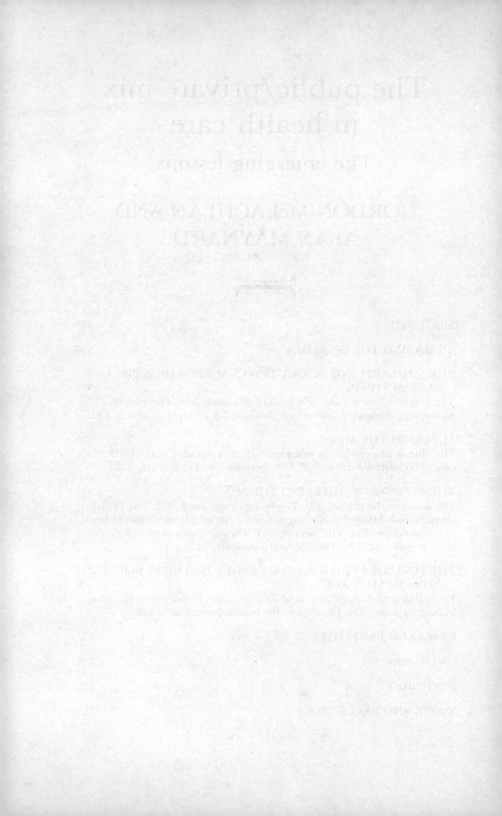

The public/private mix in
health care
The emerging lessons

ABSTRACT

In this chapter an attempt is made to draw together the
lessons which can be learnt from varying experiences of public
and private activity in health care in relation to the options
for change. Some thoughts on training and research are set
out in the belief that future research efforts in these areas will
improve the efficiency of all systems and enable them to avoid
some of the errors manifest in discussions about policies and
the way in which decisions have been made in the recent past.

The opening section sets the scene drawing on recent ema-
nations from government and the medical profession which
indicate a continuing faith in the NHS (and presumably its
ideals) effectively dismissing the 'social insurance' alternative
option for finance, and plumping for the encouragement of
private medicine to supplement the NHS, and financed by
insurance schemes. This poses the dilemma of the form of such
encouragement and of the regulation to achieve the goals of
health care which are universal in character. These problems
are of the first rank of political and administrative importance.

The *second* section emphasizes the similarity of the principal
goals of the health care systems in the countries of the
Western world. Everywhere there is a desire for greater efficiency in the use of resources, and greater equity and equality in
the distribution of health care and health.

The *third* section describes briefly the implications of altering the public/private mix in health care. These implications
are common across all health care systems despite the superficial dissimilarities in the way health care is financed and
provided. In the *fourth* section the effects of an alteration in the
public/private mix in Britain in particular, is examined and
an indication is given how 'privatization' will affect the nature
of regulation. The *fifth* section develops these general implications against the realities of medical practice, management of
resources and current problems such as the development of

prevention and the care of the elderly and outlines the long run implications of altering the public-private mix. The *sixth* section sets out a list of questions which are basic to research and which require careful investigation if managers of health care systems, public or private, are in the event to be enabled to make efficient decisions which ensure that their systems give 'value-for-money', and attain the distributional goals of policy-makers. The challenges posed by a research agenda geared to realities are significant and require a strategy to ensure the concentration of scarce intellectual resources over a considerable period if the problems common to all health care systems are to be understood better and ameliorated effectively. A *seventh* and final section summarizes the arguments and, in the context of the likelihood of a lengthy period of acute scarcity in the availability of resources to finance health care, advocates a more scientific approach to policy formulation and implementation. All systems of health care are capable of being improved. Change in the organization and finance of health care is both relevant and necessary but the nature of progress in this sector of society is evolutionary and change must be undertaken with care if the inefficiencies and inequalities which exist in all health care systems are not to be worsened. This essay concludes with a postscript underlying the editors belief in the NHS as a national asset providing basic services equitably, and economically but capable in association with the private sector of improvement if the right policies are pursued.

ANALYSING THE DILEMMA

The Trust's main purposes are the co-ordination and improvement of medical and associated services. That there is an important function in Britain today for a private independent foundation concerned with such objectives because of the existence of a near-monopoly in the public health sector, needs no labouring. By the same token there must be a place for the private practice of medicine. The Trust has therefore in its programme of research and experiment in pursuit of its purposes since its inception, continued to keep under review the effectiveness of the *total* health services available from the public/private mix. This particular study, the origins of which are given in the Prefatory Note and Introduction, has over the past two years intensified this review, and expanded into areas of enquiry which have hitherto been unplumbed, particularly by drawing on the experience of other countries on issues in the forefront of debate here. While the study started with the review of options open to government regarding the financing of services, it soon reflected the complexity of the health care field, and moved into the difficult terrain beyond, the topography of which is common to all societies and all systems whatever the mix. The main features are equity of access and distribution, regulation, the effects of financial constraints and efficiency. Thirty-years experience of the NHS has indeed shown these up in stark relief but they are not unknown abroad too, as a reading of the essays from abroad will show.

During the study there have been a number of important happenings in the UK which are in effect, sighting posts to the channels of policy lying ahead. At the end of July 1982 the Secretary of State confirmed that he was not considering the 'social insurance option'. Earlier in 1982 the Executive Committee of the BMA in a discussion document (1982) have effectively dismissed this option too. Both the Secretary of State and a spokesman for the BMA have also reaffirmed separately, the faith in the NHS, of both the government and of the profession. Both have also indicated their desire to encourage private practice, presumably through the encouragement of private insurance of one sort or another, in order to supplement the resources deployed in the NHS. This report indicates the form which such encouragement is likely to take and there is a host of conditions, political and economic, which have to be resolved. There is also a great difference in the order of resources expected. The Secretary of State holds out no promise in the foreseeable future, of extra resources in real terms to come from the Treasury; so that the encouragement of the insurance market is expected to provide what additional resources are needed. More realistically, the BMA continue to wish for more resources for the NHS from the Exchequer, as well as the resources coming from an expansion of the private sector. The fact is however, there is no evidence to suggest from experience that the supplementary resources so obtained are likely to be other than marginal to a service costing more than £14,000m p.a.

Furthermore, given the capital and the time lag involved in developing the stock of health facilities, any major supplementary resources which come available are, in reality, unlikely to be translated into service quickly and economically unless they are used in association with an expansion in the number of private beds in NHS hospitals, using existing 'stock' for which there was of course provision under Section 5 of the 1946 NHS Act. The political problems accompanying such a policy would no doubt be great, but such a move—which is as much an option as the main one of altering the total resources from public funds—could ensure the kind of partnership with the NHS in planning which is much in the forefront of the debate on the public/private mix to provide for optimum use of total resources.

Here, of course, lies the important dilemma, for the underlying notion of supplementation from insurance does not provide any signs about how or where, if forthcoming, these resources should or could be directed to ensure their optimum use. In the light of what is known of shortcomings in services, actual and forecast, it is difficult to believe that whatever the complexion of government the experience of thirty years about equity, distribution, and efficiency, to say nothing of the special needs of groups recognized as requiring priorities in services, is going to be allowed completely to go by the board. Regulation in order to direct expansion and to control any reactions from change seems therefore inevitable. The issue then becomes, what is likely to be gained by changing the mix, what are the limitations and what is involved to ensure optimum use of resources?

THE SIMILARITY OF POLICY GOALS ACROSS HEALTH CARE SYSTEMS

The major objectives

A careful analysis of the essays on the foreign systems and of other sources which set out the characteristics and problems of health care systems across the Western world (e.g. Maynard, 1975; Blanpain, 1978; and Maxwell, 1980) shows that there is a striking similarity in the problems facing most health care systems. Although the terminology differs, most policy-makers in most countries identify control of expenditure, efficiency and distributional equity as the primary problems in their health care systems.

These terms are often misused. A primary concern in Continental Europe, Australia, and North America is cost-containment which is a broad term embracing the concept of value-for-money. The latter term is one used liberally by people analysing the performance of the NHS in Britain where the system of sole-source funding makes expenditure control considerably easier than elsewhere. Cost-containment, a term most used in the USA, is a concept with two characteristics. Firstly it expresses a concern that the *total* expenditure on health care is not *limited* by effective institutional controls. Within this expression of policy-makers wishing to limit health care expenditure, there is however also a concern, sometimes implicit and sometimes explicit, whether the limited monies allocated to the provision of care, are used *in an efficient* manner.

All too often, the cost-containment debate is couched in terms of expenditure on the various elements of service (inputs) financed by expenditure. This concentration on input cost and the assertion that total and unit costs are rising too rapidly, and hence need containing, begs an association of the link between inputs and outputs. Does the emphasis on cost-containment, imply that the benefits (outputs) derived from these inputs are low? Thus, is the marginal product of health care, ('service'), lower in terms of efficiency than its marginal cost? In this case the economic argument is that expenditure should not be contained but reduced: in economic terms the ideal is to allocate resources only if their benefits in that use, exceed their costs at the margin.

The goal of efficiency

Implicit in the catch phrase 'cost-containment' is a concern about the efficiency of resource allocation: 'value for resources used'. This concern requires us to be more explicit in its use. All policy-makers, regardless of country, or public/

private sector, are seeking to ensure that resource allocation decisions minimize costs, and maximize the value (benefits) of those goods and services which are most earnestly sought after, by society. The services whose benefits are maximized, might be chosen in private markets by individuals (patients and providers if they have the power to influence patient choice), or in public (political) markets by the complex interactions of politicians, bureaucrats, (potential) patients, and providers. These choices decide the areas into which resources will be allocated. Policy-makers then have to seek to ensure that once such choices are made at the macro (decisive) level, the benefits of the services chosen are maximized at the micro (operational) level. This implies that the resources (inputs) used, have the maximum impact on the health status of the patients who consume the services (outputs), the consumption pattern of which is decided by willingness and ability to pay in the private sector, and medical (or social) need in the public sector. The maximization of benefits per unit of input, implies that costs are minimized. Thus, efficiency requires benefit maximization and cost minimization. This is a major goal common to all systems of health care, public or private, European or North American.

The goal of equity

A second major goal which pervades all health care systems, is some concern with distributional equity. Unlike efficiency which is a fixed goal through time, and across systems, the pursuit of distributional goals varies through time and across systems. 'Equality' or 'equity' like beauty is in the mind of the beholder, but despite the lack of real clarity as to meaning, such a goal is pursued in all societies regardless of public/private mix.

In the post-war period in Britain the concern about equity was set out by the Coalition (Churchill) Government in 1944 in the following way:

> the Government ... want to ensure that in the future every man and woman and child can rely on getting ... the best medical and other facilities available;

that their getting them shall not depend on whether they can pay for them or on any other factor irrelevant to real need. (Ministry of Health, A National Health Service Cmnd 6502, HMSO, 1944).

In 1946 an outline of the NHS Bill stated that the new Service would impose

> no limits on availability, e.g. limitations based on financial means, age sex, employment or vocation, areas of residence or insurance qualification. (Ministry of Health, The National Health Service: a summary of the proposed service, Cmnd 6761, HMSO, 1946).

Although these policy statements are vague and Utopian in some respects they indicate that Churchill's Coalition and Attlee's Governments shared a common concern to alter the distribution of access to health care, to reduce price barriers to care, and to increase the utilization of health care by groups who suffer great disadvantages such as the poor, the elderly, and the chronic sick.

This humanitarian desire to mitigate the effects of a totally free market is paralleled in all other health care systems. Everywhere there is a desire in government decision-makers to alter the effects of a completely free market allocation of resources in terms of facilities, in order that the less fortunate in society, who typically have inferior health status, should be given greater access to scarce health care resources. In 1972 President Nixon whose Administration in the USA is hardly renowned as exponents of welfare, expressed this policy objective in a message to Congress in terms of a national health strategy which not only gave the whole population access to the best standard of medical care but also put an end to any

> racial, economic, social or demographic barriers which may prevent adequate health protection. R. M. Nixon, Message to Congress 2 March 1972 (quoted in G. McLACHLAN, *Effectiveness and Efficiency, The Hospital as a Community Facility.* New York Academy of Medicine, 1972, New York).

The similarity of the Nixon goal and that of Bevan and the Churchill Government is striking. Similar links can however be shown to exist in the policy statements of the architects of other health care systems. The clarity of such expositions and the emphasis of subsequent practical policies working towards their attainment through planning systems does however vary over time. Policy-makers in the present British and American Governments might seem to place less emphasis on goals of distributional equity. Thus the reaction of the then Secretary of State (Jenkin) to the recommendations of the (Black) Inequalities Report as issues of practical policy, (Department of Health and Social Security, 1980, and Townsend and Davidson, 1982), was almost hostile. Yet despite this apparent reluctance to develop policies to make for better 'equity' and 'equality', both British and American Administrations have acted in ways consistent with the maintenance of a desire, at best, not to worsen the access of the poor and other groups suffering from grave disadvantages. Thus McNerney notes the decline in favour, of the pro-competition proposals in the United States and Maynard indicates the dawn of a better awareness of the costs and benefits of 'privatization' in the UK. Both processes of policy realignment have been precipitated by caution about whether competition and the private market will 'work', and alarm that if it works, its effects on the distribution of access might be politically disadvantageous (see also various articles in *New England Journal of Medicine*, 1981–2). Thus the Reagan Government is hesitating about restricting the care provided by Medicare and taking steps with regard to Medicaid which while vague as to effect, are unlikely to cut back more on that programme than the effects of the inflationary process on the means' test eligibility criteria. The Conservative Government is boasting that it has increased the real level of NHS resources each year since 1979 and shows no significant signs of wishing to reduce the level of allocation to the NHS which is based on the notion however ill-defined, of need, rather than willingness and ability to pay. The Secretary of State went on record (*The Times*, 9 July 1982) to state 'The Government is committed to the Health Service. We want to see an NHS working to the maximum effect in the service of patients'.

Personal v collectivist provision—a chimera in health

It is however true that some non-health ministers in both the UK and elsewhere still yearn after the use of prices and 'new' means of financing health care. This reflects a deep desire by Treasury Ministers to reduce public expenditure by transferring responsibility to the individual. Yet it is questionable whether the single-minded pursuit of this goal is either sensible or sophisticated in terms of recent assessments of the workings of economics—far less the economics of health services. The current 'wisdom' is that public expenditure is 'unproductive' and that in order to free resources for 'productive' private expenditure, the role of government must be reduced, public expenditure cut, and the tax burden on private initiative eased. This argument assumes certain meanings of the words 'productive' and 'unproductive' and asserts that if public activity declines, private sector activity replace it with few complications. These are assertions which require careful definition and empirical verification.

This type of argument is epitomized by Leon Brittan (1982) and is similar to that reported as being subsequently used by Sir Geoffrey Howe (1982) and their Treasury counterparts in the United States and Western Europe. These adherents to the liberal market ideology are concerned with the advancement of wealth creation and the 'long-term decline' of the economy. This 'long-term decline' manifests itself in the contraction of the (private) manufacturing base of the economy and the expansion of the (often public) service sector. As Simon Kusnets has noted this is a natural way for growing economies to develop. Analysts with this particular view of the world believe that public sector activity is wasteful at worst, or less valuable than its private counterpart. In the case of health services, some of its assumptions look less than secure. The view is curious as it seems to imply that a necessary hernia procedure done in a NHS hospital is less valuable than a similar hernia procedure completed in a private hospital. This strange view of the world, which is in essence Mercantilist and has its most recent manifestation in the work of Bacon and Eltis (1976), implies that public production, the output of health care, education and other sectors, is less valuable than private production. If this means that the value of the output of the public sector in a particular activity per unit of input cost is less than the output per unit of input cost in the private sector, it becomes a hypothesis seeking empirical verification. Such verification is difficult because of the difficulty of measuring, e.g. health care outputs (benefits) in the public and the private sector. It is certainly not clear that private production is more efficient (cost minimizing—benefit maximizing) than public production.

In the absence of such information, the view of Brittan, Howe, and others of the liberal mould, are assertions of value very much doubtful in the case of health services, rather than of identifiable facts. Assertions about the nature of the world are a poor basis on which to formulate policy and it is sobering to believe that policy initiatives in health care will possibly bear this inadequate stamp.

Another interpretation of the Bacon and Eltis position is that public activity is 'crowding out' private production. Hence Brittan and Howe (1982a) seem to have adopted the Keynesian policy of controlling inflation by deflating the economy in an effort to create 'slack' or spare capacity so providing an opportunity for the private sector to develop towards appropriate goals. Unfortunately such a development has not been forthcoming. Indeed this is not surprising as the empirical evidence that is available, indicates that private sector activity is led by public sector activity. If the latter declines it seems to take the former down with it, and the readjustments required for private sector activity to restore the economy may take decades to come to pass.

Thus, whilst it might be wise to deflate the economy to reduce the rate of growth of prices induced by the oil cartel, it is not clear that this will automatically generate more wealth creation by the private sector, and it is not clear that even if it did, the private production of health care would be superior to that of the public sector. In Britain, North America, Western Europe, and Australia, the contents of the preceding essays have shown that the 'failures' of the public sector are paralleled by similar 'failures' in the private sectors. To alter the public/private mix may well be completely irrelevant from the efficiency point of view. There are more fundamental problems which require the attention of policymakers, rather than cosmetic alterations in mix or organization which change facades but leave the essence of the market failures, public and private, unresolved. In particular the special problems of the groups in society that have grave disadvantages such as the elderly, the handicapped, etc., require special urgent attention.

It is perhaps not surprising that this conclusion seems to elude those politicians who, while commenting on the sector in general terms are not aware as they ought to be, of the complex nature of the health care market. Yet those of their colleagues who grapple with the difficulties of policy formulation and implementation in health, soon learn that there are few solutions to the common problems of reconciling the manifold inconsistencies of the elements of health care provision, not least those concerned with efficiency and inequality in the systems for which they are responsible, and which to a large extent their policies control.

ALTERING THE MIX

The illusion of over-simple solutions

Despite the fact that problems of inefficiency and inequality which demand the attention of governments pervade all health care systems, regardless of the mix of public and private activity, there is a Pavlovian tendency amongst certain theoreticians, ideologues, etc. to attempt to stampede politicians into over-simple alterations in the public/private mix in order to remedy the defects in health care systems, which in reality stem from highly complex causes, the difficulties of which are not easily removed.

Thus in Britain the Labour Party, in France the Socialist Government, in West Germany the ruling Social Democrats, in the United States the opposition Democrats, and in Australia the Labor Party, respond to the inadequacies of their domestic health care systems by pledging more public expenditure and more public regulation of the finance and provision of health care.

This somewhat naive response towards collectivism has a parallel in an opposite direction amongst the proponents of the liberal market policies. The Conservative Government in Britain, the Giscard opposition in France, the Christian Democrat opposition in West Germany, the Reagan Government in the United States, and the Fraser Liberal Government in Australia have all responded to the problems inherent in their health care systems by advocating the redesign of their public sectors which provide health care, and the 'encouragement' of the extension of private finance and provision.

The paradox of the ineffectiveness of opposite solutions

It is thus paradoxical that because of the dominance of particular ideologies, liberal or collective, in different countries, policy-makers are adopting *opposite* policies (privatization and regulation) to remedy the same problems in the health care market. Yet such policies in health care are ineffective. No government is likely to be able to avoid some obligation to provide health care to the various categories of the under-privileged at some satisfactory level. Again, all governments are concerned with the pursuit of efficiency, and value for resources. But attempts are being made to mobilize these common endeavours by policies which are sometimes completely opposite to each other and which experience shows to be less than adequate.

Thus it is less than certain that the private 'solution' to health care problems is likely to lead to the attainment of equity goals unless purposefully directed. Neither does it manifest adequacy in the pursuit of efficiency. Monopolies and cartels lead to groups of providers having the market power to raise prices and affect to their own advantages the quantity and quality of the services they provide. As a consequence the costs of health care are not minimized, the monopolies get 'rents' or surpluses in excess of the value of the services they provide. Furthermore the monopolists provide services whose benefits may be consistent with their preferences rather than those of the patients who are in their care. The distribution of these services in a 'free' competitive market, because it is largely determined by willingness and ability to pay, is unlikely to lead to the attainment of the equity goals even of the liberals. Their preference for some 'minimum' form of intervention leads them, as is clear from the US experience, down a regulatory route which is familiar to all Europeans with 'welfare' States.

Thus European experiences, as recounted in the several essays in Part 2, does, however, indicate that the public regulation of health care provided by a substantial proportion of private providers is less than effective. As Cochrane (1972) argued, one characteristic of the NHS, which is in effect no different from other health care systems public and private, is that the majority of the therapies provided by practitioners have not been evaluated scientifically and until they are, the efficiency with which the majority of services are provided can be doubted. Again the distributional achievements of the National Health Service have been widely questioned recently (Department of Health and Social Security, 1980; and Townsend and Davidson, 1982) despite the RAWP innovations in the mid 1970s. These achievements, or rather the lack of them, are paralleled in Western Europe by distributional outcomes which are less than impressive (Maynard, 1981; and Maynard and Ludbrook, 1981), also specially Lacronique and Rodwin in this collection.

Thus private markets do not achieve the goals of the liberals and are at variance with the achievement of the goals of the collectivists. Public activity in health care markets has failed to meet the objectives of the collectivists and is at variance with the goals of the liberals. Alterations in the public/private mix in health care which merely readopt tried and proven inadequate policies, may give the impression of political 'action', but the myth that this is effective action should be dispelled by the reality of the facts, that existing structures, public and private, financial and provider, are defective and require closer attention than has hitherto been given. These defects arise from the fundamental nature of health care markets, public and private, which are emphasized by Culyer and Maynard. They are also likely to be subject to an exacerbation of the sort of problems enumerated by Forsyth and Klein.

The inevitability of regulation

These inadequacies make the regulation of all health care markets inevitable. The nature of this regulation must however be clarified. Regulation usually carries with it the implication of action by the State. This is unfortunate, because regulation has a wider connotation in that it really means that activities will be controlled or moderated by rules. The acts of control and moderation can thus be exercised by public or private bodies and an important question is how such regulation bears on individuals, providers, and the profession. The private sector can be regulated by rules devised both within that sector, and from outside of it, for instance by the State. The public sector can be regulated, controlled, or moderated by rules created within the sector by public bodies or by rules devised by private bodies (for instance, by the professions). The collapse of the Voluntary Effort in the USA, despite an attempt to get the major private bodies to act together but in effect severally, to contain costs in the face of threatened Federal action is significant.

The regulation of health care markets means that public and private bodies will seek to control or moderate the effects and outcomes of the non-competitive private sector and the often monopolistic public sector. The control of these bodies will be directed at moderating the activities of decision-makers and influencing the price of services (e.g. health care) labour (e.g. doctors' pay) and capital (e.g. the rate of return on pharmaceutical or hospital investments), the quality of these services, labour and capital, and the quantity of these variables. Often controls on similar variables will be working against one another, and have countervailing effects. Thus everywhere the doctors seek to increase their income, and the paying agencies, whether sickness funds or the DHSS, will endeavour to reduce the rate of growth of expenditure—frequently attempting to put a cap on it, which in the event *will restrict incomes or employment*. (Lacronique)

Different groups in different societies adopt different policies towards health care. Whether these are of a liberal or collectivist nature they can be demonstrated to be defective, but ill considered, reactive reform through the opposite philosophy seems nevertheless still to be popular with those responsible for policy. The contending parties seem to believe as acts of faith, but with a minimum of sense, that their policies will solve—sometimes apparently at a stroke—the problems inherent in the health care market. But these beliefs are at variance with experience: always and everywhere, alternative policies can be demonstrated to generate or in some cases create and sustain inefficiency and the failure to achieve distributional goals.

It cannot be stressed too much that in the modern state to remedy these problems regulation is unavoidable. Regulation can be carried out by policy-makers in public or private institutions and will seek to moderate the outcomes or unrestricted non-competitive markets by controlling prices, quantities and qualities. These policies can be carried out in the NHS or in the private sector. As Enthoven (1980) and McNerney have argued for the United States, the market liberal 'solution' requires regulatory activity of a vigorous nature if competition is to be created and sustained in the financing and provision of health care. A reading of Culyer indicates why this is so. Similarly the Netherlands, Belgium, the Federal Republic of Germany, and France are taking, or already have taken, steps to regulate their particular health markets. In the UK, the NHS 'solution' requires more detailed regulation of budget allocation, priority setting and decision-making. Yet given the disquiet in both public (e.g. the NHS) and the private sectors, it seems necessary that new incentives have to be created to moderate (regulate) the inefficiency of particular systems (Maynard and Ludbrook, 1980).

It certainly seems unlikely that vigorous competition can be created and sustained in health care markets by simple solutions such as pluralization of insurance sources, against sole-source finance. Friedmanite pro-competition reforms would impose employment and income losses which would be likely to make government support of pro-free-market policies very expensive in terms of voting losses as indicated above (Maynard). As the distinguished Princeton economist Uwe Reinhardt has so neatly pointed out 'Friedman's vision should send shivers down the spine of any straight thinking physician' (Reinhardt, 1982). Monopolies and cartels will exist and be likely to seek to influence prices, quantities, and qualities in a way at variance to the interests of patients for the foreseeable future. To moderate outcomes in the interests of patients, public, and private regulators in public and private health care systems and sub-systems will seek to control prices, quantities and qualities. Regulation is ubiquitous and unavoidable and only a farsighted policy seeking to innovate and evaluate in all spheres of regulatory activity is likely to be productive if inefficiency is to be reduced and inequality, if it is so desired, mitigated.

THE EFFECTS OF ALTERING THE MIX

The actors in the drama

The inevitability of regulation affecting both public and private institutions poses the question what sort of regulators will be at work in each sector in differing mixes of public and private activity, and how they will affect not just the regulation, but the access to and quality of health care, as well as the effects on the cast of actors in the system.

At present the primary actors in the health care system in the UK are Government Departments. The Cabinet, Department of Health and Social Security (DHSS), the Welsh Office, the Scottish Home and Health Department (SHHD), and the Northern Ireland Ministry of Health allocate the NHS budget amongst and within the constituent parts of the UK. The Treasury monitors the performance of the NHS and seeks to influence the spending ministries in their policies and in their financial activities. The Department of Education and Science (DES) finances and oversees, together with the University Grants Committee, the General Medical Council, the Royal Colleges and the Universities, the training of doctors. The Department of the Environment (DoE) and the DHSS finance and regulate the provision of local government social services. The Exchequer and Audit Department services the Public Accounts Committee of the House of Commons and seeks to ensure that all these actors give 'value for money' in their endeavours. The Treasury are also responsible through the Finance Acts for the ways in which the private sector is allowed to develop e.g. tax reliefs to individuals, taxation of for-profit hospitals, etc.

The activities of these largely government bodies are supplemented by a variety of private bodies (e.g. professional organizations), public bodies (including statutory bodies concerned with patients' interests such as Community Health Councils,) responsible for the local provision of NHS care, the Regional and District Health Authorities. Local authorities with their social services have some part in the system too. All these 'actors' have differing roles and goals which at times may conflict with one another. Thus the DHSS and the DES argue about, and seek to implement the policies which shift the cost of training doctors from one departmental budget to another. The complexity of the interactions between policy-makers in these decision-making bodies is enormous and it is not surprising that the system is often slow and cumbersome.

At present the role of the private sector is small—much smaller and possibly less threatening than seems to be widely assumed. Although the income and expenditure of the private sector is less than two per cent of NHS activity, there are a significant number of bodies involved in the finance and provision of private acute care and with the range of purposes it is doubtful if they have common aims. The largest financing body is the British United Provident Association which has about 70 per cent of the market. The provision of care is basically institutional and in the hands of a variety of hospital 'owners', and a group of largely NHS-employed specialists who are dependent on NHS consultant contracts for basic income and whose professional body, the BMA, strongly supports the NHS (1982). There are complex interactions between these bodies and between these bodies and the State (Maynard). It would certainly be prudent to study the likely effects of appreciably altering the public/private mix in health care on the mutations of the regulatory activities of these public and private decision-makers.

The foreign experience

The chapters by the foreign experts have demonstrated that varying types of public/private mix in health care have led to varying degrees of regulatory activity, both public and private, in the countries of Europe, North America, and Australia, bearing on individuals, providers, and carriers. The clear lesson for British policy-makers is that in all these countries both private markets and public activity are inefficient in their use of scarce resources, and hardly effective in meeting whatever distributional goals have been articulated by policy-makers.

This inefficiency in resource usage and the relative failure to achieve the required degree of equality, however defined, have resulted in financiers and providers becoming motivated to regulate the general environments in which they work. Private insurers have responded to escalating health care costs, by trying to innovate with new payment systems to hospitals and doctors, the establishment and enforcement of practice norms and standards, and by varying co-payments levied on patients (a policy which the Rand Study (1982) indicates is an inadequate means of controlling hospital utilization). Public regulators have sought to control patient utilization by altering user charges (i.e. co-payments), by monitoring the performance (e.g. P.S.R.O. in the United States, 'health profiles' in France, Germany, and Australia) of health professionals, restricting the coverage of once comprehensive social insurance schemes as in Belgium, and by controlling the supply of doctors *(numerus clausus)* in most of the European countries, and hospital beds (e.g. 'health maps' in France). It is evident that regulation, the moderation or control of behaviour by the introduction and use of rules, is ubiquitous and inevitable whatever the public/private mix.

The British scenario

Fringe benefit contributions: the effects on British industry

If the experience abroad is any guide the likely effect of altering the public/private mix in Britain would seem to be that the regulation of the health care market will become more (not less) extensive and more complex. This possible outcome arises from the fact that altering the mix will change the number and the roles of the regulators, both public and private.

Which new institutions, and potential regulators, will be introduced, if the British private health care sector expands? The first set of actors already being identified, will be payers of contributions collected through pay-roll deductions and co-payments (Forsyth). Much of the existing business of BUPA and the other provident companies is with companies. If the private insurance sector expands it will collect more money from companies and individuals. As the size of company payments increase, this expanding, and increasingly costly fringe benefit will become more and more the concern of firms, industrial associations, and eventually probably, the Confederation of British Industry (CBI). McNerney notes in the United States how the Chambers of Commerce regard health care expenditure as their number one problem. Privatization is likely to create similar problems for the members of the CBI.

Yet, the CBI's realization of this problem seems to be limited at the moment. The recent arguments of its social policy division of this organization advocate the 'reduction of NHS bureaucracy' and a ten per cent cut in the labour force of the Service (1982). Even if this policy is accepted and implemented, the CBI may come to regret their failure to analyse the implications of their own proposals. Any reduction in the activities of the NHS, e.g. by reduction of services is likely to lead to an expansion in the activities of the private sector with doubtful overall economy. As Representative Henry Waxman (Chairman of the House of Representatives Energy and Commerce Committees Health Sub-Committee) has said recently to a Washington Business Group in connection with the pro-competition (privatization) movement 'Too often business leaders concern themselves with the deficit and the overall totals, without recognizing that individual budget cuts, may end up forcing the private sector to pay for what the public sector can provide more efficiently' (Waxman, 1982).

It is difficult to believe that the financial implications to businesses of the expansion of private insurance, as part of the clamour for fringe benefits, has been closely analysed as it might have been. Indeed, if the private sector does expand, it is likely that the CBI's concern will expand too! Business will have to provide the means for some care and, as in the United States, this would seem inevitably to lead them to question insurers and providers about cost and 'value for money' (McNerney). In the same way firms will be faced by choices about whether to insure for care in the market place or 'self-insure', with the firms collecting revenues and paying expenditures. If firms choose the self-insurance route, and this is attractive from the cash-flow and other perspectives, they will find themselves willy-nilly developing a regulatory capacity in the health care industry. If the experience of the United States is any guide, the activity of Divisions in businesses concerned with fringe benefits, about utilization, lengths of stay, practice standards, and costs is more than likely to increase considerably, as they seek to contain their expenditures on health care.

Consumers

The individuals who contribute to private insurance are not less likely to become concerned about 'value for money'. The payment of large and increasing insurance contributions will make potential patients aware of the costs of cover, and the consumer movement will ensure they will be anxious to identify the best cost method of acquiring care when medical need arises. This appears to be happening already (Klein) and is likely to increase. This motivation will lead to the development of consumer associations with monitoring roles and a clamour for the more active use of consumer protection legislation. Further, 'scandals' in the private sector—and experience suggests these would seem to be inevitable, will increase public pressure on governments to legislate and control the private sector. It is therefore likely that if the private/public mix did increase in Britain, it would be accompanied by much more detailed regulation of the private sector by government, as for example is still the case in Australia. (Deeble) and *Lancet* (1982).

The carriers

The anxiety of the firms and individuals who pay subscriptions to BUPA and other insurance carriers is likely to oblige these carriers to alter radically the way in which they manage the use of their resources. In early 1982 BUPA reported an operating loss for the previous financial year and indicated that it was likely in the future, by various means, to persuade its clients from using expensive facilities. This is a significant departure from BUPA's previous policy of tending to be largely a payer of clients' medical bills. If the history of insurance carriers elsewhere in the world is a guide, this change in BUPA policy is the first step on a long journey. This journey will probably oblige BUPA in its attempts to control the costs of the providers, to use co-payments, to go in for practice evaluation, standard setting, and be inclined, eventually to use its buying powers to depress fees and other payments. Thus BUPA and the other private insurers are unlikely to avoid most of the problems faced by the NHS, and will seek to resolve them by regulating the activities of providers and patients.

If private-for-profit insurers enter the British health care market in a bigger way than hitherto, it is likely that their regulatory activity will be even more extensive and vigorous. Unlike BUPA and the other provident associations, the managers of the for-profit companies generally have some property rights in any surpluses of revenue over expenditure e.g. they are paid bonuses if they make profits. The US experience is notable. This direct incentive to decision-makers to minimize cost has led such companies to grow faster than Blue Cross/Blue Shield (not-for-profit carriers) in the US and underline the significance of experience as against community rating. Thus if the private UK market on health care expands and for-profit companies enter the market on a larger scale, they are likely to challenge and perhaps might

take over the markets of the not-for-profit companies. Because this will be the result of greater management efficiency,
they are also likely to seek to regulate the health care market
more vigorously.

Thus overseas experience indicates that privatization of
health care finance, will lead to extensive private regulatory
behaviour. This regulatory behaviour will eventually restrict
the freedom of the professions and hospitals to fix the prices,
quantities, and qualities of the care they provide. Furthermore it will lead to competition between the for-profit and
not-for-profit insurance companies and this could reduce the
market share of the latter. Whether the State will be prepared to let this private regulatory activity work itself out in
the market without intervening seems, however, unlikely.

The institutional providers and State monitoring

The reason why the State may seek to oversee private
regulatory activity in the health care market is that the
workings of this market will keenly influence the prices,
quantities, and quality of care provided in the public sector.
All Western governments intervene in the health care market, ranging from, at one end of the spectrum, the USA with
its various categorical programmes—the most expensive of
which are the social ones, Medicare and Medicaid, to the
UK with the NHS. In financing and sometimes providing
care, the State will seek to minimize its costs, and maximize
the quality and quantities of the services it can buy. As we
have seen the State has hitherto not been very effective in
pursuing these goals in Western countries. Because of political and economic constraints however, it will not be diverted
from striving perhaps more strongly after such goals.

If the State is successful in depressing the prices of services
provided by doctors and hospitals, this may make the task of
the private regulators more difficult. One possible scenario is
that hospital managers could yield to government pressure
and permit below-cost fees for public contract work, compensating for those losses with above-cost fees for private work.
Alternatively the hospital managers could subsidize low private sector fees out of high public sector charges, if they feel
they can get away with these. This will have the effect in

time of stimulating counter-measures from the contractors. Doctors and other professionals will be tempted similarly to cross-subsidize and play one side off against the other. Loss-leaders are after all, a means to a profitable end in many business ventures. The process of cross-subsidization is, however, difficult to identify and reverse. It requires good data (considerably better than currently exists) and careful on-going evaluation of financial practices. If either public or private regulators identify cross-subsidies their action to reduce it may have the effect of squeezing the provider into insolvency.

The 'medical' providers

The increased regulatory activity in the health care market may change the role of the medical (doctor) providers considerably. The regulators will seek to establish 'health profiles' so that the characteristics and costs of medical practices of individual doctors can be identified and any 'deviance' from practice norms 'remedied' (cf. the Belgian, French, and Australian systems). In the future, regulatory activity, both public and private, is likely to be much more intense in this area and there will be pressures for better information. Whatever the profession does, it is likely that in the future its decisions will be questioned in much greater detail by systems of peer review by fellow-professionals as part of public and private regulation. Clinical freedom, interpreted as the freedom to do what is best and be subject to the appraisal of no-one, is probably anyway in the process of ending, with incalculable results. Medical practices, as information improves with computerization, would seem inevitably to be regulated in greater detail in the years to come.

Yet, not only is medical practice likely to be more carefully regulated than hitherto: it is also likely that the control of supply of doctors is likely to be strengthened. In theory privatization offers a threat to this control. At present it is accepted that the control of the supply of doctors is essential if health care costs are to be contained. If more doctors are trained, there will be more 'allocators' of health care available. As noted above (Maynard, *Part 4*) each UK consultant makes decisions which may cost the NHS of the order of

£500,000 per year. With the present estimated cost of producing a doctor (£56,000) it is questionable if the capital could be found to establish a new medical school. Apart from this, it is hardly something likely to be left unregulated, since to allow the private production of doctors would be for the State, a hazardous enterprise, as this may, without strict quota controls, mean the State loses control of the supply of doctors, and in the long-run, health care expenditure. In any event the approval of such schools by the authorities would require no mean effort being expended by their promotors over several years. There is also the implication with all that it entails that the entry to such schools is unlikely to be of the same quality as that to the existing medical schools where merit is the criteria. Strict quota controls does mean however that the State would be regulating the activity of the private sector.

Thus even if the State wished to encourage the privatization of the *production* of doctors, it would have to do so with careful controls of the quantity and quality of doctors. Such controls would not, however, guarantee that the State *acquired* the doctors it required to run the NHS, at whatever level of activity was chosen. Indeed this is one of the reasons that critics of the expansion of the private sector employ to denigrate such a policy. The private sector might bid labour away from the NHS by increasing the pay of private doctors. The State could respond to this by paying more for the services of doctors, with obvious public expenditure implications, or could 'tie' doctors in an informal contract to the NHS in exchange for their training. All of the speculation would however depend on a much greater expansion of the private sector in the UK than looks practicable at the moment.

Many of the same issues arise over other professionals such as nurses, although in the latter case there are at present unwritten conventions that the private hospitals restrict themselves to Whitley Council scales for nurses, and rely on better environmental conditions for supply. Whether this convention will continue to be observed is a doubtful supposition and it seems likely that controlling the pay of doctors, nurses, and other professionals would be more difficult if the public/private mix in health care altered considerably. Thus, a decision to privatize the health services even in part, could well, without controls, be a decision to increase the pay and conditions of health professionals if the total expenditure on health care was allowed to expand without check. It probably would create more difficulties for both public and private sector employers in their attempts to control the costs and the quantity and quality of health care that they provide.

Encouraging the development of private medicine could of course involve the private sector providers taking on new tasks and expanding old roles. Instead of providing mainly (cold) elective surgery, the private sector might develop its capacity to treat more complex surgical cases and other novel roles. This would however involve it 'bidding' for more labour and capital and such shifts in employment could generate problems both for the gainers (the private sector) and the losers (the NHS). Complex new regulating devices would have to be developed by the NHS, the government, and the private sector to defend their mutually conflicting interests. The experience of other countries indicates that this regulation would be both more intensive and extensive. More detail would be required for the scrutiny and control needed, and more activities would be affected by the rules of the public and private sector regulators.

Thus, to summarize, regulation by which is meant the moderation or control of prices, quantities, and qualities in the health care market, is a common resort of both public and private sectors. Whatever the public/private mix, both public and private decision-makers will seek to regulate their markets to their own advantage. Experience indicates that this regulation is extensive and complex and that these attitudes of regulation may be exacerbated by privatization: the sole buying power (monopsony) of the NHS if utilized more effectively could almost certainly be a cost-effective means of regulating the health care market and the temptation for governments to use this policy instrument, in the face of high PSBRs, will always be great. Altering the public/private mix towards more private health care is likely to increase the number of people involved in the regulation of health care and to make their roles more complex. It does not reduce the need to regulate the resultant mix, and both public and private bureaucracies will still flourish.

THE FUTURE: COMMON CHALLENGES TO THE PUBLIC AND PRIVATE SECTORS

Whatever the priorities settled on by policy-makers and whatever the nature of the public/private mix in health care in the years to come, there is a set of common challenges which must be taken up by decision-makers, public and private to make the system efficient and effective in the face of rising demands. At the forefront of these challenges is the need to improve the managerial training of doctors and develop an efficient management structure which is serviced by adequate evaluative information about the services provided from both the public and private services. In addition policy innovations particularly in prevention and in the care of the elderly are essential if services are to be efficient and humane.

The training of doctors

It is now conventional wisdom that doctors, whether they work in the public or private sectors, are the 'gatekeepers' of the health care system. It is their decisions which decide who will get access to what health care. It is their decisions also that decide who will live, who will die, and who will live in what degree of pain and discomfort. Unfortunately it is doubtful if their training in decision-making is adequate.

Despite substantial investment in medical schools, doctors tend not to acquire the habits of scientific appraisal of their performance and generally have limited skills in the management of resources. As Weed (1981), himself a physician, has argued:

> Present licensing procedures and medical school curriculum grew out of what the 'professionals' in the past identified as desirable; they do not reflect what was proved to be possible in meeting well defined goals.

Because the system has been so poorly defined over the years, there has been no way to relate the outputs of the system to inputs; conjectures piled upon conjectures have hardened into curriculums and licensing laws. Reviewing some of these conjectures in terms of the tasks of medicine, we can now see how far off the track the medical establishment has strayed.

This argument is consistent with that of Cochrane (1972) and many other observers, medical and non-medical in the UK. The failure to evaluate input/output links in health care has led to training which is not based on scientific fact but frequently on conjecture. Students are trained to behave in ways which may or may not lead to the use of scarce resources in an efficient manner. Furthermore they are not trained adequately to question existing practices and evaluate input/output links scientifically.

This inadequate training in practice and evaluative medicine, means that many doctors do not use resources efficiently. Because of their ignorance of the input (health care)—output (improved health status) link, and their inclination, due to poor training in the use of resources, not to question existing practices and links (or lack of them), doctors have neither the knowledge to use resources efficiently nor the incentive to research their practices and improve their efficiency.

The remedy for these shortcomings in doctor training is special training, but suggestions for change will be countered by the usual arguments that the syllabus is already full. Training in management, economic and statistical skills involves an opportunity cost (i.e. something will have to be given up). Such an opportunity cost may yield significant benefits if doctors can be trained to evaluate their practice, identify input/output links, and use resources efficiently. Such training would have to be sustained throughout the cycle of the doctor's life in practice, through a system of continuing education so that his evaluative and management skills are augmented regularly.

The realization of the potential contribution of economic knowledge to improving the efficiency of resource allocation in medical care seems to be growing, albeit slowly. The

Medical Research Council and the Social Science Research Council financed Drummond's work in order to provide a guide for doctors to the principles and practice of economic evaluation (Drummond, 1980, 1981). This dawning of the realization amongst doctor decision-makers that resources are scarce and must be used efficiently is being accelerated by the limits currently being imposed on expenditure. Cost containment policies abroad and cash-limits in Britain are obliging doctors to compete among themselves for resources. To make the case for acquiring resources, the doctor often as yet all too implicitly, now has to evaluate the costs and benefits of his activities relative to those of his colleagues who are competing for the same resources—and will increasingly have to do so. Thus the competition for resources, in public and private health care systems, may in time provide a spur to the doctors to identify input/output links and to use resources more efficiently. It may even give a special spur to Consultants to pick up and develop with greater vigour than hitherto the 'Cogwheel' concept (1967).

With doctors managing resources in all health care systems it is necessary to extend the training of doctors at the undergraduate and postgraduate levels and through their working lives, so that they are given the skills, particularly in economics and management, to use efficiently the scarce resources they control. Such training is necessary whatever the public/private mix and whatever the country. If doctors are not made aware of the relevant management skills they will manage health care resources inefficiently.

Enabling managers to manage

Whatever the sector, public or private, the managers of scarce health care resources must be given incentives and the means to manage. At present the doctor has an ambiguous attitude to management. *De facto* it is he who decides who will get the care, but his training and his professional ethic does not assign explicitly to him the management role. The doctor *is* and yet *is not* the manager. There still however has to be a recognition of this in the policy approaches to health care systems, public or private. This is why management concerned with health care is so suspect as to efficiency.

The key to good management is information about inputs and outputs and knowledge of the linkages between these two elements. There is however a universal reluctance at all levels of decision-making to accept the obvious that good 'intelligence' is not a cheap commodity. To argue that Medicare in the US or the NHS in the UK is 'over-bureaucratized' is rather naive. Public and private sector health care systems require an efficient bureaucracy if they are to use resources efficiently. Often health care institutions, public and private at the operating level, suffer from under-administration: the means of keeping under review the quantity and quality of their managers, medical, financial, and other, are inadequate. Yet while it is conventional wisdom that the NHS, Medicare and other public systems of health care are often inflexible, inefficient resource users, there is some diffidence about accepting that the *reason might be because of false economy in administration*.

The need to acquire better information about the costs and benefits of health care and the characteristics of decisions in health care systems is paramount. The evaluation of practice may not of course change behaviour. One can lead the horse to the water of knowledge about efficient practice, but one cannot necessarily make it drink. Good management is about 'selling' or 'packaging' this information in such a way that decision-making at the key levels is improved. Desirable outcomes may be facilitated if providers individually and institutionally are given some direct financial incentives to strive after efficient practice. Knowledge about the nature of these inducements and their effects on behaviour, is less than satisfactory but as has been indicated above (Maynard, and elsewhere) there is considerable scope for experimentation.

The problems with health care institutions is that often they fail to allocate the role of manager clearly. The tradition in the NHS has been to have medical, administrative, financial, and nursing managers, with no clear definition of who has ultimate responsibility. Above all, there is still, after 34 years of NHS experience, no adequate system of information gathering, evaluation, and dissemination, which top management can use effectively with confidence. Such carelessness in the design of the health care system has contributed considerably towards the inefficient application of resources. Managers must have clear roles, and their performance must be monitored carefully if they are to use scarce health care resources efficiently. Management is certainly a subject that merits greater attention and more than the lip service it has had hitherto, from those concerned and responsible at the top accountable level for the better use of resources.

The conclusion has to be that improved Service (NHS) management will have to be supervised by more sophisticated central management. If the DHSS geared to other tasks is incapable of providing that, some other authority is necessary. At present the capacity of the centre to monitor and evaluate the Service is inadequate—and the present much vaunted moves are widely believed to be so—and this raises the question of whether the nature of the present central management capacity, that is at Departmental level is optimally effective.

Managing what?

So far the assumption made, has been that the managers, be they doctors or administrators (acting of course with their corporate authorities), should control the allocation of health care resources. This is an adequate argument as far as it goes, but it is limited in the sense that health care is only one factor which affects the health status of the individual over his or her life. As McKeown (1977, 1979) has argued health care has probably played only a relatively minor role in causing the modern rise of population: the main causes of improved health are concerned with affluence which in various ways has financed better nutrition, and public health. Education may also be influential in encouraging better health. Private health care has little or no bearing on this particular sector of the health economy. Yet it is an area of the greatest importance, and is probably destined to come under greater attention in the future. Anything of a minor character diverting attention from it is in the long run bad politics.

Unfortunately precise knowledge about the links between

income, nutrition, public health, education and, that desired
goal, good health is absent. Prevention is a popular watch-
word in health policy discussions but what is prevention?
Which is the 'best prevention buy'? Who is responsible for
allocating resources to it? Policies concerned with persuading
individuals to reduce their consumption of tobacco and
alcohol, or to take adequate exercise—which require actions
considerably more refined than those hitherto successful in
the preventive field concerned with *public* health e.g. water
and sewage disposal, yield benefits slowly only, over decades.
Such policies, in terms, for instance, of the employment of
specialized programmes designed to alter behaviour, tend to
require fairly lengthy experimental and development runs
and are therefore costly. So prevention gives rise to immediate commitments reflected in high costs with benefits a long
way distant—just the sort of commitments which are unlikely to gain political popularity!

Other proposals, such as those advocated in the Black
Report (1980), which are not directly concerned with arrangements for health care and depend on evaluations of
social policies, are virtually assertions, which may or may not
be accurate, about the desirability of particular public policies in the uncertain future. The exact nature of the demand
for health by individuals and the relative effectiveness of
alternative policies which might affect health from conception to death, have not been the subjects of programmes of
scientific research (Muurinen, 1982). It is possible to assert
that 'prevention' is better than cure (and it is probably right
to do so) but 'prevention' encapsulates many sub-systems
which are remote from private health care, and there is as yet no
demonstration of which prevention policies are the most
efficient. The problem of course with the 'prevention industry' is that like so much in the health field it lacks a
promotional centre, for (*pace* the limited range of the DHSS),
there being no General Staff mechanism on health affairs,
there is no satellite system for prevention. Neither has it now
a great band of professional supporters. As a consequence,
prevention activities are very small, poorly organized and
expected to perform great deeds on a limited budget, and in
a short space of time. Prevention has also suffered a general

set-back in the UK in the failure to recognize with the demise of the MOH, the opening up of a serious gap. Everyone is agreed that more money should be spent on prevention, and that the policies so financed must be evaluated carefully, but at the moment the pressures are pitifully small. Politicians and the public should recognize that quick results are not to be expected.

There is much evidence that indicates that what the individual does to himself during his life has more influence on his health than health care. If one person has poor feeding habits ('junk' food, excessive alcohol, and tobacco consumption, etc.), avoids exercise, and fails to rest himself adequately, then his health will probably deteriorate more rapidly than another person who takes care in his eating, his exercise, and his rest. Informing the population about such facts is a role which the State, *via* education in childhood, youth, and throughout life, could with advantage cause to be undertaken more vigorously, and on a strategy based on scientific observation.

In the long-run the benefits of such policies, if they are successful, will be that increasing numbers of people will live longer better quality lives. Added to what has already been achieved, the policies will result in more people living into old age rather than dying painfully in middle-age from avoidable accidents, cancers, heart diseases, etc. If the objective of health (not just health care) policy is to achieve a better quality of life over the span of years, prevention may be a better use for scarce resources, than cure.

Developing the public/private mix

If prevention policies however are successful the majority of the population will survive to die in their seventies and eighties. The resource implications of this 'greying' of the population are quite significant. With care, the first ten years of retirement (65–75 years) should be active and healthy, then with differing speeds of onset, physical and mental attributes will begin to decline. After about 75 years of age there will be a need for a network of institutions of varying sorts to care for people with varying degrees of independence.

Caring services—and to some extent the curative services for the elderly—will have to be related to physical, mental, and social dependence.

A most significant provider of such care could be the private sector, and with the right policies the role of this sector could with advantage be expanded in the years to come. Thus, one particular area where there is scope for the State to encourage privatization with advantage to all is in the establishment of an insurance market for nursing care in old age (post 75 years of age). Yet the carriers shy clear of this group of people, being almost exclusively concerned with acute medicine. The financing of such an expansion into the elderly field, needs careful analysis (this is the subject of a special study by the Nuffield Provincial Hospitals Trust). It would seem sensible to encourage people (i.e. to create a market) to save specially over their working lives for specially designed care in the last decade or so of life. That there is evidence of the potential of such a market, is not in doubt. A number of private institutions for the care of the elderly of course already exist. But in the present circumstances, with what is apparently in store in the future in these affluent days, with occupational pensions and present property values, there is need to give special encouragement to people to mobilize their personal resources to provide specially for the kind of care in their declining years which they may wish to spend in a private institution. Clearly, the State could have a special function to assist in the process of experimenting with different levels of care, and helping people to maximize the use of their own resources with help from the State.

Policy initiatives in such areas as the elderly could be elaborated and experiments tried. Foreign experience on this particular issue, especially the use of cash payments to those who wanted to buy special services could be tapped for their relevance when formulating domestic policies for this particular client group, where needs are growing in a time when total resources for health are relatively scarce. The similarity of the problems faced by health care decision-makers across the Western world in this particular area are such, that a timely policy for experiments and innovations and the evaluation of such ventures would be prudent politics in all countries, regardless of their institutional structures.

RESEARCH PRIORITIES

The preceding section has indicated some special problems including those of an important group the demands of which in terms of health services, are likely to grow. Such problems have to be considered by policy-makers (with a better appreciation of the form in which the necessary intelligence is commissioned, processed and delivered) if health care systems, public and private, are to be made more efficient. This section sets out briefly a series of questions, consideration of which would establish co-ordinated action, and could lead to the establishment of research priorities irrespective of the form of health care system and the public/ private mix. Thus, regardless of the relative sizes of the public (NHS) and private (BUPA, *et al.*) sectors, what are the main issues must be addressed by policy-makers and researchers in the next two decades? The possibilities arising from the pressures which come from a wide recognition of the priorities in health assume a certain amount of flexibility in approach and in potential policies. The answers to the questions posed will differ from country to country, but they must be sought, if resource allocation decisions that take place now are to be based on a real understanding of the issues and made less wasteful. Only with such an understanding will it be possible to develop health policies, with the right degree of flexibility, to achieve the policy goals of decision-makers whatever the nature of their ideology, or objectives.

The questions comprise most of the relevant issues facing any modern industrial society and would provide an agenda to stimulate the right directions for health service research in the remaining years of this century. By the same token they assume that those in government whose responsibility (in the Rothschild manner) is to initiate programmes of scientific research and to promote and finance health services research in order to make the progress in health care we all seek, will be willing to formulate a coherent strategy for the long-term.

Thus

1. What are the objectives of the health care system, regardless of the public/private mix? What ordering or weight do these objectives get and how are these changing over time? Equity in terms of distribution and access is important and covers most systems: also, what weight is being given to the priorities which have emerged as a result of thirty years of experience of the NHS. How are they likely to be affected by change in the public/private mix? An analysis of public statements could identify the clarity or contradictions in objective setting and make possible the determination of consistent sets of possible objectives for the health care system, public and private.

2. Who is really responsible for control of the system(s): and who controls resource use at the 'margins' or boundaries of care? e.g. the boundary between hospital and primary care; the boundary between capital and current revenue allocation; the boundary between capital and labour, the boundaries between the public and private sectors, etc.? Who controls any movements in these boundaries? What criteria are used to determine policy-making at these boundaries? Why is it that insurance principles and practice, seem to gravitate only towards institutional care and particularly for acute (mainly surgical) cases, and not for general practice, prevention, the care of the elderly, and other 'Cinderella' activities?

3. What incentives (monetary and non-monetary) are there (or lack of them) to achieve efficiency for individual managers and for institutions in the public and private sectors? Why do decision-makers at the boundaries behave as they do? What incentives motivate public and private action, and the interaction between the public and private sectors? Is inefficient behaviour an inevitable product of poor incentives?

   Is it likely that research in this area could identify how behaviour in the public and private sectors could be altered with new incentives to make it more consistent with policy objectives? (as in (1) above).

4. Who rations what and how?

What criteria are used by what decision-makers in the public and private sectors to allocate scarce health care resources which have effects at the micro (operational) level? Is the allocation which results, consistent with the avowed rationing criteria of the sector and the policy objectives of that sector or system?

5. Who in effect decides, and what are the investment criteria used in the public and private health care sectors? Are the techniques of investment appraisal used? If so, how? If not, what criteria decides who will get a new hospital or a new piece of medical equipment, and are they consistent with policy objectives and the optimum use of resources?

6. What are the major unresolved problems in the health care system?

This question takes us back to (1). Are outcomes, in terms of efficiency and distributional equity, however defined, consistent with policy objectives or does the system (and its public and private sectors) fail to meet its objectives?

Indeed the questions are relevant to the Secretary of State's most recent statement on the problems of health care (*The Times* 9 July 1982) which could well be developed into a series of questions for research addressed by the DHSS and in particular by a far-seeing Chief Scientist as part of a long-term research strategy, viz:

Health care always posed a fundamental problem for government; virtually limitless demands for services which have to be set against finite resources.

The next decade will see a sharp increase in the numbers of the very old, who make particularly heavy demands on health services. We will need resources fully to exploit further advances in medicine. We must solve the medical problems of our inner cities; develop a better partnership between the NHS and the private sector; deal with long standing career problems in the medical and nursing professions; and restore NHS buildings and equipment to an acceptable standard.

The Government is committed to tackling these problems and to developing the health service . . .

This statement made by the British Secretary of State could have been made by any of his counterparts in the Western world: the challenges in all health care systems are very similar. To answer these challenges, questions 1 to 6 must be elaborated and answered, and this will require a research strategy and substantial effort; in which there is a place for both public and private sectors..

The purpose of these questions should lead to the establishment of objectives and how decisions are made. The questions are simple but the answers are not clearly known in any country. To answer them, there will need to be considerable investments in evaluative research and information generation, evaluation, and dissemination. Most health care activities, in the public and private sectors, have not been evaluated; and thus to identify efficient practice requires substantial investments in clinical and economic evaluation. If the private sector expands it must take an increasing share in financing this activity rather than, at present, taking a 'free ride' off what is regrettably inadequate public action in this neglected area.

Resolution of these questions and efficient management, requires more and better organized information and intelligence. The characteristic of much public activity is that its effects are rarely evaluated. Any 'action' by way of inputs are believed to affect outcomes beneficially, even though health care institutions in the public and private sectors have little or no evidence to substantiate such a belief. There is a need to research and determine the characteristics of the process of providing better health care and the outcomes, in terms of the effects of these provision processes on patients. This research should ultimately lead to the evaluation of procedures, and the evaluation of medical practices, e.g. what is the cost-effective way of providing primary care, solo or group practices, and in what settings?

This type of analysis will also shed light on many contem-

porary issues in health care. For instance the case for contracting out NHS ancillary services (e.g. catering, cleaning,
and laundry) is incomplete, being based on limited empirical
knowledge, and *a priori* reasoning about how things might
turn out if such services are denationalized. Experimentation
is essential. While this case rests on assertions and limited
knowledge of the facts, another quite different type of contract, the case for the NHS buying surgical services from the
private sector, is based on an assertion that the private sector
can provide supplementary services of such character more
cheaply. Again the evidence to sustain this view is absent
and if the view is wrong 'privatization' will inflate public
expenditure: a public service, might be able to provide such
services more cheaply and contain public expenditure on
health care more effectively (Waxman, 1982). Again, this
area needs experimentation and controlled trials and monitoring over a reasonable period.

   Research endeavours in these and other important areas
will require the co-operation of practitioners in many disciplines: epidemiologists, statisticians, sociologists, accountants,
and economists, and will take time to provide answers.
Follow-ups of patients for 5–10 years are required to ascertain the full effects of some medical interventions. Progress in
evaluation will be slow, costly, and difficult, but it must
figure as a priority, if scarce resources are to be used efficiently.

   The inevitable slow production of research results, is
caused by the multi-disciplinary nature of such research and
by the difficulties of defining and operationalizing measures
of output or outcome. Output measurements must be developed if health care is to be evaluated effectively. Many of the
intellectual problems in devising such measures have been
resolved. General Staff thinking, the means for which is
lacking is necessary to concentrate on a programme. Resources are required to initiate and develop it; including how
to use the results in health care systems, public and private.

   In addition to the evaluative research inherent in the
search to answer the priority questions above, there is an
associated need to investigate the behaviour of decision-
makers. To elaborate but a limited domain for such research,

modelling the behaviour of doctors, nurses, the pharmaceutical industry, and public and private hospitals, could provide explanations of existing behaviour and indicate how behaviour could be altered and made consistent with policy objectives.

The research endeavours required to answer the priority questions above, are difficult, expensive, but common across *all* health care systems *regardless* of the public/private mix. They do not involve ideological debate and grand (and foolhardy) designs to solve fundamental problems whose nature is ill-understood, and whose resolution is impossible in the present state of ignorance. The approach here is that of science rather than of rhetoric, an approach which has enabled man to get out of the caves of pre-history and help develop the sophisticated and humane society towards which we all strive today.

OVERVIEW

Policy analysis in health care is plagued by competing ideologies which tend to make the debate about options emotional, superficial, and naive. This study is concerned with the UK scene and the essays all of which were commissioned specifically are related to the major problems which have been identified here. Yet the problems are clearly of a universal character. The Pavlovian responses of liberals and socialists tends to ensure that the fundamental nature of this complex market is ignored and the relevant issues of policy, and their resolution, left to fester in a way which wastes scarce resources and fails to meet the aims of liberals and socialists alike. *It is surely time this superficial approach is abandoned so that scarce intellectual resources can be allocated in ways which resolve policy problems.*

The discussion about the public/private mix in health care is dominated by over-simplified ideological concerns. This book shows that whatever the public/private mix, be it the 50/50 role of the State and the market in the USA, the 98/2 role of the State and the market in UK, or any (e.g. Dutch) alternatives between these roles, partnership between public and private providers is inevitable but the need of cost control is a dominant factor and regulation to achieve universal goals is ubiquitous and inevitable. Regulation means that rules are used to moderate or control the outcomes of decision-making be it public or private. Shifting the public/private mix does not remove regulation; it has a marginal effect and in reality merely changes its nature. This is specially true in periods as now of great financial restraint.

Such regulation is unavoidable because of the inherent nature of the health care market: monopolies fix the prices, quantities, and qualities of the goods and services they sell in a manner advantageous to them (the providers) rather than the clients (patients); social institutions (the NHS and insurance companies, both private and social) reduce the price barriers to consumption and provide incentives for patients to over-consume (moral hazard) because a third party (the taxpayer or the insurance contributor) pays; and there are few incentives for decision-makers (doctors and managers of various sorts) to behave efficiently (i.e. to ensure costs are minimized and benefit maximized).

These market 'failures' occur in the public sector and the private sector and both sectors are manifestly inadequate in the way they identify the goals of policy, and identify and evaluate the alternative means by which policy objectives can be pursued. Resources always and everywhere are scarce. Change in the way in which health care resources are used is necessary, but such changes unless in the context of a deliberate strategy which draws on the lessons of the past will not improve matters merely by alterations to the public/private mix. The 1948, 1974, and 1982 reorganizations of the NHS, and the expansion of BUPA and the rest of the private sector recently in the UK, has not remedied the failures of the health care market, public and private. Rather have NHS reorganizations and the rhetoric involved in minor alterations to the public/private mix diverted attention (and energies) away from the fundamental problems of providing health care and towards superficial issues, which have all too little bearing on efficiency and equity.

Whatever the public/private mix, the structure of the NHS in Britain, the structure of the Funds in Europe, the structure of Government funding and the insurance market in the United States, and other organizational forms elsewhere, the fundamental failures of the health care market, public and private, to achieve the objectives we all desire will thrive, unless attention is paid to developing a strategy to secure the optimum use of resources for the production of health care services in the form of both public and private services. The resolution of the questions involved will take many decades of careful research, experiments, and developments contributing to policy formation. It would be folly not to recognize the extent of the time-scale required and the need for careful planning of this activity, in which government has a key role.

POSTSCRIPT

In the preceding essays the authors have expressed their own views about the public/private mix in health care in their own countries and in this essay we, as editors, have sought to draw attention to common major issues which have been revealed. At this stage it is appropriate for the editors to make their position about the mix and the NHS quite clear. After reviewing the evidence we have accumulated over these past months, as well as from our collective experience and observations, we both feel that despite its faults, the variety of complex services which is termed the 'National Health Service' constitutes a unique and precious national asset which provides basic services of a high standard at a very low proportion of GDP compared to other countries. According to OECD data it has a relatively low cost of administration too (Maynard, Part 4). Above all it still retains a vital core of the ideal regarding equity in service, with which it was launched in 1948 and the importance of this should not be overlooked. One does not have to be a collectivist ideologue to appreciate the advantages of the NHS, since neither the present Conservative Secretary of State for Health nor the Executive Committee of the Council of the BMA would probably wish to be so described. Yet such an appreciation seems a belief fundamental to recent expressions of policies adopted by both towards the public/private mix for health. It is also our observation that those of our current troubles such as financial constraint—or one of its major resultants, industrial unrest in the hospital service caused by restric-

tions in the raising of salaries and wages—are not unique to the way in which the services in the UK are financed, or organized.

That perceptive economist Uwe Reinhardt (1982a) has observed that there are currently three desiderata which universally dominate health goals: equity; provider freedom to price and practice; and budgetary and economic control. The political scientist might well wonder with him, whether it is possible to achieve more than two of these goals at any one time. If, as we believe, that the vast majority of the population would elect for equity to be the prime consideration, the only subject for debate is which of the two other goals should be pursued. It is doubtful if the choice of the second goal for the UK leaves decision-makers much discretion: surely they will elect for the efficient use of resources and the control of provision.

This is not to say that all things are perfect here or that we should be complacent in any way in considering how matters could be improved by way of policy initiatives for the ultimate benefit of services; but it is sad that somehow or other we have got the reality of health affairs out of perspective, by giving too much credence to the 'ultras' on either side—the 'no-private-practice-at-any-cost' brigade at one end of the spectrum, to the reckless denigrators of an intensely personal human service served by a vast army of dedicated people at the other. It is inconceivable that there should be any sanctions on personal choice and therefore private medicine is likely to flourish. The fears of any 'dismantling' of the NHS, or the slipping eventually into a 'two-tier' system, whatever that may mean, are to our minds ill-founded, given the present proportions of the mix, and the nature and the order of private service likely to be developed in the foreseeable future. In any event, it surely must be asked whether it can be believed that the prime actors, the doctors or nurses, will vary their skills towards patients simply because they are practising in different environments—their time, perhaps for some, their attitudes, but surely never their skills. We should therefore be concentrating on how to get the most out of the partnership.

The challenge is to those responsible in the present circumstances for making the rules and regulations, to find the right mix with the right degree of flexibility, to allow those many idealistic people engaged in the British health services to apply their skills and endeavours to the maximum. It requires and one hopes for a coherent strategy from statesmen, who are capable of taking a long-term view of the field and of producing policies which will improve the health of this nation.

NOTES AND REFERENCES

BACON, R., and ELLIS, W. (1976). *Britain's Economic Problem: Too few producers.* (Macmillan).

BLANPAIN, J., DELESIE, L., and NYS, H. (1978). *National Health Insurance and Health Resources: the European Experience.* (Harvard University Press).

BMA (1982) 'Health Services Financing'. Discussion document.

BRITTAN, L. (1982). 'The Government's economic strategy', in J. KAY (ed.) *The 1982 Budget.* (Institute for Fiscal Studies: London).

COCHRANE, A. L. (1972). *Effectiveness and Efficiency: Random reflections on health services.* (Nuffield Provincial Hospitals Trust: London).

DEPARTMENT OF HEALTH AND SOCIAL SECURITY (The Black Report) (1980). *Inequalities in Health, a report of a working party.* (HMSO: London).

DRUMMOND, M. (1980). *Principles of Economic Appraisal in Health Care.* (Oxford University Press: Oxford).

— — (1981). *Studies in Economic Appraisal in Health Services.* (Oxford University Press: Oxford).

ENTHOVEN, A. (1980). *Health Care Plan.* (Addison-Wesley; New York).

HOWE, G. (1982). 'Health and the economy: the British view'. *Health Affairs,* 1(1), 30–9.

— — (1982a). Lecture to Conservative Political Centre Summer School, Cambridge, 3 July 1982, (Central Conservative Office News Service).

KNIGHT, JOHN (1982). 'Australian headlines on the Hayden Plan', *Lancet,* i, 1009.

MAXWELL, R. J. (1980). *Health and Wealth: an International Study of Health Care Spending.* (Lexington).

MAYNARD, A. (1975). *Health Care in the European Community.* (Croom Helm and University of Pittsburg Press).

— — (1981). 'The inefficiency and inequalities of the health care systems of Western Europe' *Social Policy and Administration,* 15(2), 145–63.

— — and LUDBROOK, A. (1980). 'What's wrong with the NHS?, *Lloyds Bank Review,* October.

— —, — — (1981). 'Thirty Years of Fruitless Endeavour? an analysis of government intervention in the health care market', in J. VAN DER GAAG and M. PERLMAN (eds.), *Health, Economics and Health Economics.* (North Holland: New York and Oxford).

MCKEOWN, T. (1977). *The Modern Rise of Populations.* (Arnold: London).

— — (1979). *The Role of Medicine.* (Blackwells, 2nd edition: London).

MINISTRY OF HEALTH, (The 'Cogwheel' Report) (1967). *First Report of the Joint Working Party on Organization of Medical Work in Hospitals.* (HMSO: London).

MUURINGN, J. M. (1982). 'The Demand for Health: a generalised Grossman model, *Journal of Health Economics,* 1.

NUFFIELD PROVINCIAL HOSPITALS TRUST (1980). *Tenth Report, 1975–80.*

REINHARDT, U. E. (1982). 'Tablemanners at the health care feast', in D.

YAGGY and W. A. ANYLAN (eds.), *Financing Health Care: Competition versus regulation.* (Ballinger: Cambridge, Mass.).

— — (1982a). Uwe Reinhardt's observations on the *desiderata* concerning health care goals mentioned on p. 530 have been elaborated in a number of conversations between him and McLachlan. They are likely to be published shortly: but the principle enunciated is impressive enough to be elevated as a Law!

ROTHSCHILD, LORD (1972). *A Framework for Government Research and Development.* Cmnd. 5046. (HMSO: London).

— — (1982). *An Enquiry into the Social Science Research Council.* Cmnd. 8554. (HMSO: London).

TOWNSEND, P., and DAVIDSON, N. (1982). *Inequalities in Health.* (Penguin: London).

WAXMAN, H. (1982). 'Private sector to pay for budget cuts', *Hospital Week,* **18,** 26, 2 July.

WEED, L. L. (1981). 'Physicians of the Future', *New England Journal of Medicine, 15,* 304, 903–7.

Author, country, and subject index

The compilation of an index for a collection of this nature presents a
great number of problems because of the diversity of the subjects
touched upon within different contexts. This is not only because
foreign countries are included, but because even in the papers
written by the British authors, many elements discussed have their
own hues when viewed separately. The index may be used
differently by scholars interested in compiling their own lists from
readings of the essays, but the collection is intended by the editors as
a guide to the common problems of health care systems in a group of
nations where high standards of medical practice are expected, and
whose general objectives as far as health is concerned are broadly
similar. The distinction of the authors gives it a special flavour.
Because of this it is only worthwhile giving in this index, a series of
cross references to authors, titles and headings to enable readers to
pick out from the references and bibliographies the issues and
themes they wish to follow up in the context of the particular lines
being pursued.

564 *Author, country and subject index*